Gender, Ethnicity, and Health Research

Gender, Ethnicity, and Health Research

Sana Loue

Case Western Reserve University
Cleveland, Ohio

Kluwer Academic / Plenum Publishers
New York, Boston, Dordrecht, London, Moscow

ISBN 0-306-46172-2

©1999 Kluwer Academic / Plenum Publishers
233 Spring Street, New York, N.Y. 10013

10   9   8   7   6   5   4   3   2

A C.I.P. record for this book is available from the Library of Congress

Printed in the United States of America

Preface

Health researchers routinely evaluate health and illness across subgroups defined by their sex, gender, ethnicity, and race. All too often, these classifications are proffered as an explanation for any differences that may be detected, for example, in access to care, frequency of disease, or response to treatment. Relatively few researchers, however, have examined what these classifications mean on a theoretical level or in the context of their own research.

Assume, for example, that a researcher concludes from his or her data that African-Americans utilize certain surgical procedures less frequently than whites. This conclusion may mean little without an examination of the various underlying issues. Is there such a construct as race at all? How were whites and African-Americans classified as such? Does this finding reflect inappropriate overutilization of the specific procedures among whites or inappropriate underutilization among African-Americans? To what extent are socioeconomic status and method of payment related to the less frequent use? Are there differences in the manner in which health care providers present the various treatment options to whites and to African-Americans that could account for these differences in utilization? Are there differences in health care-seeking and health care preferences between the two groups that would explain the difference in utilization? Is the racial classification a surrogate measure for another variable that has remained unidentified and unmeasured? All too often, unfortunately, such issues are ignored or lightly dismissed with an entreaty for additional research.

This text represents an effort to address these and other issues. The text uses a multi-disciplinary approach, integrating concepts from a variety of disciplines including anthropology, epidemiology, ethics, history, law, public health, and sociology. The text is designed to encourage critical thinking about the meaning of these constructs; our past, current, and future use of these concepts; and the implications and consequences of such use. Consequently, the text does not set forth answers to these issues, but rather focuses on a process of inquiry that can be used to find answers. This approach is critical because how we resolve such issues is likely to vary over time, place, and population.

Acknowledgments

Several people deserve special mention for their thoughtful and critical review of earlier drafts of this text. Linda Lloyd of Alliance Healthcare Foundation and Beth Quill of the University of Texas at Houston, School of Public Health, provided me with invaluable feedback. Two former students who had taken my course on Gender, Ethnicity, and Health Research, Lynn Sivinski and Siran Karoukian, provided me with insightful comments from the viewpoint of graduate students utilizing the text as a text. Jill Korbin and Atwood Gaines, both of Case Western Reserve University, are to be thanked for our many discussions relating to issues examined in this text.

Hal Morgenstern of the University of California at Los Angeles, School of Public Health, kindly granted permission for the use of diagrams pertaining to study design and confounding, which have been incorporated into Chapter 2. Southern Illinois University Press also granted permission for portions of Chapter 2, which appear as Chapter 3 in *Forensic Epidemiology*, Southern Illinois University Press (1998).

Fatoumata Traore, Jay F. Fiedler, and Sandra M. Ferber provided me with invaluable research assistance. Mariclaire Cloutier of Kluwer Academic / Plenum Publishers deserves accolades, as always, for her editorial support and encouragement.

Contents

Part III. Case Studies of Disease

Gender, Ethnicity,
and Health Research

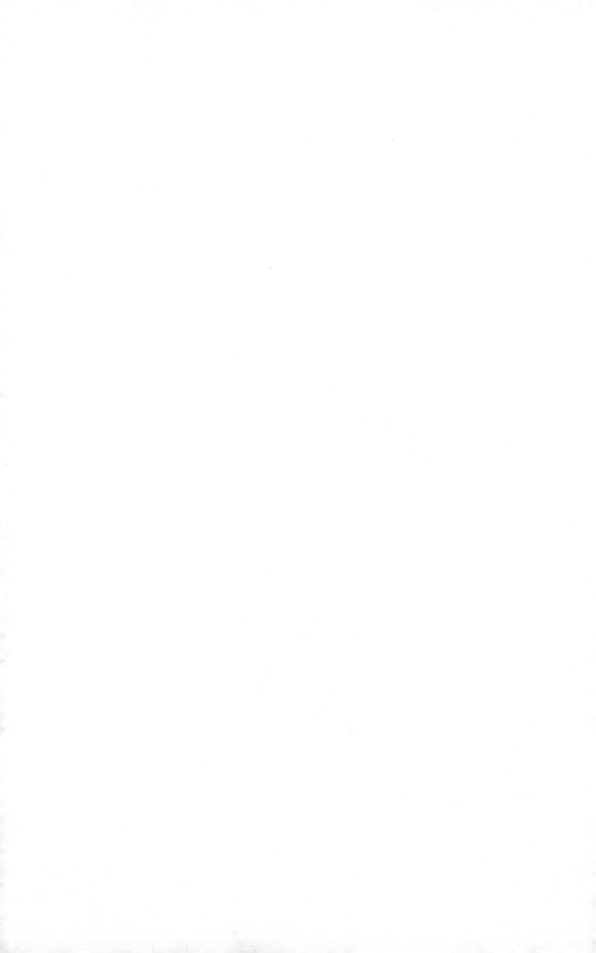

Prologue
Understanding Social Constructs

Why some groups or individuals appear to be more or less susceptible to specific diseases or illnesses has been and continues to be an area of active inquiry and is the focus of this text. Attention to this question necessitates input from and understanding across multiple disciplines including, but not limited to, epidemiology, sociology, anthropology, history, medicine, and genetics. Our ability to investigate and to answer questions of disease susceptibility, causation, and prevention is clearly limited by the boundaries of our knowledge in each relevant discipline, as well as our ability to integrate our understandings across disciplines.

This text proceeds from a biocultural approach to the examination of health and illness in specific groups in the United States. This approach requires an examination of cultural and historical factors that affect the distribution and the natural history of diseases, such as methods of food preparation, beliefs about the cause of illness, and the availability of various medications and substances. The first portion of the text establishes the foundations for this inquiry, with chapters focusing on research ethics, research study design, and an examination of basic constructs such as race, ethnicity, gender, sex, sexual orientation, health care utilization, and health care-seeking behavior.

The second portion of this text focuses on health and illness in specific subgroups: African-Americans, Asians and Pacific Islanders, Latinos, Native Americans, women, and communities with varying sexual and gender orientations. This emphasis may appear to be in contradiction to one of the basic premises of the first portion of the text: that we must move away from the use of race as a marker in health research and utilize, instead, a biocultural approach, which relies more heavily on ethnicity as a construct. Similarly, our construction of both sex and gender as polarized concepts, often inextricably linked together, demands extension if we are to find alternative explanations for our questions.

A biocultural approach requires that we attempt to integrate not only the biology, the "hard science," into our search for answers, but also the history, the culture, and the experience of each group. This is clearly not an easy task. How can one generalize across the many diverse subgroups that we now classify as "Asian and Pacific Islander?" How can we continue to disregard the broad spectrum of history and culture within what we now call "African-American" or "black American," which encompasses individuals of Caribbean, African, and Latin American heritage, to name but a few? This task is rendered all the more difficult because much health research to date continues to report findings on the basis of race, ethnicity, or sex, without a deeper exploration of what revealed associations may signify.

Reliance on this biocultural approach reveals, perhaps surprisingly to some and regrettably to others, our propensity to characterize and/or respond to various subgroups as being in some way deviant. Our construction of this deviance is often reflected in our characterization of the health and, at times, the moral nature of the subgroup at issue and our subsequent approach to the investigation of health status. This tendency is more clear in some instances, as with African-Americans and certain Asian groups, and less clear in others, as with Latinos. It is difficult to determine the extent to which these characterizations have had a short- or long-term effect on the health of the subpopulation, the perception of its health, or on its ability to access care. How and why this characterization of subgroups as deviant is not easily answered and requires a brief review of various approaches to deviance.

A 1965 (U.S.) study of public perceptions of deviance revealed wide diversity in what people classify as deviant: homosexuals (49% of responses), drug addicts (47%), alcoholics (46%), prostitutes (27%), murderers (22%), lesbians (13%), the mentally ill (12%), perverts (12%), communists (10%), and atheists (10%), to name a few (Simmons, 1965). Various approaches have been offered in an attempt to better understand the nature of deviance and why there exists both variation and similarity in perceptions of deviance. Orcutt (1983) has suggested that deviance can be viewed alternatively as: (1) behavior that violates social norms or (2) behaviors that are defined as deviant by the social audiences viewing them. The former definition is termed the "normative" perspective, while the latter is termed "relativistic."

The normative view of deviance is premised on the observation that rules or expectations for behavior (i.e. norms) are shared by members of a group or society (Orcutt, 1983). Although Edgerton (1985) premises his discussion of deviance on rule violation, the concept of the norm is closely related. Edgerton (1985:24), for instance, has defined a rule as "a shared understanding of how people ought to behave and what should be done if someone acts in a way that conflicts with that understanding." Edgerton (1985:24) further explains that

> rules may differ in the extent to which they are known, recognized, accepted as just or proper, and uniformly applied to members of the society. Rules may also vary in the severity of the sanctions that may be incurred by their violations as well as in their consistency of enforcement. They may vary in the degree to which they are internalized, in the mode of their transmission, and in the amount and kind of conformity they receive.... [S]ome rules are relatively explicit while others are implicit, and some clear while others are ambiguous. Some rules contradict others, while others stand for the most part unchallenged.

A "norm" has been variously defined as

> a rule or a standard that governs our conduct in the social situations in which we participate. It is a societal expectation. It is a standard to which we are expected to conform whether we actually do so or not. (Bierstedt, 1963:222)

> shared convictions about the patterns of behavior that are appropriate or inappropriate for the members of a group; what group members agree they can, should, might, must, cannot, should not, ought not, or must not do in any given situation. (DeFleur et al., 1977:620)

> a rule which, over a period of time, proves binding on the overt behavior of each individual in an aggregate of two or more individuals. It is marked by the following characteristics: (1) Being a rule, it has a content known to at least one member of the social aggregate.

(2) Being a binding rule, it regulates the behavior of any given individual in the social aggregate by virtue of (a) his having internalized the rule; (b) external sanctions in support of the rule applied to him by one or more other individuals in the social aggregate; (c) external sanctions in support of the rule applied to him by an authority outside the social aggregate; or any combination of these circumstances. (Dohrenwend, 1959:470)

a rule, standard, or pattern for action ... Social norms are rules for conduct. The norms are the standards by reference to which behavior is judged and approved or disapproved. A norm in this sense is not a statistical average of actual behavior but rather a cultural (shared) definition of desirable behavior. (Williams, 1968:204)

Several elements emerge from these definitions that permit us to better define what is meant by deviance: (1) consensus, both as to what constitutes a rule and a violation of that rule and (2) agreed upon consequences in response to that violation. A review of several definitions of deviance supports this conclusion:

[D]eviance constitutes only those deviations from norms which are in a disapproved direction and of sufficient degree to exceed the tolerance limits of a social group such that the deviation elicits, or is likely to elicit if detected, a negative sanction. (Clinard and Meier, 1979:14)

Deviance is the name of the conflict game in which individuals or loosely organized small groups with little power are strongly feared by a well-organized, sizable minority or majority who have a large amount of power. (Denisoff and McCaghy, 1973:26)

[D]eviant behavior refers to conduct that departs significantly from the norms set for people in their social statuses. (Merton, 1966:805)

[W]e may define deviant behavior in terms of public consensus. We may define it as *any behavior considered deviant by public consensus that may range from the maximum to the minimum.* (Thio, 1978:23)

However, these definitions leave numerous questions unresolved: Whose consensus? Whose opinion is to be considered in "calculating" consensus and what weight is it to be given in that "calculation"? How many/what proportion of a group must agree for there to be consensus? Does the absence of a consequence to an act or behavior validate that behavior as a norm? What kind of reaction must occur for an act to be defined as or considered deviant? If norms change over time, does "deviance" also change? If so, what drives these changes? Additional issues are raised by the definitions of deviance. Deviance, according to some of these definitions, is linked to power (those who define deviance) or its absence (those who are defined as "deviant"). What constitutes deviance is linked to social status, and deviance may exist at the far end of a spectrum of tolerance. However, if classification of a behavior as deviant is linked to social status and power, then can the same behavior be classifiable as "not deviant" based on context and/or observer? If there exists a spectrum of tolerance with respect to individuals' acts or behaviors, is there also a spectrum of tolerance relating to the consequences that can be meted out in response to an act that is termed deviant?

LeVine (1982) has argued that deviance may result not only from norm or rule violation, but also from norm exaggeration. He posits that a cultural environment may induce individuals to behave in a manner that exaggerates "normal" and culturally distinctive behavior. He argues, for instance, that the relatively high rate of suicide among the Japanese may, in fact, be an exaggeration of the cultural value of self-sacrifice.

The degree to which individuals conform to a norm may vary. LeVine (1982), for instance, developed the idea of the J-curve. At the lower (left) side of the curve is a small percentage of individuals who regularly violate the norm. The center portion of the curve represents the percentage of individuals who have infrequently violated the norm and, for the most part, have conformed to it. The right side of the curve reflects the largest proportion of the population, those who have consistently conformed to the norm.

Edgerton (1985) explored situations in which rule violations are not deemed to be acts of deviance. He noted, for example, that some rules have exceptions. Others are only loosely enforced, while still others are enforced with surprising rigidity. How is it that some rule violations will provoke a consequence while others are not enforced? How is it that some rules have exceptions? To some extent, this depends on the nature of the rule, as indicated, and on the status of the violator. However, the consequences may also turn on the account of the violation that is proffered by the violator (Edgerton, 1976). That account, or explanation, can exacerbate the violator's situation, excuse it, or justify it (Edgerton, 1976; Scott and Lyman, 1968). The process of account giving and consequence "is usually more akin to a negotiation than to a mechanical or impartial effort to support propriety or administer justice" (Edgerton, 1976:30).

Under the normative approach, then, behaviors or statuses that are outside the boundaries or push the boundaries of what is considered "normal" by consensus will be considered deviant and subject to consequences. This could include, for example, numerous health-related behaviors such as the use of alcohol (MacAndrew and Edgerton, 1969), violent behavior (Edgerton, 1976), and some forms of sexual behavior and gender role differences, such as homosexuality and transgenderism. Deviance, according to this approach, also encompasses departures from an "ideal" or normative status, so that those who look different or speak differently are to be considered deviant and, potentially, suspect. We see this theme repeated across numerous ethnic groups including, for example, the Chinese, who were perceived as purveyors of leprosy and uncleanliness, and Haitians, who were labeled as a risk group for the transmission of human immunodeficiency virus (HIV).

The "social audience" approach defines deviance quite differently, with an emphasis on those viewing the behavior rather than on a violation of a norm:

> Basically the ultimate measure of whether or not an act is deviant depends on how others who are socially significant in power and influence define the act.... One could commit any act, but it is not deviant in its social consequences if no elements of society react to it. (Bell, 1971:11)

> [A]cts and actors violating the norms of society will be termed "rule-breaking behavior" and "rule breakers," while the terms "deviant behavior" and "deviant" will be reserved for acts and actors labeled as deviant by a social audience. (Cullen and Cullen, 1978:8)

> Deviance is not a property *inherent* in certain forms of behavior; it is a property *conferred upon* these forms by the audience which directly or indirectly witnesses them. (Erikson, 1962:308)

Lemert (1951) has explained how this dynamic comes about. He notes that norms vary across time and place and that members of society become aware of norms only after they have been violated. Such deviation can be measured objectively:

> [T]he sum total of deviation in a given situation will consist of the variance of the actions
> from the prescribed social norms multiplied by the number of persons who engage in such
> actions. (Lemert, 1951:51)

The societal response to this deviation corresponds to the degree and visibility of the deviation. In some cases, the response is extreme in proportion to the actual breach. Lemert (1951:56) explains such "spurious" reactions as the result of "rivalry or conflict of groups ... as they aspire to power or struggle to maintain their position."

Lemert distinguished between primary deviation, which refers to instances of norm violation in which individuals do not view themselves as deviant, and secondary deviation. Secondary deviance arises from the societal response to primary deviance:

> When a person begins to employ his deviant behavior or a role based upon it as a means of
> defense, attack, or adjustment to the ... problems created by the consequent societal reaction
> to him, his deviation is secondary. (Lemert, 1951:76)

Becker (1973) expanded on Lemert's theory by identifying distinct aspects of the social audience's role: (1) the formulation of rules, (2) the application of these rules, and (3) the labeling of particular individuals as outsiders or deviants. The process through which individuals are so labeled often depends more on who is doing the labeling and who is being labeled than on the nature of the behavior involved. Consequently, behavior cannot be labeled as deviant until after the response has occurred. Becker (1963:9) explains:

> Social groups create deviance by making the rules whose infraction constitutes deviance,
> and by applying those rules to particular people and labeling them as "outsiders." From this
> point of view, deviance is not a quality of the act the person commits, but rather a conse-
> quence of the application by others of rules and sanctions to an offender. The deviant is one
> to whom that label has successfully been applied; deviant behavior is that people so label.

Kitsuse (1962) posited that audiences create deviance through a three-stage process: (1) interpretation of behavior as deviant; (2) definition of individuals who engage in that behavior as deviant; and (3) response to the individual(s) in a manner considered appropriate to the specific type of deviance. An individual is not considered deviant until the third stage, when he or she is subject to the verbal or physical repercussions of the behavior.

Ben-Yehuda (1990:36) has argued that "who interprets whose behavior, why, where, and when is very crucial." He offers two specific examples, those of Joan of Arc and the Nobel laureate chemist Linus Pauling. Joan of Arc, convicted of being a heretical deviant and executed in 1431, was later canonized by Pope Benedict XV. Pauling, supported by thousands of scientists from all over the world, lobbied the United Nations in the late 1950s to end nuclear weapons testing. His efforts led to an interrogation by the U.S. Senate and he was prohibited from attending various international scientific meetings. In 1962, he was awarded the Nobel Prize for his efforts in promoting peace (Ben-Yehuda, 1990).

Like the normative approach, however, the "social audience" definition is also unable to address all issues satisfactorily. Kitsuse's (1962:253) definition of deviance underscores some of the difficulties with this approach:

> Forms of behavior *per se* do not differentiate deviants from non-deviants; it is the responses
> of the conventional and conforming members of the society who identify and interpret
> behavior as deviant which sociologically transform persons into deviants.

It is unclear, however, what kind of response, both in nature and degree, is either necessary or sufficient to merit classification of a particular behavior as deviant. It is also unclear what kind of acts, both in nature and degree, are necessary or sufficient to provoke a necessary and sufficient response. If there is no response to acts such as murder and torture, can it be said that these acts are not "deviant?" Conversely, if these acts are inherently "deviant," regardless of audience response, can it really be said then that classification as "deviant" rests entirely on definition by the audience, without reference to a norm?

In examining health and illness among specific groups then, we must be cognizant of whether and how specific groups and illnesses have come to be associated with each other. We must ask ourselves whether such apparent associations are real, or whether we have disproportionately focused our attention on a specific illness or disease within a specific community due to our often unvoiced conceptualizations of what is normal or acceptable. Have these underlying biases driven our interpretation of our data, including our "hard science"? When our research indicates differences in health or health care access across groups, we must continuously seek the underlying reasons for these apparent differences, while simultaneously recognizing that our classification of individuals into such groups may, itself, be faulty.

Viewed synchronically, our approach to questions related to sexual orientation and gender role differences is illustrative of these issues. "Sexual deviance" has been defined as "the inappropriate or flawed performance of a conventionally understood sexual practice" (Simon, 1994). Particular forms of sexual deviance have been classified as perversions, defined as

> a disease of sexual desire not only in the sense that it appears to violate the sexual practices of a time and place, but also because it constitutes a violation of common understandings that render current sexual practice plausible. (Simon, 1994:5)

Oral sex, for instance, has at various times in history been considered deviant and/or perverse, while it is now (in the United States) considered conventional (Gagnon and Simon, 1987). "Deviance" has been used to refer to a broad range of sexual behaviors, including exhibitionism (Marshall, Ecles, and Barbaree, 1991), masturbation, homosexuality, pedophilia, sadomasochism (Simon, 1994), prostitution (James and Davis, 1982) and solicitation of a prostitute (Salamon, 1989), transsexuality (Nanda, 1991), nymphomania, "sex addiction," and table-top dancing (Nelson and Robinson, 1994).

These behaviors are generally outside the norm or perceived to be outside of the norm, or statistical average, in the context in which they occur. Various hypotheses have been offered to explain their origin, including chromosomal abnormality and hormonal abnormality. Outside of the medical arena, however, there seems to be general consensus that much of what is considered "deviant" in the context of sexual behavior has attained that status due to social audience response. Young (1977) has argued that the media has promoted a dichotomized view of majority and deviant minority, often employing stereotyped images of "deviance." Reiss (1986) has further argued that such discussions actually, then, become the vehicle for the reinforcement of culturally normative ideas about sex.

Gender deviance has been defined as

> behavior that violates the norms for gender-appropriate behavior; this deviance is to be distinguished from sexual deviance, which may or may not also be gender deviant. Thus, while transvestites and homosexuals are gender deviant, prostitutes and rapists are sexual deviants who are quite gender conventional. (Harry, 1983:350)

(Contrast Harry's classification of homosexuality as gender deviance with those of other writers, indicated earlier, who have classified it as a form of sexual deviance.)

Two examples of gender or sexual deviance are those of the berdache and the *hijra*. (Note that depending upon the author, they may be considered examples of sexual or gender deviance.) The berdache is a status that has existed within numerous Native American tribes. Berdaches are perceived as neither men nor women, but as an alternative gender (Callender and Kochems, 1985), and may refer to themselves as "halfmen–halfwomen" (Williams, 1992). Berdaches often do the work that is normally assigned to women, but may combine the behavior, social roles, and dress of both men and women. Although the berdache may become asexual or assume a passive sexual relationship with a man, the sexual relationship is seen as a secondary characteristic of this status (Callender and Kochems, 1985). The *hijras* of India have been termed "neither man nor woman and man and woman" (Nanda, 1990). The term *hijra* includes both "born *hijras*" (hermaphrodites) and "made *hijras*" (eunuchs). The surgical removal of the male genitals is considered a religious obligation of those who are not born *hijras* (Nanda, 1990).

A variety of responses are available to both the "deviant" individual and to those witnessing the "deviance." Responses of the "deviant" may include the proffering of an account, secondary deviance, and/or attempts to cover deviance.

Scott and Lyman (1968:46) have defined an "account" as "a linguistic device employed whenever an action is subjected to valuative inquiry." They elaborate:

> By an account, then, we mean a statement made by a social actor to explain unanticipated or untoward behavior—whether that behavior is his own or that of others, and whether the proximate cause for that statement arises from the actor himself or from someone else. An account is not called for when people engage in routine, common-sense behavior in a cultural environment that recognizes that behavior as such.

Scott and Lyman (1968) distinguish between accounts that are excuses and those that constitute justifications. Excuses will mitigate or relieve the actor from his or her responsibility. Excuses include appeals to accidents, defeasibility, biological drives, and scapegoating. Justifications will not only neutralize an act or its consequences, but will also assert the positive value of the act. Justifications include denial of injury, denial of the victim, condemnation of the condemners, and appeal to loyalties. Whether any account will be honored will depend on the character of the social circle in which it is utilized and the expectations of the audience receiving the account.

The response of the audience may well depend on the nature of the account that is offered. For instance, where the audience response is likely to be one of deterrence (i.e., punishment), the account given to explain a criminal act may determine (1) whether there will, in fact, be any punishment and (2) the extent of that punishment, if imposed. Homosexual intercourse provides one example of where an account may be critical to the response. For instance, a military person's explanation of why he engaged in intercourse with another man may be a decisive factor in the determination of actions to be taken against him and the decision to retain him in the military.

Secondary deviance arises from the societal response to primary deviance, which refers to instances of norm violation in which individuals do not view themselves as deviant:

> When a person begins to employ his deviant behavior or a role based upon it as a means of defense, attack or adjustment to the … problems created by the consequent societal reaction to him, his deviation is secondary. (Lemert, 1951:76)

Covering refers to attempts to hide the deviance from others, in an attempt to "blend" with the nondeviant (French, Wilke, Mayfield, and Woolley, 1985). Covering attempts may include the use of a wig to hide baldness due to chemotherapy or elaborate routines to "cover" one's mental retardation. Goffman (1963) documented, for example, one blind man's attempts to hide his blindness from a date. Throughout numerous dates and several movies, this gentleman held the hand of his date, so that she unwittingly led him where he needed to go, giving her the perception that he was a sighted person. Edgerton (1993) documented in detail the efforts of formerly institutionalized mentally retarded adults to "pass" by lying about where they were from to avoid discovery of the prior institutionalization; by marrying to appear normal and to emphasize their status as a free person; by acquiring "memorabilia" so as to have a history; by finding excuses to explain their lack of a car; and by devising mechanisms to simplify others' responses, such as asking whether it is 9:00 yet (responses: almost, no, just after) rather than asking the exact time (responses: 8:40, 20 minutes to 9, etc.). Covering, or "passing," has been used by members of communities of color to gain access to privileges and benefits once accorded to only whites and by gays to avoid social and economic sanctions for being homosexual (Chauncey, 1994; Lopez, 1994; Polednak, 1997).

Gove (1982) has delineated various classes of audience response to deviance: social reaction, deterrence, prevention, incentives, treatment, amelioration, and self-curative. To these can be added acceptance (Bogdan and Taylor, 1987). The literature relating to each of these strategies is extensive and will only be touched upon briefly.

Social reaction advocates the redefinition of a situation so that the behavior initially viewed as a problem is no longer viewed as such. The proposed removal of transsexuality as a form of mental disorder from the *Diagnostic and Statistical Manual of Mental Disorders* provides one such example of redefinition (Loue, 1996).

Punishment or deterrence is one of the most common strategies for dealing with deviant behavior. The use of a deterrence approach is premised on operant theory, which posits that individuals perform an act when the rewards of that act exceed the costs (Gove, 1982). Operant theory suggests, then, that punishment, as in the criminal justice system, must be systematically and rapidly applied. Increased efforts to address drunken driving are illustrative of this approach (Robertson, 1997). Neither, however, may occur, due to a variety of reasons, including overburdening of the courts and plea bargaining (Gove, 1982).

Prevention focuses on the identification of what is perceived to be the weak link in a complex causal process and the manipulation of that link in order to prevent the potentially developing deviance. This strategy, commonly used in the health context, encompasses a broad range of interventions, including legislation, such as gun control measures (Gove, 1982) and tobacco control (Cummings, 1997), education (Gove, 1982), and screening (Champion and Miller, 1997).

Gove (1982) notes that the use of incentives to reward nondeviant behavior, thereby encouraging nondeviant behavior while simultaneously discouraging deviant behavior, is rarely utilized. One example is the use of employee incentive programs to encourage attendance and discourage absences due to illness.

Treatment is one of the most common responses to deviance and often occurs in response to deviance forms that have become medicalized, such as transsexuality and homosexuality. The form of the treatment necessarily depends on the form of deviance or malady.

Gove (1982) indicates that some forms of deviance are believed to be self-curative, that is, an individual will "grow out of it." As an example, this author has been informed by various physicians in Laos and Thailand that homosexuality is normal through adolescence, and that individuals are expected to "grow out of it" by the time they reach their late teens. The behavior is seen as deviant only after mid- to late adolescence when the "self-cure" has not taken root.

Bogdan and Taylor (1987:35) define acceptance as a

[relationship] … between a person with a deviant attribute and another person, which is of long duration and characterized by closeness and affection and in which the deviant attribute does not have a stigmatizing, or morally discrediting, character. Accepting relationships are not based on a denial of difference, but rather on the absence of impugning the different person's moral character because of the variation.

Such relationships are generally founded on feelings of family, a sense of religious obligation or commitment, humanitarian orientation, and feelings of friendship. Accepting relationships are often characterized by formation in stages over a period of time; increasing levels of trust and comfort as the relationship develops; shared contempt between the "deviant" and the nondeviant for "outsiders" who manifest their discomfort; de-emphasis of the differences and emphasis on the positive aspects of the relationship; and empathy from the nondeviant individual with the discrimination or rejection experienced by the "deviant."

References

Becker, H.S. (1973). *Outsiders: Studies in the Sociology of Deviance*. New York: Free Press.

Bell, R.B. (1971). *Social Deviance*. Homewood, IL: Dorsey.

Ben-Yehuda, N. (1990). *The Politics and Morality of Deviance: Moral Panics, Drug Abuse, Deviant Science, and Diverse Stigmatization*. Albany, NY: State University of New York Press.

Bierstedt, R. (1963). *The Social Order* (2nd ed). New York: McGraw-Hill.

Bogdan, R., & Taylor, S. (1987). Toward a sociology of acceptance: The other side of the study of deviance. *Social Policy, 18*, 34–39.

Callender, C., & Kochems, L.M. (1985). Men and not-men: Male gender-mixing statuses and homosexuality. *Journal of Homosexuality, 11*, 165–178.

Champion, V.L., & Miller, A. (1997). Adherence to mammography and breast self-examination regimens. In D.S. Gochman (Ed.), *Handbook of Health Behavior Research II: Provider Determinants* (pp. 245–267). New York: Plenum Press.

Chauncey, G. (1994). *Gay New York: Gender, Urban Culture, and the Making of the Gay World, 1890–1940*. New York: BasicBooks.

Clinard, M.B., & Meier, R.F. (1979). *Sociology of Deviant Behavior* (5th ed.). New York: Holt, Rinehart, and Winston.

Cullen, F.T., & Cullen, J.B. (1978). *Toward a Paradigm of Labeling Theory*. Lincoln, NE: University of Nebraska.

Cummings, K.M. (1997). Health policy and smoking and tobacco use. In D.S. Gochman (Ed.), *Handbook of Health Behavior Research IV: Relevance for Professionals and Issues for the Future* (pp. 231–251). New York: Plenum Press.

DeFleur, M.L., Antonio, W.V., DeFleur, L.B., Nelson, L., & Adamic, C.H. (1977). *Sociology: Human Society* (2nd ed.). Glenview, IL: Scott, Foresman.

Denisoff, R., & McCaghy, C.H. (1973). *Deviance, Conflict, and Criminality*. Chicago: Rand McNally.

Dohrenwend, B.P. (1959). Egoism, altruism, anomie and fatalism: A conceptual analysis of Durkheim's types. *American Sociological Review, 24*, 466–473.

Edgerton, R.B. (1976). *Deviance: A Cross-Cultural Perspective*. Menlo Park, CA: Benjamin Cummings Publishing Company.

Edgerton, R.B. (1985). *Rules, Exceptions, and Social Order*. Berkeley, CA: University of California Press.

Edgerton, R.B. (1993). *The Cloak of Competence* (rev. ed.). Berkeley, CA: University of California Press.

Erikson, K.T. (1962). Notes on the sociology of deviance. *Social Problems, 9*, 307–314.

French, F., Wilke, A.S., Mayfield, L., & Woolley, B. (1985). The physician's role in covering deviance: Assisting the physically handicapped. *Psychological Reports, 57*, 1255–1259.

Gagnon, J.H., & Simon, W. (1987). The sexual scripting of oral genital contacts. *Archives of Sexual Behavior, 16*, 1–25.

Goffman, E. (1963). *Stigma: Notes on the Management of Spoiled Identity*. New York: Simon and Schuster, Inc.

Gove, W.R. (1982). The formal reshaping of deviance. In M.M. Rosenberg, R.A. Stebbins, & A. Turowetz (Eds.), *The Sociology of Deviance* (pp. 175–201). New York: St. Martin's Press.

Harry, J. (1983). Parasuicide, gender, and gender deviance. *Journal of Health and Social Behavior, 24,* 350–361.

James, J., & Davis, N.J. (1982). Contingencies in female sexual role deviance. The case of prostitution. *Human Organization, 41,* 345–350.

Kitsuse, J.I. (1962). Societal reaction to deviant behavior: Problems of theory and method. *Social Problems, 9,* 247–256.

Lemert, E.M. (1951). *Social Pathology.* New York: McGraw Hill.

Levine, B.A. (1982). *Culture, Behavior, and Personality* (2nd ed.). New York: Alsine Publishing Company.

Lopez, I.F.H. (1994). The social construction of race: Some observations on illusion, fabrication, and choice. *Harvard Civil Rights—Civil Liberties Law Review, 29,* 1–62.

Loue, S. (1996). Transsexualism in medicolegal limine: An examination and proposal for change. *Journal of Psychiatry and Law, Spring,* 27–51.

MacAndrew, C., & Edgerton, R.B. (1969). *Drunken Comportment: A Social Explanation.* Chicago: Aldine Publishing Company.

Marshall, W.L., Ecles, A., & Barbaree, H.E. (1991). The treatment of exhibitionists: A focus on sexual deviance versus cognitive and relationship features. *Behavior Research and Therapy, 29,* 129–135.

Merton, R.K. (1966). Social problems and sociological theory. In R.K. Merton & R. Nisbet (Eds.), *Contemporary Social Problems* (2nd ed., pp. 775–823). New York: Harcourt, Brace, and World.

Nanda, S. (1990). *Neither Man Nor Woman: The Hijras of India.* Belmont, CA: Wadsworth Publishing Company.

Nanda, S. (1991). Deviant careers: The *hijras* of India. In M. Freilich, D. Raybeck, & J. Savishinsky (Eds.), *Deviance: Anthropological Perspectives* (pp. 149–171). New York: Bergin and Garvey.

Nelson, E.D.A., & Robinson, B.W. (1994). "Reality talk" or "telling tales"? The social construction of sexual and gender deviance on a television talk show. *Journal of Contemporary Ethnography, 23,* 51–78.

Orcutt, J.D. (1983). *Analyzing Deviance.* Homewood, IL: Dorsey Press.

Polednak, A.P. (1997). *Segregation, Poverty, and Mortality in Urban African Americans.* New York: Oxford University Press.

Reiss, I. (1986). *Journey Into Sexuality.* Englewood Cliffs, NJ: Prentice-Hall.

Roberston, L.S. (1997). Health policy, health behavior, and injury control. In D.S. Gochman (Ed.), *Handbook of Health Behavior Research IV: Relevance for Professionals and Issues for the Future* (pp. 215–230). New York: Plenum Press.

Salamon, E. (1989). The homosexual escort agency: Deviance disavowal. *British Journal of Sociology, 40,* 1–21.

Scott, M.B., & Lyman, S.M. (1968). Accounts. *American Sociological Review, 35,* 46–62.

Simmons, J.L. (1965). Public stereotypes of deviants. *Social Problems, 13,* 223–232.

Simon, W. (1994). Deviance as history: The future of perversion. *Archives of Sexual Behavior, 23,* 1–20.

Thio, A. (1978). *Deviant Behavior.* Boston: Houghton Mifflin.

Williams, R.M., Jr. (1968). The concept of norms. In D.L. Sills (Ed.). *International Encyclopedia of the Social Sciences* (Vol. 11, pp. 204–208). New York: Macmillan.

Williams, W.L. (1992). *The Spirit and the Flesh: Sexual Diversity in American Indian Culture.* Boston: Beacon Press.

Young, J. (1977). The police as amplifiers of deviancy. In P. Rock (Ed.), *Drugs and Politics* (pp. 99–134). New Brunswick, NJ: Transaction Books.

I

Foundations

1

Ethical Principles Governing Research Involving Human Participants

The ethical conduct of research is grounded in the principles of respect for persons, justice and fairness, beneficence, and nonmaleficence. This chapter provides a brief overview of the development, enunciation, and application of these principles.

Historical Foundations

Health research involving human experimentation has been conducted in the United States for over a century. Such research has been and continues to be subject to specified standards. For example, during the early years of the 20th century, humans were not to be used in experiments until after the safety of the new drug or procedure had been established in animals (Osler, 1907). Second, "full consent" of a patient was a prerequisite to application of the new therapy. Patients entrusted to the care of the physician were not to be recruited for experimentation unless the new therapy would potentially result in a direct benefit to the individual patient. Third, the participation of healthy volunteers in experimentation was permissible, subject to the requirement of full knowledge of the circumstances and agreement to participate (Osler, 1907).

Despite these enunciated standards, research involving human experimentation was conducted under sometimes questionable circumstances. One experiment involving the injection of sterilized gelatin into two young boys and a "feeble-minded girl" resulted in "prostration and collapse" (Abt, 1903). Other researchers studying the ability of several new tests to detect tuberculosis injected tuberculin solution into more than 164 children under the age of 8, most of whom were residents of an orphanage. The experiment often resulted in discomfort, eye lesions, or eye inflammations (Belais, 1910; Hamill, Carpenter, and Cope, 1908). Other questionable experiments related to the etiology, diagnosis, and/or prevention of other diseases, including syphilis, yellow fever, typhoid, and herpes, were often conducted on children, prisoners, soldiers, or the mentally ill (Lederer, 1997).

It was the events of World War II, however, that provided the impetus for the development of formal international standards to guide experimentation involving human participants: the Nuremberg Code. During World War II, prisoners in Nazi concentration camps were "recruited" for participation in experimentation without either advance knowledge of the procedures to be performed or consent. These experiments, which included the exposure of prisoners to cold water and low air pressure (Appelbaum, Lidz, and Meisel, 1987), the injection of dye into eyes in an attempt to change the eye color, and the inoculation of prisoners with typhus bacilli (Grodin, 1992), often resulted in injury or death.

The Nuremberg Code (1949) enumerates ten basic principles that are deemed to be universally applicable to research involving human subjects:

1. The prospective participant's voluntary consent is essential.
2. The results to be obtained from the experiment must be beneficial to society and those results cannot be obtained through any other means.
3. The study must have as its foundation the results of animal experiments and a knowledge of the natural history of the disease so that the anticipated results justify the conduct of the experiment.
4. All unnecessary physical and mental injury or suffering must be avoided during the course of the experiment.
5. No experiment should be conducted if it is believed that death or disabling injury will occur, except where the research physicians also serve as research participants.
6. The degree of risk should not exceed the humanitarian importance of the problem being addressed.
7. Adequate facilities and preparations should be used to protect the participant against death or injury.
8. Only scientifically qualified persons should conduct the experiment.
9. The participant has a right to end his or her participation at any time if he or she reaches a point where continuation seems to be impossible.
10. The scientist in charge must be prepared to end the experiment if there is probable cause to believe that continuing the experiment will be likely to result in the injury, disability, or death of the research participant (World Medical Association, 1991b; Annas and Grodin, 1992).

The Nuremberg Code has been subject to a great deal of criticism, particularly for its failure to distinguish between therapeutic clinical research and clinical research on healthy participants and to provide a review mechanism for researchers' actions (Perley, Fluss, Bankowski, and Simon, 1992). These deficiencies and the resulting discussions ultimately led to the formulation and adoption of the Declaration of Helsinki.

The Declaration of Helsinki was initially adopted by the World Medical Association in 1964. Unlike the Nuremberg Code, the Declaration (1) allows participation in research through the consent of a surrogate, where the actual participant is legally or physically unable to consent to his or her participation and (2) distinguishes between clinical research combined with professional care and nontherapeutic clinical research. Later revisions in 1975, 1983, and 1989 further emphasized the need for an individual's voluntary informed consent to participate in research (World Medical Association, 1991a; Perley *et al.*, 1992; Christakis and Panner, 1991).

International documents were later developed to provide further guidance in the conduct of research involving humans. The *International Guidelines for Ethical Review of Epidemiological Studies* were compiled by the Council for International Organizations of Medical Sciences (CIOMS, 1991) specifically to aid researchers in the field of epidemiology to resolve moral ambiguities that may arise during the course of their research. The *International Ethical Guidelines for Biomedical Research Involving Human Subjects* (1993), prepared by CIOMS and the World Health Organization (WHO), set forth a statement of general ethical principles, 15 guidelines, and relevant commentary reflecting both the majority and minority points of view. The WHO's *Guidelines for Good Clinical Practice for Trials on Pharmaceutical Products* (1995) provides additional guidelines for the conduct of clinical trials.

In addition to the principles and guidelines enunciated by these international organizations, U.S. researchers conducting studies involving human subjects must be aware of the regulations promulgated by the U.S. government. Unlike the principles and guidelines, which provide ethical guidance to researchers, these regulations, which reflect the U.S. interpretation and application of the principles and guidelines, constitute a legal obligation.

The initial regulations were promulgated in 1974 by what was then the Department of Health, Education, and Welfare. These regulations stipulated that research would not be funded by the agency unless the prospective grant recipient had submitted the research proposal for review and approval to an institutional review board (IRB). The regulations provided that the IRB was to consist of at least five individuals with specifically enumerated skills; that the IRB members were to ensure that the anticipated benefits of the research outweighed the risks of the research; that the participants' rights and welfare would be adequately protected; and that the participants' informed consent would be obtained by adequate and appropriate means (45 Code of Federal Regulations section 46.102(b), currently at 45 Code of Federal Regulations sections 46.107, 46.111, 1996). Informed consent was defined to include an explanation of (1) the procedures that would be utilized in the study, (2) the risks and benefits to the research participant, (3) any alternative procedures or treatments that were available if the prospective participant did not wish to join the study, and (4) the right of the participant to withdraw from the study at any time, without fear of repercussions (45 Code of Federal Regulations section 46.103(c)(6), currently at 45 Code of Federal Regulations section 46.116, 1996).

A number of states have also promulgated legislation regulating the conduct of research involving humans, including Virginia, New York (Glantz, 1992), and California (California Health and Safety Code sections 24170–24179.5, 1997). Other states have implemented procedures for obtaining informed consent from surrogate decision-makers in situations where the prospective participant is unable to give his or her own consent (R.J. Levine, 1991).

Governing Principles

Respect for Persons

Respect for persons encompasses respect for autonomy which, in turn, relates to informed consent, voluntariness, and the maintenance of confidentiality and privacy. Each of these issues is discussed in greater detail below.

Informed Consent

The informed consent process requires that (1) an individual be competent to give consent, (2) the individual be provided with adequate information to make a decision regarding his or her participation, (3) the individual have understood the information provided, and (4) the consent to participate has been given voluntarily (Grodin, Kaminow, and Sassower, 1986; Mendelson, 1991). Maintaining integrity during this process is critical for various reasons. First, the process minimizes the harm that may result to the research participant from the research (Capron, 1991). Second, because all of the risks of the experimentation may not be known in advance, the participant must be able to decide whether or not to proceed. Third, unlike a clinical setting, the researcher cannot say with certainty which treatment or procedure will be more likely to benefit the prospective participant or cause discomfort, so that the participant is the best person to decide whether or not to proceed. Fourth, participation in the research may or may not provide a direct benefit to the participant. Finally, the prospective participant is in the best position to protect his or her own interests in situations where the researcher and the participant have conflicting interests or differing values which would lead them to assess the benefits of the research quite differently (Delgado and Leskovac, 1986).

Consent. In general, individuals' consent to participate in research is express, that is, the individual provides a clear statement, whether orally or in writing, that he or she is willing to participate in the research. In some circumstances, however, express consent may not be possible. Some researchers might argue that a comatose patient's presentation at the emergency department constitutes implied consent to be furnished the most effective treatment and, absent knowledge as to which treatment is most effective, that consent extends to participation in a trial to determine which procedure is most effective. Whether or not such a presentation at the emergency department constitutes consent remains controversial.

Concern also exists regarding the nature of the consent given and the duration of its validity. The concept of autonomy rests on a concept of individual sovereignty. However, many cultures subordinate the wishes of the individual to those of the immediate or extended family, or even to those of the community. Consequently, in some cultures, the ability of an individual to consent to participate in research may be dependent on the acquiescence or lack of disagreement from a particular family member or community individual (Lane, 1994; Loue, Okello, and Kawuma, 1996).

Whether consent once given remains valid through time is also related to issues of individual identity. For instance, an individual while mentally competent may agree to participate in a study that requires that he or she undergo various medical tests or procedures. However, during the course of the study, the individual may lose his or her capacity to make such decisions. The question then arises as to whether the decision to participate should be honored, even though the individual may no longer be aware of the implications of that decision or of the procedures that he or she is undergoing and may not have contemplated or anticipated such loss of capacity.

Capacity to Consent. Capacity to give consent may be equally difficult to determine. In many cases, governing laws provide initial guidance as to who is and who is not competent to consent to participate in research. For example, minors generally cannot consent to participate, nor can mentally ill persons or mentally retarded persons. Others, however, may be competent to consent at one point in time, but not at others, as may be the case with individuals suffering from dementia.

Generally, a person is deemed to have capacity to consent if he or she is able to understand the nature of the research, the nature of his or her participation in the research, the risks and benefits that may result from participation in the research, and the alternatives to participation (High, 1992; Lo, 1990). Various tools are available to aid the researcher in assessing a prospective participant's competence to consent when it is suspect, including dementia rating scales and mental status examinations. A mental status examination, for example, will provide the researcher with very basic information relating to the individual's orientation to time and place, his or her capacity for immediate recall, his or her long- or short-term memory, and his or her ability to perform simple calculations (Lo, 1990). Such instruments must be chosen carefully, particularly if the test is administered in a language that is not the prospective participant's first language or in situations where the questions on the examination are culture-based.

Information.   Researchers may differ in the quantity and detail of information that they believe a prospective research participant should have or would want prior to deciding whether or not to enroll in a particular research study. Researchers may fear that full written disclosure that details all the possible risks will ultimately discourage individuals from enrolling in the study, consequently resulting in the prolongation of the recruitment period or the abandonment of the research altogether (Lara and de la Fuente, 1990; Thong and Harth, 1991). However, government regulations now specify the minimum information that must be provided in most instances to prospective research participants as a prerequisite for their consent. Briefly, the participant must be told that the study involves research, the purpose of the research and the expected duration of the individual's participation in the research, the procedures involved in the research, the reasonably foreseeable risks or discomforts that the participant may experience, the benefits to the individual or to others that may result from the individual's participation in the research, the alternative procedures or treatments that might be advantageous to the participant, the extent to which the records identifying the participant will be confidential, the availability and nature of compensation and any medical treatment in case of injury, which individual(s) may be contacted by the participant for answers to questions about the research or in case of a research-related injury to the participant, that the individual's participation is voluntary and that a refusal to participate will not result in a penalty or loss of benefits to which the participant is otherwise entitled, and that the participant may discontinue his or her participation at any time without a penalty or loss of benefits to which he or she would otherwise be entitled (45 Code of Federal Regulations section 46.116, 1996). Other statements may also be included, such as statements related to unforeseeable risks, the involuntary termination of the individual's participation, additional costs to the participant, the consequences of a participant's decision to withdraw from the study and the procedures to be followed to do so, significant new findings that are developed during the course of the study that may relate to the individual's willingness to continue his or her participation in the study, and the approximate number of participants in the study (45 Code of Federal Regulations section 46.116, 1996).

Understanding.   Difficulties in understanding the information presented may arise due to problems of information processing, false belief, or nonacceptance (Beauchamp and Childress, 1994). Difficulties in understanding the information presented may be related to the reading level at which the informed consent form is written (Young, Hooker, and Freeberg, 1990; Meade and Howser, 1992), the time at which the information is presented (Lavelle-Jones, Byrne, Rice, and Cuschieri, 1993), the format in which the information is presented (Peterson, Clancy, Champion, and McLarty, 1992), and the accuracy with which the consent form is translated into the appropriate language (Peterson *et al.*, 1992).

Various techniques have been identified that will facilitate comprehension, including use of a readability scale to reduce the reading level of the informed consent form to the eighth grade level or below (LoVerde, Prochazka, and Bynny, 1989; Silva and Sorrell, 1988; Young *et al.*, 1990); presentation of the information on the consent form in a simple, clear, and concise manner (Epstein and Lasagna, 1969; Simel and Feussner, 1992); providing the participant sufficient time to study the form prior to signing it (Lavelle-Jones *et al.*, 1993; Morrow, Gootnick, and Schmale, 1978; Tankanow, Sweet, and Weisikoff, 1992); use of organizational modifications, such as varying the size of the type and the spacing of the information (Taub, 1986); use of graphics and summary declarative statements (Peterson *et al.*, 1992); and use of a video (Benson *et al.*, 1988).

Voluntariness

The issue of voluntariness of participation most frequently arises in situations where an individual's ability to freely consent is called into question. These situations are often characterized by the vulnerability of particular research participants such as children, due to their young age, lack of mental or legal capacity to consent, and relative inability to comprehend; the mentally retarded and mentally ill, due to their relative inability to comprehend; and prisoners, due to the inherently coercive nature of their confinement. Other circumstances, such as the provision of an incentive to participate, may transform an apparently voluntary decision into one that borders on the coercive.

Children have been found to be more likely to understand the very concrete aspects of research, such as the time involved, but generally less likely to understand more abstract concepts, such as the nature of the research (Susman, Dorn, and Fletcher, 1992). Federal regulations that recognize both the child's limited ability to understand as well as the need to involve the child in the decision-making process to the extent possible, require that a child "assent," or affirmatively agree to participate in the research as a prerequisite to participation (45 Code of Federal Regulations sections 46.404.–46.408, 1996). The process of obtaining the child's assent includes the provision of both information to the child and the opportunity to participate in the decision-making process, which includes honoring a child's refusal to assent (Leiken, 1993).

To be valid, the assent must reflect the child's understanding of what he or she must do and of what will be done to him or to her as part of the research (Weithorn and McCabe, 1988). Clearly, a child's cognitive abilities will affect his or her ability to understand the information provided (Leiken, 1993). The child's willingness to withhold assent or to dissent may be affected by his or her cultural, ethnic, or economic background (Weithorn and Scherer, 1994). Obtaining assent may be particularly difficult with children who are especially vulnerable, such as children whose parents are divorced, abusive, mentally ill or mentally retarded; children who are migrant, homeless, or living in an impoverished environment; and children who are members of particular ethnic or religious groups (Cooke, 1994).

In addition to the child's assent, federal regulations also require the consent of one or both of the parents to the child's participation. The requirement of parental consent appears to stem from the traditional view of parental authority, as well as the need to protect children (Leiken, 1989). These regulations classify research involving children into four categories that are delineated by the level of risk associated with the research, the level of the child's participation in the decision-making process, and the need for parental consent from one or both of the parents (45 Code of Federal Regulations sections 46.102, 46.404–46.408, 1996). These regulations should be consulted prior to formulating research involving children.

Particular problems relating to consent and assent may exist in situations where the child is in the care of foster parents, is a ward of the state, or is an emancipated minor, or where the child's parent or parents are unavailable or are legally, mentally, or physically unable to give consent (Ackerman, 1990; Gray, 1989; Grodin and Alpert, 1988; C. Levine, 1991). A number of states, including California, Georgia, Massachusetts, New Jersey, North Carolina, Pennsylvania, and Texas have attempted to address this issue by appointing a medical guardianship for foster parents and by instituting a central review board for the approval of protocols and enrollment of children (C. Levine, 1991). Federal regulations now provide that children who are wards of the state or any agency, institution, or entity may participate in research only if the research is related to their status as wards or if the research is conducted in a setting, such as a school, in which the majority of children are not wards (45 Code of Federal Regulations section

46.409, 1996). In addition, an advocate must be appointed for each such child. The advocate may not be associated with the investigator, the research, or the guardian organization (45 Code of Federal Regulations section 46.409, 1996).

The voluntariness of prisoners' consent to participate in research may be questionable because the research itself may provide a benefit not otherwise available to them. For example, where prison health care services are inadequate, participation in research may be the only identifiable mechanism to receive adequate care (Dubler and Sidel, 1989; Siegel *et al.*, 1993). The voluntariness of consent is also questionable if prisoners are explicitly offered an otherwise unavailable benefit in exchange for their participation. For example, the then-governor of Mississippi in 1915 offered male prisoners pardons in exchange for their participation in a study designed to test the hypothesized association between diet and pellagra (Etheridge, 1972). Accordingly, federal regulations enumerate specific provisions for the inclusion of prisoners in research, in an effort to ensure that the procedures to be used are fair to all prisoners and that the risks to be borne by the prisoner-participants are commensurate with the risks that would be borne by nonprisoner research participants (45 Code of Federal Regulations sections 46.301–46.306, 1996).

First, the membership of the IRB reviewing research that involves prisoners must include at least one prisoner or a representative of prisoners' interests. A majority of the IRB members may not have any association with the prisoners involved, apart from their membership on the IRB (45 Code of Federal Regulations section 46.304, 1996). Secondly, the research must fall into one of the categories of research permitted by regulation. These include studies of (1) the possible causes, effects, and processes of incarceration, and of criminal behavior; (2) prisons as institutional structures or of prisoners as incarcerated persons; (3) conditions particularly affecting prisoners as a class; and (4) practices that may improve the health or well-being of the subject (45 Code of Federal Regulations section 46.306(a)(2), 1996). The IRB is also required to provide certification relating to the balancing of risks and benefits, the selection procedures for study enrollment, the clarity of the protocol and informed consent procedures, and the availability of adequate follow-up care (45 Code of Federal Regulations section 46.305, 1996).

The use of payments to encourage participation in research has been called a paradox: "The higher the monetary payment, the greater is the benefit [of the research to the participant]; the greater the benefit, the more acceptable is the research. However, the greater the monetary benefit, the more potential subjects are unduly influenced to participate; the more coercive the recruitment, the more unacceptable is the research" (Macklin, 1989). This is not merely a theoretical concern. Researchers have found that financial reward is the primary factor that motivates healthy individuals to participate in research (Bigorra and Banos, 1990).

Even nonmonetary rewards may be coercive if their value far exceeds the risk of the research. For example, the provision to a homeless research participant of a bicycle in exchange for his or her participation in a survey may be too good an offer to turn down, regardless of any concerns relating to the research itself.

Confidentiality and Privacy

Concern for participants' confidentiality and privacy stems from the basic principle of autonomy, which includes the individual's right to control information about him or her and to protect his or her privacy. Bayer, Levine, and Murray (1984) have noted the tension that exists between the need to protect the privacy of research participants and the need for information in research.

Both state and federal law may limit a researcher's ability to maintain the confidentiality of research records (Loue, 1995). State law may impose such limitations through laws that require the reporting of specified infectious diseases, the reporting of certain forms of family violence, and the notification of certain individuals whose sexual partners are infected with specified sexually transmitted diseases. Both state and federal courts may compel the disclosure of otherwise confidential information through the issuance of a subpoena. Information that an individual might believe to be confidential may, in fact, be accessible to others through the federal Freedom of Information Act (5 United States Code section 552, West 1977 & Supp. 1997) or its state equivalents (Loue, 1995).

Various federal legislative provisions can be used in specific situations to enhance the confidentiality of information obtained during the course of research. These include the Privacy Act (5 United States Code Annotated section 552a, 1997 & Supp. 1993), the Public Health Services Act (42 United States Code Annotated section 241(d), 1994), the Drug Abuse Office and Treatment Act of 1972 (42 United States Code Annotated section 290dd-2, 1994), the Crime Control Act of 1973 (42 United States Code Annotated section 3789g(a), 1994), and the Controlled Substances Act (21 United States Code Annotated section 872(c), 1981). In addition, a motion to quash a subpoena can be brought in the appropriate state or federal court to contest the issuance of a subpoena that mandates the disclosure of otherwise confidential research records.

A number of security measures can be implemented during the course of a study, as well, to further protect participants' privacy and the confidentiality of the information that they have provided. This includes the use of unique numeric identifiers for each participant, rather than his or her name (Loue, 1995); restricting employee access to both stored files and computer data through the use of locks and passwords (Torres, Turner, Harkess and Istre, 1991); training employees to follow laws and internally developed protocols relating to the preservation of confidentiality and the disclosure of information (Loue, 1995); protecting transmitted data (Koska, 1992; Loue, 1995); and obtaining certificates of confidentiality where appropriate and available (Avins and Lo, 1989; Bayer *et al.*, 1984; Loue, 1995).

Justice and Fairness

The obligation to ensure that the benefits and the burdens of research are distributed equitably arises from the ethical principle of justice (Coughlin, 1996). Researchers have been criticized in the past for their exclusion of women, minorities, and other subgroups from research (Mastroianni, Faden, and Federman, 1994). Questions have also arisen regarding the obligation of investigators studying a potential intervention to provide that intervention, if effective, to all participants in the study following the conclusion of the research (Glanz, Rimer, and Lerman, 1996).

Beneficence and Nonmaleficence

Beneficence refers to the provision of benefits and to the balancing of those benefits against the risks of participation (Beauchamp, 1996). The principle of nonmaleficence requires that researchers attempt to avoid causing harm (Coughlin, 1996). The balancing of risks and benefits requires an examination not only of the potential physical risks and benefits of participation in research, such as adverse effects of a drug or treatment or an improvement in health status, but also the risks and benefits of participation that may not be directly measurable. Such risks could include a loss of housing, insurance, or employment; stigmatization; social isolation; and civil or criminal consequences for activities disclosed during the course of the research. Nonmeasurable benefits might include a feeling of personal satisfaction or acceptance of one's disease status.

Risks attending participation can be minimized through the adoption and implementation of protocols appropriate to the study and the potential risk. For example, risks inherent in participation in a clinical trial of a new drug might be minimized by observing the participant for a short period after administration to verify that there are no immediate adverse effects and by having skilled staff and the necessary equipment and treatment available to treat such a reaction if it does occur. Risks related to a breach of confidentiality and unauthorized disclosure of information can be minimized by formulating, adopting, and enforcing strict confidentiality protections. Referral for counseling or crisis intervention may reduce the intensity or duration of psychological distress.

The Role of the Institutional Review Board

The Institutional Review Board (IRB) is charged with the responsibility of reviewing all proposed research to be undertaken by or at an institution to determine whether the risks of participation are in relation to the benefits, whether the selection of participants is equitable, that informed consent will be obtained and will be documented, that procedures are in place to protect the participants' privacy and maintain their confidentiality, and that data will be monitored where appropriate (45 Code of Federal Regulations section 46.111, 1996). The IRB may also require that the researcher provide additional information to the prospective research participant, including the possibility of unforeseeable risks, circumstances in which the individual's participation may be terminated without his or her consent, costs to the participant of participating in the research, and the potential impact of the participant's decision to withdraw from the research (45 Code of Federal Regulations section 46.116, 1996). The IRB may review the procedures that have been implemented to protect participants' privacy and the confidentiality of the data.

An IRB must adopt and follow written procedures for various functions. These include (1) the initial and continuing review of the research; (2) the reporting of its findings and actions to the principal investigator and the research institution; (3) the determination of which projects require review more frequently than once a year; (4) the determination of which projects require verification from persons other than the investigators to the effect that no material changes have occurred since the last IRB review; (5) the prompt reporting of proposed changes in the research activity to the IRB; and (6) the prompt reporting to the IRB and officials of the research institution of any serious or continuing noncompliance by the investigator with the requirements or determinations of the IRB (45 Code of Federal Regulations section 46.103, 1996).

IRBs meet at regular intervals to review proposed and ongoing research projects. Members of the IRB cannot have competing interests, so that they can perform their duties without risk of bias. Membership of the IRB must reflect a cross-section of the scientific and lay communities (45 Code of Federal Regulations section 46.107, 1996).

The IRB must maintain written documentation of its activities and meetings, where applicable. This documentation should include copies of all research proposals that have been reviewed; scientific evaluations accompanying the proposals; approved sample consent forms; investigators' progress reports; reports of injuries to research participants; copies of all correspondence between the IRB and investigators; minutes of IRB meetings, including a list of attendees and the votes on each item; a list of IRB members and their credentials; and a copy of the IRB's written procedures (45 Code of Federal Regulations section 46.115, 1996).

Despite the laudatory goals underlying the formulation and implementation of IRBs, IRBs have been criticized for being overly permissive in their approval of proposed research (Classen, 1986), their apparent lack of impact on the readability and understandability of informed consent forms by uneducated research participants (Hammerschmidt and Keane, 1992), and their relative inability to ensure that the researchers actually use only the forms and procedures that have been approved for use (Delgado and Leskover, 1986). The lack of standardization between IRBs (Castronovo, Jr., 1993) may create the appearance of injustice (Rosenthal and Blanck, 1993). Procedures have also been criticized for their lack of a remedy to a researcher's violation of a protocol, apart from termination of funding (Delgado and Leskovac, 1986). Conversely, other critics have charged that IRBs are often overzealous in acting as gatekeepers, at the expense of scientists, who are ethically bound to do good research (Rosenthal and Rosnow, 1984). In practice, IRBs of medical schools are more likely to review the science more critically than are IRBs located in liberal arts colleges (Rosnow, Rotheram-Borus, Blanck, and Koocher, 1993).

Several writers (Reiser and Knudson, 1993) have suggested the development of a position of "research intermediary" as a possible solution to some of the IRB's systemic shortcomings. The research intermediary would ensure that the research participants understand the research process by discussing the informed consent forms with the participants before and after they have signed them. The intermediary would also monitor how well the research protocol was being followed. The intermediary would be hired and trained by the IRB, and would be charged with the responsibility of reporting directly to the IRB.

IRBs are now facing particularly difficult questions. Many new therapies and clinical trials involve individuals with life-threatening diseases. The principle of fairness mandates that individuals meeting the scientific eligibility criteria for a clinical trial, for example, be invited to participate in clinical trials without regard to ethnicity, gender, or socioeconomic status (Mitchell and Steingrub, 1988). Yet, there are numerous examples of reasonable exclusions based on these factors. For example, researchers may want to limit their own liability by excluding from participation individuals who do not have a regular physician or medical insurance, which could be needed in the event of an adverse drug reaction. Researchers may wish to exclude individuals whose native language is not English not for scientific reasons, but because staffing becomes more difficult and costly once interpretation and translation services are required. The question of what constitutes an incentive to participate in research, versus a coercive inducement, has also become more complex as research studies increasingly include individuals from diverse cultural backgrounds and lower socioeconomic strata.

Exercises

1. It has been observed clinically that some individuals with HIV infection develop an HIV-related dementia. This level of impairment seems to vary between individuals. It is unclear what causes the dementia and what the risk factors are for the dementia, since it is clear that it does not affect all HIV-infected individuals. You have decided that you would like to determine what the risk factors are for the development of dementia.
   a. What ethical issues must be resolved in order to conduct your proposed study?
   b. Explain how you will recruit your study participants.
2. Alan Cantwell, Jr., M.D., has stated: "To those perceptive enough to discern it, the mass deaths of homosexuals from AIDS was similar to the mass deaths of Jews in the Holocaust."
   a. Compare and contrast HIV-related human research with the human research conducted

with the Jews during the Holocaust. Include in your response a discussion of the following items as they relate to both gay–AIDS research and Jewish–Holocaust era research:

i. *the nature of the research conducted;*

ii. *the procedures used to enroll participants in the research;*

iii. *the historical and social contexts in which the research occurred and is occurring.*

b. Assume that you are conducting a study that is examining the relationship between various types of social support and actual reductions in HIV risk behaviors.

i. *To what extent, if any, might the attitude/approach reflected in Cantwell's statement influence your ability to recruit and retain participants in your research study? Support your response using historical examples.*

ii. *If you believe that this attitude will influence your recruitment efforts, what strategies will you utilize to mediate the impact of this view on your recruitment of participants? If you do not believe that there will be an impact, or that any particular strategies are required, state so and support your answer.*

References

Abt, I. (1903). Spontaneous hemorrhages in newborn children. *JAMA*, *40*, 284–293.

Ackerman, T.F. (1990). Protectionism and the new research imperative in pediatric AIDS. *IRB*, *12*, 1–5.

Annas, G.J., & Grodin, M.A. (Eds.). (1992). *The Nazi Doctors and the Nuremberg Code: Human Rights in Human Experimentation*. London: Oxford University Press.

Appelbaum, P.S., Lidz, C.W., & Meisel, A. (1991). *Informed Consent: Legal Theory and Clinical Practice*. London: Oxford University Press.

Avins, A.L. & Lo, B. (1989). To tell or not to tell: The ethical dilemmas of HIV test notification in epidemiologic research. *American Journal of Public Health*, *79*, 1544–1548.

Bayer, R., Levine, C. & Murray, T.H. (1984). Guidelines for confidentiality in research on AIDS. *IRB*, *6*, 1–7.

Beauchamp, T.L. (1996). Moral foundations. In S.S. Coughlin & T.L. Beauchamp (Eds.), *Ethics and Epidemiology* (pp. 24–52). New York: Oxford University Press.

Beauchamp, T.L., & Childress, J.F. (1994). *Principles of Biomedical Ethics* (4th ed.). New York: Oxford University Press.

Belais, D. (1910). Vivisection animal and human. *Cosmopolitan*, *50*, 267–273.

Benson, P.R., Roth, L.H., Appelbaum, P.S., Lidz, C.W., & Winslade, W.J. (1988). Information disclosure, subject understanding, and informed consent in psychiatric research. *Law and Human Behavior*, *12*, 455–475.

Bigorra, J. & Banos, J.E. (1990). Weight of financial reward in the decision by medical students and experienced healthy volunteers to participate in clinical trials. *European Journal of Clinical Pharmacology*, *38*, 443–446.

California Health and Safety Code sections 24170-24179.5 (1997).

Capron, A.M. (1991). Protection of research subjects: Do special rules apply in epidemiology? *Journal of Clinical Epidemiology*, *44 (Suppl.)*, 81S-89S.

Castronovo, F.P. Jr. (1993). An attempt to standardize the radiodiagnostic risk statement in an institutional review board consent form. *Investigative Radiology*, *28*, 533–538.

Christakis, N.A., & Panner, M.J. (1991). Existing international ethical guidelines for human subjects research: Some open questions. *Law, Medicine & Health Care*, *19*, 214–221.

Classen, W.H. (1986). Institutional review boards: Have they achieved their goal? *Medicine and Law*, *5*, 387–393.

Cooke, R.E. (1994). Vulnerable children. In M.A. Grodin & L.H. Glantz (Eds.), *Children as Research Subjects: Science, Ethics, and Law* (pp. 193–214). London: Oxford University Press.

Coughlin, S. (1996). Ethically optimized study designs in epidemiology. In S.S. Coughlin & T.L. Beauchamp (Eds.), *Ethics and Epidemiology* (pp. 145–155). New York: Oxford University Press.

Council for International Organizations of Medical Sciences (CIOMS). (1991). *International Guidelines for Ethical Review of Epidemiological Studies*. Geneva: CIOMS.

Council for International Organizations of Medical Sciences (CIOMS), World Health Organization (WHO). (1993). *International Ethical Guidelines for Biomedical Research Involving Human Subjects*. Geneva: CIOMS and WHO.

Delgado, R., & Leskover, H. (1986). Informed consent in human experimentation: Bridging the gap between ethical thought and current practice. *UCLA Law Review, 34,* 67–130.

Dubler, N.N., & Sidel, V.W. (1989). On research on HIV infection and AIDS in correctional institutions. *Milbank Quarterly, 67,* 171–207.

Epstein, L.C., & Lasagna, L. (1969). Obtaining informed consent. *Archives of Internal Medicine, 123,* 682–688.

Etheridge, E. (1972). *The Butterfly Caste: A Social History of Pellagra.* Westport, CT: Greenwood.

Freedom of Information Act, 5 United States Code section 552 (West 1977 & Supp. 1997).

Glantz, L.H. (1992).The influence of the Nuremberg Code on U.S. statutes and regulations. In G.J. Annas & M.A. Grodin (Eds.), *The Nazi Doctors and the Nuremberg Code: Human Rights in Human Experimentation* (pp. 183–200). New York: Oxford University Press.

Glanz, K., Rimer, B.K., & Lerman, C. (1996). Ethical issues in the design and conduct of community-based intervention studies. In S.S. Coughlin & T.L. Beauchamp (Eds.), *Ethics and Epidemiology* (pp. 156–177). New York: Oxford University Press.

Gray, J.N. (1989). Pediatric AIDS research: Legal, ethical, and policy influences. In J.M. Siebert & R.A. Olson (Eds.), *Children, Adolescents, and AIDS* (pp. 179–227). Lincoln, NE: University of Nebraska Press.

Grodin, M.A. (1992). Historical origins of the Nuremberg Code. In G.J. Annas & M.A. Grodin (Eds.), *The Nazi Doctors and the Nuremberg Code: Human Rights in Human Experimentation* (pp. 121–144). New York: Oxford University Press.

Grodin, M.A., & Alpert, J.J. (1988). Children as participants in medical research. *Pediatric Clinics of North America, 35,* 1389–1401.

Grodin, M.A., Kaminow, P.V., & Sassower, R. (1986). Ethical issues in AIDS research. *Quality Review Bulletin, 12,* 347–352.

Hamill, S.M., Carpenter, H.C., & Cope, T.A. (1908). A comparison of the von Pirquet, Calmette and Moro tuberculin tests and their diagnostic value. *Archives of Internal Medicine, 2,* 405–447.

Hammerschmidt, D.E., & Keane, M.A. (1992). Institutional review board (IRB) review lacks impact on the readability of consent forms for research. *American Journal of the Medical Sciences, 304,* 348–351.

High, D.M. (1992). Research with Alzheimer's subjects: Informed consent and proxy decision making. *Journal of the American Geriatrics Society, 40,* 950–957.

Koska, M.T. (1992, January 5). Outcomes research: Hospitals face confidentiality concerns. *Hospitals,* 32–34.

Lane, S.D. (1994). Research bioethics in Egypt. In R. Gillon (Ed.), *Principles of Health Care Ethics* (pp. 885–894). New York: John Wiley.

Lara, M.D.C., & de la Fuente, J.R. (1990). On informed consent. *Bulletin of Pan-American Health Organization, 24,* 419–424.

Lavelle-Jones, C., Byrne, D.J., Rice, P., & Cuschieri, A. (1993). Factors affecting quality of informed consent. *British Medical Journal, 306,* 885–890.

Lederer, S.E. (1997). *Subjected to Science: Human Experimentation in America Before the Second World War.* Baltimore: Johns Hopkins University Press.

Leiken, S. (1993). Minors' assent, consent, or dissent to medical research. *IRB, 15,* 1–7.

Leiken, S.L. (1989). Immunodeficiency virus infection, adolescents, and the institutional review board. *Journal of Adolescent Health Care, 10,* 500–505.

Levine, C. (1991). Children in HIV/AIDS clinical trials: Still vulnerable after all these years. *Law, Medicine & Health Care, 19,* 231–237.

Levine, R.J. (1991). Informed consent: Some challenges to the universality of the western model. *Law, Medicine, & Health Care, 19,* 207–213.

Lo, B. (1990). Assessing decision-making capacity. *Law, Medicine, & Health Care, 18,* 193–201.

Loue, S. (1995). *Legal and Ethical Aspects of HIV-Related Research.* New York: Plenum Press.

Loue, S., Okello, D., & Kawuma, M. (1996). Research bioethics in the Ugandan context: A program summary. *Journal of Law, Medicine, and Ethics, 24,* 47–53.

LoVerde, M.E., Prochazka, A.V., & Bynny, R.L. (1989). Research consent forms: Continued unreadability and increasing length. *Journal of General Internal Medicine, 4,* 410–412.

Macklin, R. (1989). The paradoxical case of payment as benefit to research subjects. *IRB, 11,* 1–3.

Mastroianni, A.C., Faden, F., & Federman, D. (Eds.). (1994). *Women and Health Research: Ethical and Legal Issues of Including Women in Clinical Studies.* Washington, DC: National Academy Press.

Meade, C.D., & Howser, D.M. (1992). Consent forms: How to determine and improve their readability. *Oncology Nursing Forum, 19,* 1523–1528.

Mendelson, J.H. (1991). Protection of participants and experimental design in clinical abuse liability testing. *British Medical Journal, 86,* 1543–1548.

Morrow, G., Gootnick, J., & Schmale, A. (1978). A simple technique for increasing cancer patients' knowledge of informed consent to treatment. *Cancer, 42,* 793–799.

Osler, W. (1907). The evolution of the idea of experiment in medicine. *Transactions of the Congress of American Physicians and Surgeons, 7*, 7–8.

Perley, S., Fluss, S.S., Bankowski, Z., & Simon, F. (1992). The Nuremberg Code: An International Overview. In G.J. Annas & M.A. Grodin (Eds.), *The Nazi Doctors and the Nuremberg Code: Human Rights in Human Experimentation* (pp. 149–173). New York: Oxford University Press.

Peterson, B.T., Clancy, S.J., Champion, K., & McLarty, J.W. (1992). Improving readability of consent forms: What the computers may not tell you. *IRB, 14*(6), 6–8.

Reiser, S.J., & Knudson, P. (1993). Protecting research subjects after consent: The case for "research intermediary." *IRB, 15*, 10–11.

Rosenthal, R., & Blanck, P.D. (1993). Science and ethics in conducting, analyzing, and reporting social science research: Implications for social scientists, judges, and lawyers. *Indian Law Journal, 68*, 1209–1228.

Rosenthal, R., & Rosnow, R.L. (1984). Applying Hamlet's question to the ethical conduct of research: A conceptual addendum. *American Psychologist, 39*, 561–563.

Rosnow, R.L., Rotheram-Borus, S.J., Blanck, P.D., & Koocher, G.P. (1993). The institutional review board as a mirror of scientific and ethical standards. *American Psychologist, 48*, 821–826.

Siegel, H.A., Carlson, R.G., Falck, R., Reece, R.D., & Perlin, T. (1993). Conducting HIV outreach and research among incarcerated drug abusers: A case study of ethical concerns and dilemmas. *Journal of Substance Abuse and Treatment, 10*, 71–75.

Silva, M.C., & Sorrell, J.M. (1988). Enhancing comprehension of information for informed consent: A review of empirical research. *IRB, 10*, 1–5.

Simel, D.L., & Feussner, J.R. (1992). Suspended judgment: Clinical trials of informed consent. *Controlled Clinical Trials, 13*, 321–324.

Susman, E.J., Dorn, L.D., & Fletcher, J.C. (1992). Participation in biomedical research: The consent process as viewed by children, adolescents, young adults, and physicians. *Journal of Pediatrics, 121*, 547–552.

Tankanow, R.M., Sweet, B.V., & Weisikoff, J.A. (1992). Patients' perceived understanding of informed consent in investigational drug studies. *American Journal of Hospital Pharmacy, 49*, 633–635.

Taub, H.A. (1986). Comprehension of informed consent for research: Issues and directions for future study. *IRB, 8*, 7–10.

Thong, Y.H., & Harth, S.C. (1991). The social filter effect of informed consent in clinical research. *Pediatrics, 87*, 568–569.

Torres, C.G., Turner, M.E., Harkess, J.R., & Istre, G.R. (1991). Security measures for AIDS and HIV. *American Journal of Public Health, 81*, 210–211.

Weithorn, L.A., & McCabe, M.A. (1988). Emerging ethical and legal issues in pediatric psychology. In D. Routh (Ed.), *Handbook of Pediatric Psychology* (pp. 567–606). New York: Guilford Press.

Weithorn, L.A., & Scherer, D.G. (1994). Children's involvement in research participation decisions: Psychological considerations. In M.A. Grodin & L.H. Glantz (Eds.), *Children as Research Subjects: Science, Ethics, and Law* (pp. 133–179). London: Oxford University Press.

World Health Organization. (1995). *Guidelines for Good Clinical Practice for Trials on Pharmaceutical Products.* Geneva: WHO.

World Medical Association. (1991a). Declaration of Helsinki. *Law, Medicine & Health Care, 19*, 264–265.

World Medical Association. (1991b). The Nuremberg Code. *Law, Medicine & Health Care, 19*, 266.

Young, D.R., Hooker, D.T., & Freeberg, F.E. (1990). Informed consent documents: Increasing comprehension by reducing reading level. *IRB, 12*(3), 1–5.

45 Code of Federal Regulations section 46.102 (1996).

45 Code of Federal Regulations section 46.107 (1996).

45 Code of Federal Regulations section 46.111 (1996).

45 Code of Federal Regulations section 46.116 (1996).

45 Code of Federal Regulations section 46.301–46.306 (1996).

45 Code of Federal Regulations section 46.404–46.406 (1996).

45 Code of Federal Regulations section 46.408–46.409 (1996).

2

Principles of Research Design

Every discipline that concerns itself with health research—sociology, anthropology, epidemiology, psychology, and health promotion, for example—maintains a lexicon specific to that field that constitutes, in effect, a shorthand for describing the study designs, relevant measures and measurements, and issues that constitute the core of that discipline's research methodology. It is, consequently, impossible to address specifically the concerns across all relevant disciplines or to use each discipline's language in discussing issues pertaining to study design. Accordingly, study design and issues affecting the interpretation of one's results are discussed here using epidemiology as a framework, with the understanding that many of the broader concepts, if not the language itself, are applicable across disciplines. Because relevant measures and measurements differ so greatly across fields, they are not discussed here. Rather, readers are urged to consult references in their specific disciplines.

Causation and Causal Inference

Epidemiology seeks to answer such questions as "Why do some people contract certain illnesses more frequently than others?" and "Why does a specific illness progress more rapidly in some people compared to others?" The simplest approach to causality in such circumstances is that of pure determinism.

Pure determinism posits specificity of cause and specificity of effect, that is, that the factor being examined as a cause is the one and only cause of the disease under examination, and that the disease under investigation is the only effect of that factor (Kleinbaum, Kupper, and Morgenstern, 1982). This implies that the factor under examination is both a necessary and sufficient cause of that disease.

Robert Koch's formulation of the criteria for disease causality, in essence, operationalized pure determinism (Kleinbaum *et al.*, 1982). Koch's work on tuberculosis provided the basis for his refinements of causation criteria to include five elements:

1. An alien structure must be exhibited in all cases of the disease.
2. The structure must be shown to be a living organism and must be distinguishable from all other microorganisms.
3. The distinction of microorganisms must correlate with and explain the disease phenomena.

4. The microorganism must be cultivated outside the diseased animal and isolated from all disease products which could be causally significant.

5. The pure isolated microorganism must be inoculated into test animals and these animals must then display the same symptoms as the original diseased animal. (Carter, 1985)

Koch's causational model has been criticized for its various limitations, including its failure to recognize (1) the multifactorial etiology of many diseases, (2) the multiplicity of effects associated with specific factors, (3) the complexity of many causal factors, (4) our incomplete understanding of disease and disease processes, and (5) the limitations inherent in our ability to measure the causal process (Kleinbaum *et al.*, 1982).

Modified determinism addresses the limitations of Koch's model. Rothman explains this model as follows:

> A *cause* is an act or event or a state of nature which initiates or permits, alone or in conjunction with other causes, a sequence of events resulting in an *effect*. A cause which inevitably produces the effect is *sufficient*....
>
> A specific effect may result from a variety of different sufficient causes ... If there exists a component cause which is a member of every sufficient cause, such a component is termed a *necessary* cause ...

Hence, this model recognizes that a cluster of factors, rather than a single agent, may produce an effect, and that a specific effect may be the product of various causes. The strength of a specific causal factor depends on the relative prevalence of component causes. A factor, even though rare, may constitute a strong cause if its complementary causes are common (Rothman, 1986). Two component causes of a sufficient cause are said to be synergistic, in that their joint effect exceeds the sum of their separate effects (Rothman, 1976). As an example, individuals exposed to asbestos are at increased risk of cancer if they also smoke (Hammond, Selikoff, and Seidman, 1979).

This modified deterministic model, however, also has its limitations. We are often unable to identify all the components of a sufficient cause (Rothman, 1986). Consequently, epidemiologists use probability theory and statistical techniques to assess the risk of disease resulting from exposure to hypothesized causal factors (Rothman, 1986). Causation may be inferred by formulating general theories from observation (induction) or by testing general theories against observation (deduction) (Weed, 1986).

Using an inductive approach, Hill has enunciated the criteria to be considered in identifying causal associations: (1) strength, (2) consistency, (3) specificity, (4) temporality, (5) biological gradient, (6) plausibility, (7) coherence, (8) experimental evidence, and (9) analogy (Morabia, 1991). Each of these criteria is discussed briefly below.

The *strength* of an association between the putative causal factor and the effect depends on the relative prevalence of other component causes. This criterion encompasses two separate issues: the frequency with which the factor under investigation is found in cases of a specific disease and the frequency with which the factor occurs in the absence of the disease (Sartwell, 1960). *Consistency* refers to the repeated observation of an association between the putative causal factor and the effect in varied populations at varied points in time and under different circumstances (Susser, 1991). Inconsistency, however, does not necessarily negate a causal relationship because all causal components must exist to bring about the effect, and some may be absent. *Specificity* refers to the association between a postulated cause and a single effect

(Rothman, 1986). Hill specifically cautions against overemphasizing the importance of this particular element (Hill, 1965).

Temporality requires that the cause precede the effect in time (Rothman, 1986). Although a dose–response curve, or "biological gradient," is to be considered, it does not necessarily indicate causation due to the effects of confounders. *Plausibility* requires that the hypothesized relationship between the causal factor and the effect be biologically plausible. This is clearly limited by the state of our knowledge at any point in time. *Coherence* requires that a postulated causal association be consistent with our knowledge of the natural history and biology of the disease in question. Experimental evidence is rarely available for human populations. *Analogy* posits that reference to known examples, such as a causal association between one drug and birth defects, may provide insights into other causes of birth defects, such as another drug (Rothman, 1986).

Research Design

Research design provides a way to examine the relation of cause and effect in a specific population (Susser, 1991). This section explores the basic study designs used in epidemiological research, as well as several hybrid designs. Other resources should be consulted for a more extensive discussion.

Types of Research

Epidemiologic research can be classified into three major types: experimental, quasi-experimental, and observational. With each type of research, a variety of different designs can be used. Each of these types is described briefly here, followed by a discussion of specific study designs.

Experimental Research

Experimental research involves the randomization of individuals into treatment groups, also known as study arms. Individuals are randomly allocated to receive a particular treatment under investigation (treatment group) or an alternative treatment or placebo (control group). Randomization is considered essential as a safeguard against selection bias and as insurance against accidental bias (Gore, 1981), that is, to ensure that both groups are representative of the population as a whole or that both groups are similar in all respects except in the treatment received. Experimental studies conducted in the laboratory are usually of relatively short duration and are often used to test etiologic hypotheses, to estimate treatment effects, or to examine the efficacy of an intervention (Kleinbaum *et al.*, 1982).

Clinical trials are experimental studies of much longer duration. They have been referred to as "the epidemiologic 'gold standard' for causality inference" (Gray-Donald and Kramer, 1988:885). They are usually conducted to test the efficacy of a specific intervention, to test etiologic hypotheses, or to estimate long-term health effects. Both the experimental group and the control group consist of patients who have already been diagnosed with the disease of interest or are at risk of the disease of interest in a clinical trial involving a prevention. In addition, the patients must have agreed to be randomized to one of the study arms. Clinical trials often use double blinding, whereby neither the individuals conducting the study nor the participants in the study know who is in the treatment group and who is in the control group (Senn, 1991).

Community interventions are also usually of longer duration. They are often initiated to test the efficacy of a particular health intervention.

Experimental studies offer numerous advantages, including the ability, through random-ization, to control for extraneous factors that may be related to the outcome under examination. Unfortunately, the study population ultimately selected through this process may not be com-parable to the target population with respect to important characteristics.

Quasi-Experiments

Quasi-experiments involve the comparison of one group to itself or of multiple groups. Although this study design permits the investigator to manipulate the study factor, as in an experiment, randomization is not used. Quasi-experiments are most often conducted in a clinic or laboratory setting to test etiologic hypotheses, to evaluate the efficacy of an intervention, or to estimate the long-term health effects of an intervention. Those conducted in the program and policy arenas are often devoted to the evaluation of programs or interventions or to an analysis of the costs and benefits of an intervention (Kleinbaum *et al.*, 1982). Quasi-experiments are generally of a smaller scale and less expensive than experimental studies. However, the investigator has less control over the influence of extraneous risk factors due to the lack of randomization (Kleinbaum *et al.*, 1982).

Observational Studies

Observational studies are the most frequently used study designs in epidemiology. Unlike experimental and quasi-experimental studies, they do not involve the manipulation of the study factor. The goal of observational studies is to arrive at the same conclusions that would have resulted from an experiment (Gray-Donald and Kramer, 1988). Observational studies may be descriptive or etiologic in nature. Descriptive studies are often used to estimate the frequency of a specific disease in a population or to generate hypotheses or ideas for new interventions. Etiologic studies can be used not only to generate etiologic and preventive hypotheses, but also to test specific hypotheses and estimate health effects. Observational studies afford the investigator much less control over extraneous risk factors than do experimental or quasi-experimental studies because they are conducted in a natural setting (Kleinbaum *et al.*, 1982).

Observational studies can use any of numerous study designs, depending on how the research question is framed, the current state of knowledge with respect to the disease or exposure/risk factor in question, the costs of the proposed study, and various other considera-tions. Observational study designs include cohort study design, case–control design, and cross-sectional design. Other common observational designs include the etiologic study, the propor-tional study, space–time cluster studies, and the family cluster study (Kleinbaum *et al.*, 1982).

Clinical trials and observational studies are particularly central to epidemiology. For this reason, clinical trials and various types of observational study designs are addressed in further detail below.

Clinical Trials

Clinical trials of new drugs are conducted in three phases. The first phase consists of the initial introduction of the drug into humans. Phase I studies are conducted to assess the metabolic and pharmacologic actions of the drugs in humans, the side effects of the drug, and the effectiveness of the drug. Phase I studies, which are closely monitored, are generally limited to 20 to 80 participants (21 Code of Federal Regulations section 312.21(a), 1998).

Phase II studies build on the knowledge that was obtained from Phase I studies. Phase II studies are carried out in patients with the disease under study for the purpose of assessing the drug's effectiveness for a particular indication and for determining the drug's short-term side effects and risks. Typically, Phase II studies involve up to several hundred participants (21 Code of Federal Regulations section 312.21(b), 1998).

Phase III studies incorporate the knowledge gained through Phase I and Phase II trials. Phase III trials focus on gathering additional data relating to the drug's effectiveness and safety. Phase III studies are potentially quite large, sometimes involving thousands of participants (21 Code of Federal Regulations section 312.21(c), 1998).

In planning a clinical trial, the treatment(s) to be studied and the eligibility criteria for individuals to participate in the trial must first be determined (Rosner, 1987). Clinical trials designed to answer questions relating to biological response generally enroll a rather homogeneous participant population, in order to reduce the variability between participants and simplify the analysis of the results. Patients enrolled in such a study must be sufficiently healthy so that they do not die before the end of the study, but not so well that they recover from the disease.

Larger clinical trials, particularly multi-site trials, often enroll more heterogeneous participants. This situation more closely mirrors everyday clinical practice with diverse patients and also comforms to ethical considerations and federal regulations regarding the equitable distribution of the benefits and the burdens of research.

Researchers must also decide which endpoint(s) to use as a basis for evaluating participants' response to the treatment (O'Brien and Shampo, 1988). The endpoint(s) will vary depending on the disease and the treatment under investigation, but may include recurrence of an event, such as myocardial infarction; quality of life; functional capacity; or death. Clinical trials are often concerned not only with whether an endpoint occurs, but also with the length of time until its occurrence. As an example, a clinical trial for a cancer treatment may be concerned not only with the recurrence of the malignancy, but also the time between the treatment and the reappearance of the disease.

Ethical concerns have been raised about classic clinical trials on a number of grounds. Clinicians may believe that patients should not be randomized because it may deprive them of an opportunity to receive a new alternative drug (Farrar, 1991). Others believe that randomization is inappropriate in situations in which the patient has exhausted all available therapies or one in which the standard therapy has provided no benefit (Rosner, 1987).

Crossover designs have also been proposed as an alternative to classic clinical trials and as a mechanism for addressing variations between patients in response to treatment. With a crossover design, half of the patients are randomized to Group 1 and the second half to Group 2. Following administration of Treatment A to Group 1 and Treatment B to Group 2, the allocation of treatment is reversed. Generally, crossover designs incorporate an appropriate "washout period" between administration of the treatment to each group, in order to reduce the possibility of a carryover effect from the first treatment period to the second (Hills and Armitage, 1979). Crossover designs are most useful in situations in which the treatment under investigation alleviates a condition, rather than effects a cure.

Observational Designs

Cohort Studies

Cohort studies can be conducted prospectively or retrospectively. Prospective cohort studies require the identification and classification of initially disease-free individuals into categories according to whether they have or have not been exposed to the factor under study.

Each group is followed over time in order to observe the number of new cases of the disease under investigation that occurs in each group in a specified period of time (Kelsey, Thompson, and Evans, 1986).

Numerous difficulties may attend prospective studies. First, individuals may already have been exposed to the factor under study, and the length and intensity of that exposure may be difficult to ascertain. As an example, a cohort study to examine the effects of an occupational exposure would consist of a group exposed to the substance under study and a group that was not exposed. Depending on the particular industry and configuration of the workplaces, however, some members of the group classified as unexposed may, in fact, have been exposed to small amounts of the substance. Second, although individuals enrolled in the study may be believed to be free of the disease, the disease process may, in fact, have commenced in some but may be undetectable by diagnostic methods and tools then available. This could be true, for example, in studies involving cancer or schizophrenia. Third, a minimum length of time following exposure may be required to allow a biologically appropriate induction time, as well as a subsequent period of time after causation but before disease detection (latent period). In situations where we do not have complete knowledge of the induction and latency periods, we must make assumptions about the lengths of these times (Rothman, 1986). Fourth, prospective cohorts also require large sample sizes and are often quite costly (Kelsey et al., 1986). (What is considered a large sample size varies depending on the disease under study, the exposure under study, and various other factors.) Fifth, the choice of a comparison group of unexposed individuals may be quite difficult. We also tend to think of disease as being present or absent, but some diseases, such as high blood pressure, may occur along a spectrum, making classification of individuals as diseased or not diseased more complex (Kelsey et al., 1986).

Individuals in a prospective cohort study are to be followed over time, as is indicated in Figure 2.1. However, some individuals may drop out of the study or be lost to follow-up. These losses may be related to disease status, thereby producing a bias in the measurement of disease (Kelsey et al., 1986). It is easy to imagine that as someone becomes progressively more ill, he or she may not want to undergo a physical examination or respond to questions relating to the illness. Information on other extraneous variables that may affect the results may not be available (Kelsey et al., 1986).

Retrospective cohort studies, also known as historical cohort studies, require the identification of individuals based on their past exposure and the reconstruction of their disease experience up to a defined point in time. Retrospective cohort designs are often useful for examining the effects of occupational exposures. Unlike prospective cohort studies, they often

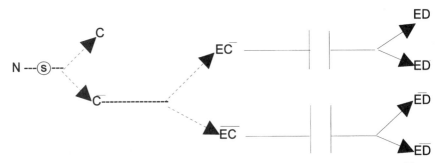

Figure 2.1. Diagrammatic representation of a cohort study. N, Source or base population; C/C̄, prevalent cases/noncases; D/D̄, incident cases/noncases or deaths/survivors; E/Ē, subjects with/without the exposure; Ⓢ, random sampling.

rely on existing records and may consequently be completed in less time and at a lower cost than a prospective cohort study. Retrospective cohort studies do, however, share some of the same difficulties as prospective studies, including difficulties in the ascertainment and measurement of extraneous relevant characteristics (confounding variables), and difficulties tracing individuals through time. Despite the difficulties inherent in cohort designs, cohort studies offer a major benefit: the ability to calculate incidence rates for the exposed and the unexposed groups.

Case–Control Studies

Unlike cohort studies which follow individuals through time after classifying them based on their exposure status, case–control studies require the classification of individuals on the basis of their current disease status and then examine their past exposure to the factor of interest (see Fig. 2.2). Case–control design has been used to investigate disease outbreaks (Dwyer, Strickler, Goodman, and Armenian, 1994); to identify occupational risk factors (Checkoway and Demers, 1994); in genetic epidemiologic studies (Khoury and Beaty, 1994); for indirect estimation in demography (Khlat, 1994); to evaluate vaccination effectiveness and vaccine efficacy (Comstock, 1994); to evaluate treatment and program efficacy (Selby, 1994); and to evaluate the efficacy of screening tests (Weiss, 1994). Case–control studies are most useful in evaluating risk factors for rare diseases and for diseases of rapid onset. With diseases of slow onset, it may be difficult to ascertain whether a particular factor contributed to disease or arose after the commencement of the disease process (Kelsey *et al.*, 1986).

The conduct of a case–control study requires selection of the cases (the diseased group) and the controls (the nondiseased group) from separate populations. Prior to selecting the cases, the investigator must define what constitutes a case conceptually. This is not as simple a task as it first appears, particularly when the disease condition is a new and relatively unstudied entity (Lasky and Stolley, 1994). Causal inference is possible only if one assumes that the controls are "representative of the same candidate population ... from which the cases ... developed ..." (Kleinbaum *et al.*, 1982:68). Consequently, the selection of appropriate cases and controls is crucial to the validity of the study.

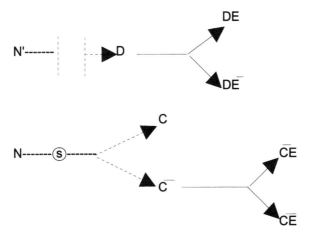

Figure 2.2. Diagrammatic representation of a case–control study. N, Source or base population; C/C̄, prevalent cases/noncases; D/D̄, incident cases/noncases or deaths/survivors; E/Ē, subjects with/without the exposure; Ⓢ, random sampling.

Methods and criteria for the selection of appropriate cases and controls have been discussed extensively in the literature and will only be summarized here. Cases are often selected from patients seeking medical care for the condition that is being investigated. It is preferable to include as cases individuals who have been recently diagnosed with the illness rather than individuals who have had the disease for an extended period of time, in order to discriminate between exposure that occurred before disease onset and exposure that occurred after. Other sources of cases include disease registries, drug surveillance programs, schools, and places of employment (Kelsey *et al.*, 1986).

Controls must be "representative of the same base experience" as the cases (Miettinen, 1985:545). "[T]he control series is intended to provide an estimate of the exposure rate that would be expected to occur in the cases if there were no association between the study disease and exposure" (Schlesselman, 1982:76). It is important to recognize that controls are theoretically continuously eligible to become cases. An individual who is initially selected as a control and who later develops the disease(s) under study, thereby becoming a case, should be counted as both a case and a control (Lubin and Gail, 1984). Controls are frequently selected from probability samples of the population from which the cases arose; from patients receiving medical care at the same facilities as the cases, but for conditions unrelated to the cases' diagnoses; or from neighbors, friends, siblings, or coworkers of the cases (Kelsey *et al.*, 1986). Dead controls may also be used in studies where the researcher wants to compare individuals who died from one cause with individuals who died from other causes (Lasky and Stolley, 1994).

Case–control studies are valuable because they permit the evaluation of a range of exposures that may be related to the disease under investigation. They are generally less expensive to conduct than cohort studies, in part because fewer people are needed for the study. However, it may be difficult to determine individuals' exposure status (Rothman, 1986).

Cross-Sectional Studies

Unlike cohort studies or case–control studies, cross-sectional studies measure exposure and disease status at the same point in time (see Fig. 2.3). This approach results in a serious limitation, in that it may be difficult to determine whether the exposure or the disease came first, since they are both measured at the same time. In addition, because cross-sectional studies include prevalent cases of a disease (i.e., new cases and existing cases), a higher proportion of cases will have had the disease for a longer period of time. This may be problematic if people who die quickly or recover quickly from the disease differ on important characteristics from

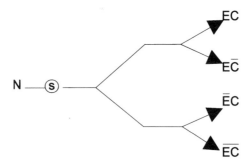

Figure 2.3. Diagrammatic representation of a cross-sectional study. N, Source or base population; C/C̄, prevalent cases/noncases; E/Ē, subjects with/without the exposure; Ⓢ, random sampling.

those who have the disease over a long period of time. Moreover, individuals whose disease is in remission may be erroneously classified as nondiseased (Kelsey *et al.*, 1986).

Ecological Studies

In the study designs previously discussed, the individual was the unit of observation. Ecological designs, however, use a group of people, such as a census tract, as the unit of observation (Rothman, 1986). An example of an ecological study would be an examination of oral cancer rates against the use of chewing tobacco in each state. Ecological studies are often conducted to observe geographic differences in the rates of a specific disease or to observe the relationship between changes in the average exposure level and changes in the rates of a specific disease in a particular population. They are useful in generating etiologic hypotheses and for evaluating the effectiveness of a population intervention. Because data is available only at the group level, however, inferences from the ecological analysis as applied to individuals within the groups or to individuals across groups may be seriously flawed (Morgenstern, 1982). This often results from an inability to assess and measure extraneous factors on an individual level that may be related to the disease and the exposure under examination (see Fig. 2.4).

Interpreting the Results

Statistical Significance and Confidence Intervals

In testing a hypothesis of association between exposure and disease, the investigator often begins with the hypothesis that there is no association between the exposure and the disease (null hypothesis). If the data do not support the null hypothesis, it can be rejected. The investigator must specify the level of statistical significance (alpha), which will indicate that any association that is found is unlikely to have occurred by chance. Although this alpha level is usually set at .05, this is completely arbitrary (Rothman, 1986). It is important to remember that statistical significance does not equate to clinical significance; a result may be clinically significant even in the absence of statistical significance.

A *p*-value is a statistic used to test the null hypothesis. It refers to the probability that the data will depart from an absence of association, to an extent equal to or greater than that observed, by chance alone, assuming that the null hypothesis is true. A lower *p*-value indicates a higher degree of inconsistency between the null hypothesis of no association and the data. Stated more simply, the *p*-value is the probability that we will make a mistake and reject the

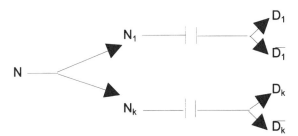

Figure 2.4. Diagrammatic representation of an ecological study. N, Source or base population; D/$\overline{\text{D}}$, incident cases/noncases or deaths/survivors.

hypothesis of no association when, in fact, it is true. We want the p-value to be very small. The smaller the p-value, the more certain we are that the null hypothesis is not true.

An alpha, or Type I, error occurs when the null hypothesis is erroneously rejected, that is, it is true and it is rejected as false. If the p-value was set to .05, an alpha error will occur approximately 5% of the time. Conversely, a beta, or Type II, error will occur if the null hypothesis is false and is not rejected.

Reliance on p-values has been criticized because p-values fail to provide information about the magnitude of an effect estimate or its variability (Rothman, 1986). Rothman has encouraged, instead, the use of interval estimation (confidence intervals). A point estimate, which is a single best estimate of the parameter (e.g., an effect measure such as an odds ratio), is derived from the data. A confidence interval, equivalent to one minus the alpha level, is calculated around the point estimate. As an example, if the alpha level is .05, the confidence interval to be constructed is a 95% confidence interval.

Internal and External Validity

The scientific validity of a study depends on its internal validity and its external validity, or generalizability. Internal validity refers to the validity of the inferences drawn that relate to the study participants. External validity refers to the validity of the inferences drawn as they relate to groups other than the study population, such as all adults, or all children with a particular disease.

Internal Validity

Biases in research can affect a study's internal validity by affecting the accuracy of measurement. The *Dictionary of Epidemiology* defines "bias" as "any trend in the collection, analysis, interpretation, publication or review of data that can lead to conclusions that are systematically different from the truth" (Last, 1988:13–14). There are many types of bias, but they are often classified into three general categories: selection bias, information bias, and confounding.

Selection bias may result from flaws in the procedures used to select participants for the study. These flaws lead to a distortion in the estimate of effect (Kleinbaum *et al.*, 1982). Various common forms of selection bias are noted in Table 2.1.

Information bias results in a distortion of the effect estimate due to misclassification of the research participants on one or more variables. The misclassification may result from measurement errors or recall bias. Misclassification is said to be nondifferential if the misclassification on one axis (exposure or disease) is independent of misclassification on the other axis. Differential misclassification occurs when misclassification on one axis is not independent of misclassification on the other axis (Rothman, 1986). Differential misclassification can result in an over- or underestimation of the effect measure (Copeland, Checkoway, McMichael, and Holbrook, 1977). Recall bias is one form of differential misclassification that may occur in a case–control study that relies on participants' memories of their exposure experiences. Memory may differ between the exposed cases and the nondiseased controls for a variety of reasons. As an example, particular exposures may become more significant to the cases in retrospect because of an attempt to identify a cause or reason for the illness.

Confounding can occur if the exposure of interest is closely linked to another variable and to the disease of interest. For instance, if one were to study the association between alcohol use and a specific form of cancer without collecting data on levels of smoking, the results would be confounded if that form of cancer were associated with tobacco usage.

Table 2.1. Common Forms of Selection Bias[a]

Berkson's bias	Occurs most frequently through seletion of hospitalized patients as controls; controls selected based on the fact that they have a condition other than the one that is under investigation in the study
Diagnostic access	Differential access to diagnostic procedures due to differences in geographic location, socioeconomic status, or other characteristics
Diagnostic suspicion	Differential intensity and/or outcome within the diagnostic process due to knowledge of previous exposure
Healthy worker effect	Occurs in occupation-based studies; relatively healthy people remain in the work force and less healthy individuals leave due to poorer health
Nonrespondent/latecomer/ newcomer bias	Latecomers or newcomers have exposures or outcomes that differ from the earlier enrollees in the study
Self-selection	Individuals refer themselves to study for reasons related to the outcome under investigation

[a]Sources: Coughlin (1990); Feldman, Finch, and Dowd (1989); Greenland (1977); Jooste *et al.* (1990); Sackett (1979); Sterling, Weinkam, and Weinkam (1990).

To be a confounder, a factor (1) must be associated with both the exposure under study and the disease under study; (2) must be associated with the exposure among the source population for cases; and (3) may not be a step in the causal chain between exposure and disease (Rothman, 1986). It is important to note that, just as with exposure and disease status, confounders are subject to misclassification. Under some circumstances, such misclassification can seriously distort the results (Greenland and Robins, 1985). Figures 2.5 through 2.19 illustrate the various properties of confounders (Morgenstern, 1996).

Confounding is often confused with effect modification. Unlike confounding, which refers to a bias in the estimate of effect that results from a lack of comparability between the groups in the study, effect modification refers to a heterogeneity of effect. As an example, if the effect of smoking on cervical cancer differs by ethnicity, we would say that ethnicity in this case is an effect modifier. Ethnicity could also, however, be a confounder if there is an association between ethnicity and smoking among the controls.

External Validity

Scientific generalization is "the process of moving from time- and place-specific observations to an abstract universal statement" (Rothman, 1986: 96). As an example, the applicability to women of the results of clinical trials relating to heart disease and HIV in men, for example, has been called into question (Mastroianni *et al.*, 1994).

Strategies to Increase Validity

A variety of options are available to control for potential bias. One such option, randomization, was discussed previously in the context of clinical trials. Other options include restriction, matching, stratification, and mathematical modeling.

Restriction is used in the design phase of a study to limit inclusion in the study to individuals who meet certain predetermined eligibility criteria. In this way, individuals who possess certain characteristics may be excluded, thereby reducing the potential of bias due to the presence of those extraneous factors (Gray-Donald and Kramer, 1988). For example, investigators studying the etiology of HIV-associated dementia would exclude from the study individuals who possess other risk factors for dementia or dementia-like conditions, such as

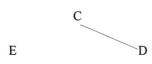

Figure 2.5. Factors C and D are associated in the study population, but not necessarily in the base population. This may result from selection procedures. In this situation, C is not a confounder. C, covariate; D, disease; E, exposure.

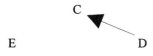

Figure 2.6. The C–D association results from the effect of D on C. C is not a confounder. C, covariate; D, disease; E, exposure.

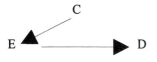

Figure 2.7. The effect of C on D in the base population is not independent of the exposure. C is not a confounder. C, covariate; D, disease; E, exposure.

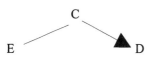

Figure 2.8. C is associated with exposure status in the base population and C is a risk factor for D in the unexposed base population. C is a confounder. C, covariate; D, disease; E, exposure.

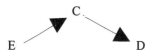

Figure 2.9. C is an intermediate (intervening) variable in the causal pathway between E and D. C is not a confounder. C, covariate; D, disease; E, exposure.

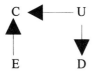

Figure 2.10. Both C and D are affected by the same unmeasured risk factor U. C is affected by E. C is not a confounder. C, covariate; D, disease; E, exposure.

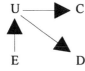

Figure 2.11. Both C and D are affected by another unmeasured risk factor U. U is affected by E. C is not a confounder. C, covariate; D, disease; E, exposure.

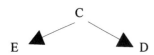

Figure 2.12. C is a risk factor for both E and D. C is a causal confounder. C, covariate; D, disease; E, exposure.

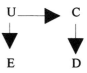

Figure 2.13. U is a causal confounder. C is in the causal pathway between U and D. By controlling for C, all confounding due to U will be eliminated, if there are no measurement errors. C, covariate; D, disease; E, exposure.

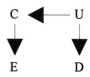

Figure 2.14. U is a causal confounder. C is in the causal pathway between U and E. By controlling for C, all confounding due to U will be eliminated, if there are no measurement errors. C, covariate; D, disease; E, exposure.

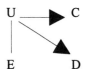

Figure 2.15. U is a causal or proxy confounder. C is associated with U. C is not in every causal pathway between U and E or between U and D. Controlling for C will not eliminate confounding by U. C, covariate; D, disease; E, exposure.

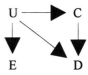

Figure 2.16. U is a causal or proxy confounder. C is associated with U, but is not in every causal pathway between U and E or U and D. Controlling for C could result in either increased or decreased bias because the direct and indirect effects of U on D could be in opposite directions. C, covariate; D, disease; E, exposure.

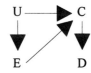

Figure 2.17. C is a proxy for the unmeasured confounder U. Confounding due to U will be eliminated by controlling for U if C is an intermediate variable and U is a confounder. If we have no information on U, C is a proxy confounder in addition to being an intermediate variable. Our estimate of E will be biased whether or not we control for C. C, covariate; D, disease; E, exposure.

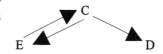

Figure 2.18. C is a time-dependent variable and is both a confounder and an intermediate between E and D. Conventional statistical methods will not produce an unbiased estimate of the effect of E. C, covariate; D, disease; E, exposure.

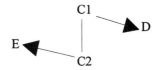

Figure 2.19. C2, a confounder, is a proxy for C1, a confounder. C1 and C2 are redundant confounders. Analysis must control for either C1 or C2 to eliminate bias. C, covariate; D, disease; E, exposure.

current alcohol or drug abuse or certain forms of mental illness. As a technique, restriction is relatively inexpensive and facilitates the analysis and interpretation of the results. However, generalization to populations other than those included in the study may not be valid. Also, restriction may not control completely for confounding (Kleinbaum *et al.*, 1982). Restriction may also raise ethical issues due to the routine exclusion of specific groups, such as women, from participation in research studies (Mastroianni *et al.*, 1994).

Matching refers to the selection of a comparison group that is comparable to the study group with respect to certain prescribed characteristics that could potentially confound or bias the results, such as age or sex. Matching reduces or eliminates the potential variability between the study and comparison groups with respect to the matched variables. Consequently, the factors selected as the basis for matching should not be factors of interest that the investigator wants to examine further (Kelsey *et al.*, 1986). For example, an investigator may be interested in factors that affect the quality of care received by HIV-infected patients. If the investigator matches on insurance status, he or she will be unable to investigate the effect that insurance has on whether or not the patient receives a particular treatment or undergoes a particular procedure. Although matching can be used with cohort, case–control, and cross-sectional designs (Kelsey *et al.*, 1986), it is most often used in case–control designs. Matching is often not feasible in cohort and cross-sectional studies due to lack of information on the potentially confounding factors (Kelsey *et al.*, 1986).

The variables on which cases and controls are to be matched must be thought to be related to both disease and exposure, that is, they must be confounders that must be controlled for in the design or the analysis. In addition, matching should not be unduly costly (Kelsey *et al.*, 1986). Cost may become a particular issue if matched controls are difficult to locate due to the closeness of the matching that is required (Smith, 1983). Matching brings several advantages, including the ability to more adequately control for confounding variables, the ability to obtain time comparability between cases and controls for exposures that may vary over time, and a gain in statistical power (Wacholder, Silverman, McLaughlin, and Mandel, 1992).

Stratification means dividing the analysis into two or more groups, such as males and females, to permit separate analysis of each. Stratified analysis can be used in cohort, case–control, and cross-sectional studies. This technique requires that levels of the confounding variables be defined and the exposure–disease association estimated within each level. Stratification is appropriate if (1) there is a sufficient number of individuals in each level; (2) the choice of control variables is appropriate; and (3) the definition of levels for each of the confounding variables is appropriate (Kleinbaum *et al.*, 1982). For example, smoking could be a confounding variable in a study examining the relationship between asbestos exposure and certain lung diseases. Consequently, the investigator would want to stratify the analysis by level of smoking (e.g., lifetime levels of smoking).

Mathematical modeling involves the use of analyses that relate exposure, outcome, and extraneous variables. These analyses are said to be multivariate because they include multiple factors in the model. In cohort studies, the illness or disease outcome or status is often the dependent variable, while either the exposure status or disease outcome may be the dependent variable in case–control studies. Mathematical modeling has many advantages, including ease of use with small numbers; the ability to predict individual risk; and the ability to use this technique with continuous variables and with multiple exposure variables.

Mathematical modeling also has several disadvantages. All models require that certain assumptions be made about the data prior to the application of the model. The selection of the model requires an evaluation of these underlying assumptions. If the assumptions do not hold, another modeling technique must be used. Mathematical modeling may also present difficulty in the interpretation of the results (Kleinbaum *et al.*, 1982).

Sampling and Sample Size

Many epidemiologic studies use data from existing data sources, often collected on a routine basis, such as data from various disease registries or hospital discharge records. This type of data is known as secondary data. It is crucial that these data sources be as accurate as possible and that minimal misclassification exists.

Most epidemiologic studies, however, rely on primary data collected from the original source, such as individuals with a particular disease or exposure of interest. This often requires the identification of the individuals who will participate, the development of questionnaires, or conducting interviews. In most cases, a sample of such individuals must be used, rather than an entire population. Reliance on a sample of the population helps to reduce study costs and, to some extent, may increase the accuracy of the measurements since more time can then be focused on fewer people.

When assembling a sample population, the sampling unit will depend on the particular study. Most often, the unit will be an individual or a household, although it may also be a neighborhood center, school, or other entity. A listing of the sampling units constitutes the sampling frame.

Sampling Techniques

The manner by which sampling is conducted is critical. Appropriate sampling techniques will reduce random error, which can reduce the precision of the epidemiologic measurements that are obtained (Rothman, 1986). Probability sampling is one method of reducing random error. Probability sampling refers to sampling by which "each sampling unit has a known, nonzero probability of being included in the sample" (Kelsey *et al.*, 1986). There are various techniques available for probability sampling, including simple random sampling, systematic sampling, stratified sampling, cluster sampling, and multi-stage sampling. Other sampling techniques, such as snowball sampling, can be used when probability sampling is not possible.

Simple Random Sampling

With simple random sampling, each sampling unit in the eligible population has an equal chance of being included in the study. In order to conduct random sampling, the investigator must know the complete sampling frame, that is, everyone who is potentially eligible to be in the study. Sampling can occur with or without replacement. With replacement sampling, selected sampling units, such as the individuals selected for participation in the study, are returned to the pool from which the sample is being taken. Most epidemiologic studies rely on sampling without replacement, which yields more precise estimates.

Systematic Sampling

With systematic sampling, sampling units are selected from regularly spaced positions in the sampling frame, such as every tenth patient admitted to an inpatient facility. Systematic sampling is relatively easy to implement and does not require *a priori* knowledge of the sampling frame.

Stratified Sampling

Stratified sampling requires that the population be divided into predetermined strata. Within each stratum, the sampling units share particular characteristics, such as sex. The study participants are then selected by taking a random sample from within each stratum. Stratified sampling is particularly useful to ensure that all subgroups of interest are represented in the study population. Stratified sampling may also yield more precise estimates of the population parameters since the overall variance is based on the within-stratum variances (Kelsey *et al.*, 1986).

Disproportionate stratification refers to the disproportionate sampling of strata, such as specific neighborhoods, which contain high concentrations of the population of interest. For instance, if an investigator were interested in studying the effect of culture on nutritional intake, he or she might oversample certain groups to ensure that there is a sufficient number of such individuals in the study to be able to analyze the data. This technique results in unequal selection probabilities for members of the different strata, and requires weighting adjustments in the analysis of the data (Kalton, 1993).

Cluster Sampling

Cluster sampling involves the selection of clusters from the population. Observations are then made on each individual within a cluster. As an example, one may wish to identify certain neighborhoods (clusters) and then sample all households within those selected neighborhoods.

Multi-Stage Sampling

Multi-stage sampling is similar to cluster sampling in that it first requires the identification of primary sampling units, such as neighborhoods. Unlike cluster sampling, however, multi-stage sampling uses a sample of secondary units with each primary unit, rather than a sample of all of the secondary units. For example, multi-stage sampling would require the sampling of households within the selected neighborhoods, such as every tenth house in the selected neighborhoods, rather than reliance on all of the households within each selected neighborhood (Kalton, 1993).

Location Sampling

Location sampling refers to the selection of participants through recruitment at locations and times when numbers of the target population are expected to be high. Locations could include, for instance, bars, grocery stores, bookstores, or churches, depending on the population to be sampled. This type of sample is generally considered a convenience sample.

Time/space sampling is conducted at specified locations and times when population flows are expected to occur, such as voting booths on Election Day. A sampling frame consisting of time/location combinations is constructed and a sample of individuals is then selected from these sampling units. This method of sampling produces a probability sample of visits, rather than individuals (Kalton, 1993).

Snowball Sampling

Snowball sampling is based on the premise that members of a particularly rare population know each other. Individuals are identified within the targeted rare population. These individuals are asked to identify other individuals within the same target group. This technique can be used to generate the sample ("snowball sampling") or, alternatively, to construct a sampling frame for the rare population, from which the sample is then selected. For example, if an investigator wanted to examine the prevalence of needle-sharing behaviors among injection drug users, snowball sampling would permit the investigator to identify eligible participants by relying on previously identified eligible participants. This could be more efficient than attempting to identify individuals through hospitals or clinics. Snowball sampling is a non-probability sampling procedure. Snowballing for frame construction does not suffer from this weakness, but carries the possibility that socially isolated members of the rare population will be missing from the frame (Kalton, 1993).

Sample Size and Power

The epidemiologist is concerned not only with the appropriateness of the sampling method used, but also with the size of the sample. Increasing the size of the sample may reduce random error and increase precision.

Power calculations are often used to determine the requisite sample size. *Power* has been defined as "the probability of detecting (as 'statistically significant') a postulated level of effect" (Rothman, 1986). In order to calculate power, one must specify the (statistical) significance, or alpha level; the magnitude of the effect that one wishes to detect, such as an odds ratio of 2; the sample size of the exposed group in a cohort or cross-sectional study or the sample size of the diseased group in a case–control study; and the ratio of the size of the comparison group to the size of the exposed group in a cohort or cross-sectional study or to the size of the diseased group in a case–control study (Kelsey *et al.*, 1986).

An alternative approach to assessing the adequacy of the sample size is to calculate the requisite size using one of the accepted sample size formulas. These formulas require that the investigator specify the level of statistical significance (alpha error); the chance of missing a real effect (beta error); the magnitude of the effect to be detected; the prevalence of the exposure in the nondiseased or the disease rate among the unexposed; and either the ratio of the exposed to the unexposed or the ratio of the cases to the controls (Rothman, 1986). Reliance on such formulas has been criticized because they create the illusion of a boundary between an adequate and inadequate sample size when, in fact, the variables specified to determine the sample size are often set either arbitrarily or by relying on estimates (Rothman, 1986).

Meta-analysis offers "[a] quantitative method of combining the results of independent studies (usually drawn from the published literature) and synthesizing summaries and conclusions which may be used to evaluate therapeutic effectiveness, [amd] plan new studies ..." (Olkin, 1995:133). Meta-analysis refers to not only the statistical combination of these studies, but also to "the whole process of selection, critical appraisal, analysis, and interpretation" (Liberati, 1995:81). Because meta-analysis permits the aggregation of studies' results, it may be useful in detecting effects that have been somewhat difficult to observe due to the small sample size of individual studies. Its use, however, is not uncontroversial, and various approaches to meta-analysis have been subject to criticism, including the use of quality scores for the aggregation of studies of both good and poor quality and over-reliance on *p*-values (Olkin, 1995). In addition, because "[t]he validity of a meta-analysis depends on complete sampling of all the studies performed on a particular topic" (Felson, 1992:886), the results of meta-analysis may be biased due to various forms of sampling bias, selection bias, or misclassification (Felson, 1992). The establishment of more or less rigid inclusion and exclusion criteria can considerably affect the results of a meta-analysis.

Exercises

1. You are the editor of a scientific journal. You must make the final decision regarding publication of a paper addressing the relationship between nutritional status and probability of mortality. The paper has been recommended for publication by the two peer reviewers. The study was conducted from 1968 to 1973 in the Punjab region of India. The researchers used a cohort design and followed 2,800 minor children for a period of 3 years each. The researchers found an inverse linear relationship between nutritional status and the probability of mortality: the lower the nutritional status, the higher the probability of mortality.

   a. At the time that the study was conducted, were there any ethical concerns regarding the conduct of the study? If so, what were they? Refer to then-existing precepts and regulations, if any, to support your answer.

   b. At the present time are there any ethical concerns regarding the conduct of this study? If so, what are they? Refer to any currently existing precepts and regulations, if any, to support your answer.

   c. In what ways could the design of the study have been modified to avoid the ethical concerns, if any, that you noted? If you believe that no modifications are necessary, state so and support your answer.

   d. In what ways could the study have been modified to avoid the ethical concerns, if any, that you have addressed? If you believe that no modifications are necessary, state so and support your answer.

   e. What are the implications of publishing or not publishing this study?

   f. Would you, as the senior editor of the journal, recommend the publication of this article? Explain your response.

2. You are the head of the Department of Health of State Woeisme. You have become increasingly dismayed with what appears to be the interminable process required by the FDA for the approval and marketing of drugs designed to delay the progression of HIV infection. You have decided to present draft legislation to a state legislator to implement a drug research and approval process in your state.

   a. Outline the elements of your proposed legislation. Include in your response a discussion of the phases of your approval process; limitations, if any, on the types of drugs or the nature of the manufacturers that are encompassed by your process; ethical considerations implicit in your proposed research and approval process; and the similarities and differences between your proposed plan and that currently in existence under the FDA.

   b. State Woeisme is suffering from severe budgetary problems, and the governor had mandated that you slash the health department's budget, threatening to do it for you if you didn't do it yourself. At the time of that discussion, you had devised a plan to restructure the state's system of health insurance coverage, in view of the large number of state residents who are uninsured under any health care plan, and the large number of individuals who do not qualify on a continuous basis for publicly funded medical care. In view of your state's budgetary crisis, explain the following.

      i. *How will this drug research/approval process be funded?*

      ii. *Considering both scientific and ethical concerns, what are the limitations, if any, on who is eligible to participate in research conducted under your new procedures?*

   c. The state of Woeisme has a remarkably diverse population, with some school districts' students speaking 43 different primary languages. How does this linguistic and cultural diversity affect the ethical components of your process, if at all? If you do not believe that there is or should be any impact, state so and support your response.

References

Carter, K.C. (1985). Koch's postulates in relation to the work of Jacob Henle and Edwin Klebs. *Medical History, 29,* 353–374, 356–357.

Checkoway, H., & Demers, D.A. (1994). Occupational case—control studies. *Epidemiologic Reviews, 16,* 151–162.

Comstock, G.W. (1994). Evaluating vaccination effectiveness and vaccine efficacy by means of case–control studies. *Epidemiologic Reviews, 16,* 77–89.

Copeland, K.T., Checkoway, H., McMichael, A.J., & Holbrook, R.H. (1977). Bias due to misclassification in the estimation of relative risk. *American Journal of Epidemiology, 105,* 488–495.

Coughlin, S.S. (1990). Recall bias in epidemiologic studies. *Journal of Clinical Epidemiology, 43,* 87–91.

Dwyer, D.M., Strickler, H., Goodman, R.A., & Armenian, H.K. (1994). Use of case-control studies in outbreak investigations. *Epidemiologic Reviews, 16,* 109–123.

Farrar, W.B. (1991). Clinical trials: Access and reimbursement. *Cancer, 67,* 1779–1782.

Feldman, F., Finch, M., & Dowd, B. (1989). The role of health practices in HMO selection bias: A confirmatory study. *Inquiry, 26,* 381–387.

Felson, D.T. (1992). Bias in meta-analytic research. *Journal of Clinical Epidemiology, 45,* 885–892.

Gore, S.M. (1981). Assessing clinical trials—why randomise? *British Medical Journal, 282,* 1958–1960.

Gray-Donald, K., & Kramer, M.S. (1988). Causality inference in observational vs. experimental studies: An empirical comparison, *American Journal of Epidemiology, 127,* 885–892.

Greenland, S. (1977). Response and follow-up bias in cohort studies. *American Journal of Epidemiology, 106,* 184–187.

Greenland, S., & Robins, J.M. (1985). Confounding and misclassification. *American Journal of Epidemiology, 122,* 495–506.

Hammond, E.C., Selikoff, I.J., & Seidman, H. (1979). Asbestos exposure, cigarette smoking, and death rates. *Annals of the New York Academy of Science, 330,* 473–490.

Hill, A.B. (1965). The environment and disease: Association or causation? *Proceedings of the Royal Society of Medicine, 58,* 295–300.

Hills, M., & Armitage, P. (1979). The two-period cross-over clinical trial. *British Journal of Clinical Pharmacology, 8,* 7–20.

Jooste, P.L., Yach, D., Steenkamp, H.J., Botha, J.L., & Rossouw, J.E. (1990). Drop-out and newcomer bias in a community cardiovascular follow-up study. *International Journal of Epidemiology, 19,* 284–289.

Kalton, G. (1993). Sampling considerations in research on HIV risk and illness. In D.G. Ostrow & R.C. Kessler (Eds.), *Methodological Issues in AIDS Behavioral Research* (pp. 53–74). New York: Plenum Press.

Kelsey, J.L., Thompson, W.D., & Evans, A.S. (1986). *Methods in Observational Epidemiology.* New York: Oxford University Press.

Khlat, M. (1994). Use of case-control methods for indirect estimation in demography. *Epidemiologic Reviews, 16,* 124–133.

Khoury, M.J., & Beaty, T.H. (1994). Applications of the case-control method in genetic epidemiology. *Epidemiologic Reviews, 16,* 134–150.

Kleinbaum, D.G., Kupper, L.L., & Morgenstern, M. (1982). *Epidemiologic Research: Principles and Quantitative Methods.* New York: Van Nostrand Reinhold.

Lasky, T., & Stolley, P.D. (1994). Selection of cases and controls. *Epidemiologic Reviews, 16,* 6–17.

Last, J.M., (Ed.). (1988). *A Dictionary of Epidemiology* (2nd ed.). New York: Oxford University Press.

Liberati, A. (1995). "Meta-analysis: statistical alchemy for the 21st century": Discussion. A plea for a more balanced view of meta-analysis and systematic overviews of the effect of health care interventions. *Journal of Clinical Epidemiology, 48,* 81–86.

Lubin, J.H., & Gail, M.H. (1984). Biased selection of controls for case-control analyses of cohort studies. *Biometrics, 40,* 63–75.

Mastroianni, A.C., Faden, R., & Federman, D. (Eds.) (1994). *Women and Health Research: Ethical and Legal Issues of Including Women in Clinical Studies,* vol. 1. Washington, DC: National Academy Press.

Miettinen, O.S. (1985). The case-control study: Valid selection of subjects. *Journal of Chronic Disease, 38,* 543–548.

Morabia, A. (1991). On the origin of Hill's causal criteria. *Epidemiology, 2,* 367–369.

Morgenstern, H. (1996, Spring). *Course Materials, Part II: Class Notes for Epidemiologic Methods II, Epidemiology 201B,* 54–82.

Morgenstern, H. (1982). Uses of ecologic analysis in epidemiologic research. *American Journal of Public Health, 72,* 1336–1344.

O'Brien, P.C., & Shampo, M.A. (1988). Statistical considerations for performing multiple tests in a single experiment. 5. Comparing two therapies with respect to several endpoints. *Mayo Clinic Proceedings, 63,* 1140–1143.

Olkin, I. (1995). Statistical and theoretical considerations in meta-analysis, quoting the National Library of Medicine. *Journal of Clinical Epidemiology, 48,* 133–146.

Rosner, F. (1987). The ethics of randomized clinical trials. *American Journal of Medicine, 82,* 283–290.

Rothman, K.J. (1976). Causes. *American Journal of Epidemiology, 104,* 587–592.

Rothman, K.J. (1986). *Modern Epidemiology.* Boston: Little, Brown and Company.

Sackett, D.L. (1979). Bias in analytic research. *Journal of Chronic Diseases, 32,* 51–63.

Sartwell, P.E. (1960). On the methodology of investigations of etiologic factors in chronic disease—further comments. *Journal of Chronic Disease, 11,* 61–63.

Schlesselman, J.J. (1982). *Case Control Studies.* New York: Oxford University Press.

Selby, J.V. (1994). Case-control evaluations of treatment and program efficacy. *Epidemiologic Reviews, 16,* 90–101.

Senn, S.J. (1991). Falsification and clinical trials. *Statistics in Medicine, 10,* 1679–1692.

Smith, P.G. (1983). Issues in the design of case-control studies: Matching and interaction effects. *Tijdschrift voor Sociale Gezondheidszorg, 61,* 755–760.

Sterling, T.D., Weinkam, J.J., & Weinkam, J.L. (1990). The sick person effect. *Journal of Clinical Epidemiology, 43,* 141–151.

Susser, M. (1991). What is a cause and how do we know one? A grammar for pragmatic epidemiology. *American Journal of Epidemiology, 133,* 635–648.

Wacholder, S., Silverman, D.T., McLaughlin, J.K., & Mandel, J.S. (1992). Selection of controls in case–control studies. III. Design options. *American Journal of Epidemiology, 135,* 1042–1050.

Weed, D.L. (1986). On the logic of causal inference. *American Journal of Epidemiology, 123,* 965–979.

Weiss, N.S. (1994). Application of the case–control method in the evaluation of screening. *Epidemiologic Reviews, 16,* 102–108.

21 Code of Federal Regulations section 312.21(a) (1998).

21 Code of Federal Regulations section 312.21(b) (1998).

21 Code of Federal Regulations section 312.21(c) (1998).

3

Race and Ethnicity

Racial and ethnic classifications are frequently used when describing health differences between groups. For example, race has been associated with reactivity for syphilis (Hahn *et al.*, 1989), an increased risk of pelvic inflammatory disease (Lee, Rukin, and Grimes, 1991), incidence of *Chlamydia trachomatis* (Ryan *et al.*, 1990), and high blood pressure (Harburg *et al.*, 1978a, 1978b; Klag *et al.*, 1991). Apparent racial effects are often attributed to unexplained genetic and biological variations (Kaufman, Cooper, and McGee, 1997). Differences by race have also been noted in the utilization of diagnostic and therapeutic procedures, including coronary angioplasty, bypass grafting procedures (Carlisle, Leake, and Shapiro, 1995), and cardiac catheterization (Peterson, Wright, Daley, and Thibault, 1994). These disparities in utilization of health care procedures have often been explained by reference to inadequately measured differences in socioeconomic status or by unmeasured environmental factors (Byrne, Nedelman, and Luke, 1994). Similar disparities in health status and utilization of treatments have been noted across groups differentiated by "ethnicity" (Black, 1984; Qureshi, 1989). Apparent "ethnic" effects are often explained as the result of culture or ethnicity, operationalized as a single demographic variable that fails to encompass, explain, or define the complexities and nuances that underlie such classification (Blane, 1993). This chapter examines the concepts of race and ethnicity, their usage in the context of health research, and the appropriateness of that usage.

Race

The concept of race has been used to explain differences in appearance and in behavior across individuals and groups of individuals (Gaines, 1994). A variety of criteria have been used to define race, including region or geographical area of origin (King and Stansfield, 1990), nationality (Taylor, 1988), language, skin color, and religion (Gaines, 1994). These distinctions have provided the foundation for numerous suppositions about race in the United States: (1) the existence of a fixed number of distinct races (Becker and Landav, 1992; Campbell, 1981; Segen, 1992), (2) some of which are superior to others and (3) each of which is characterized by distinct physical, mental, or behavioral attributes (4) that are reproduced over time (Boas, 1940; Gould, 1981; Montagu, 1964a). As an example, consider the following "scientific" distinctions drawn between white and black individuals on the basis of skin color, made by a physician in 1851:

> Before going into the peculiarities of these diseases, it is necessary to glance at the anatomical and physiological differences between the negro and the white man; otherwise their diseases cannot be understood. It is commonly taken for granted, that the color of the skin constitutes the main and essential difference between the black and the white race; but there are other differences more deep, durable and indelible in their anatomy and physiology, than that of mere color. It is not only in the skin that a difference of color exists between the negro and the white man, but in the membranes, the muscles, the tendons, and in all the fluids and secretions. Even the negro's brains and nerves, the chyle and all the humors, are tinctured with a shade of the pervading darkness. His bile is of a deeper color, and his blood is blacker than the white man's. (Cartwright, 1851)

With respect to the reproducibility of such characteristics, consider the statements of the scientist Nott (1843), who argued against the intermarriage of the races based on his observation that (1) mulattoes live shorter lives in comparison with other classes of humans; (2) mulatto women are more likely to suffer from chronic diseases and inability to reproduce than are other women; and (3) the children of mulatto women are more likely to die at a young age. (Nott clearly failed to consider that mulattoes' relatively darker skin color might have affected individuals' ability to obtain care which might, in turn, have affected morbidity and mortality.)

The lack of conceptual clarity in defining "race" is evident from the variation in definition and classification over time, place, and purpose of designation (Gaines, 1994; LaVeist, 1994; Osborne and Feit, 1992). The United States alone has used a multitude of definitions and terms in an attempt to distinguish "whites" from "nonwhites" (Davis, 1991). For example, the censuses of 1840, 1850, and 1860 counted mulattoes, but failed to explain the term's meaning. The 1870 and 1880 censuses specifically defined "mulattoes" as "quadroons, octoroons, and all persons having any perceptible trace of African blood" (Davis, 1991). The 1890 census required that *enumerators* record the exact proportion of "African blood," while the 1900 census required that "pure Negroes" be distinguished from mulattoes, defined as persons "with some trace of black blood" (Davis, 1991). The scientist Lawrence (1819) had earlier devised an informal test for use in the West Indies to detect the "blackness" of any such individuals who may have become indistinguishably white through the successive intermarriages of previous generations:

> Europeans and Tercerons produce Querterons or Quadroons (ochavones, octavones, or alvinos), which are not to be distinguished from whites; but they are not entitled, in Jamaica at least, to the same privileges as the Europeans or the white Creoles, because there is still a contamination of dark blood, although no longer visible. *It is said to betray itself sometimes in a relic of the peculiar strong smell of the great-grandmother.* (Italics added)

As of the 1930 census, "black" was defined as an individual with any black blood. In 1960, the basis for enumeration changed again, to permit the head of each household, rather than the enumerator, to identify the race of its members (Davis, 1991). This system of designating race was embedded in the protocol used for the assignment of race on birth certificates prior to 1989: a child was considered "white" only if both parents were considered "white" (LaVeist, 1994). An individual with one "white" parent and one "black" parent, then, would have been classifiable as a mulatto in 1900 and as a black in 1930. The 1990 census requested that each respondent report his or her racial classification as the one that he or she most closely identified with, but failed to provide a definition of race, resulting in confusion and "misreporting" (McKenney and Bennett, 1994).

Designation of an individual's race has been shown to vary by place as well. Even among the various states, the racial classification of an individual could differ. For example, the "privileges of whites" were extended to a "quadroon" female by the Supreme Court of Ohio in 1831 due to "the difficulty of ... ascertaining the degree of duskiness which renders a person liable to such disabilities" (Gray v. Ohio, 1831). By contrast, the California Supreme Court construed the word "white" as excluding "black, yellow, and all other colors.... The term 'black person' is to be construed as including everyone who is not of white blood" (People v. Hall, 1854). The black/mulatto child born in the United States would be classified as a mulatto in Brazil, and further categorized by the degree of darkness or lightness of the skin color as a *preto* (black), *preto retinto* (dark black), *cabra* (slightly less black), *escuro* (lighter), *mulato esuro* (dark mulatto), *mulato claro* (light mulatto), *sarara*, *moreno*, *blanco de terra*, or *blanco* (LaVeist, 1994). Prior to 1989 in the United States, a child born to a "white" father and a Japanese mother was classified as Japanese on his or her birth certificate. The same child would have been classified as white on his or her birth certificate in pre-1985 Japan (LaVeist, 1994).

The purpose or process of racial designation may also affect the ultimate classification of an individual. For example, a child's race on his or her birth certificate is designated by that infant's mother, whereas the assignment of race at death is often made by the funeral director for completion of the death certificate. It is not inconceivable that an individual classified as a member of one race at birth will be classified as a member of another race at death (Hahn, 1992). Interviewer-reported race has been shown to vary significantly from respondent-reported race. A study conducted by the National Center for Health Statistics found that 5.8% of the individuals who reported themselves as "black" were classified as "white" by the interviewer, while 32.3% of self-reported Asians and 70% of self-reported Native Americans were classified by the interviewer as "white" or "black" (Massey, 1980). Misclassification has been noted, as well, in data collected by the Health Care Financing Administration relating to elderly Medicare enrollees (Lauderdale and Goldberg, 1996). Finally, shifting perceptions of self-identity may result in inconsistent self-designation across time and circumstance (Johnson, 1974; Siegel and Passel, 1979; Snipp, 1986).

These classification schema and the discrepancies that they create underscore the difficulty of applying the concept of race, however it is defined. They also lend credence to the observation that "race is a societally constructed taxonomy that reflects the intersection of particular historical conditions with economic, political, legal, social, and cultural factors, as well as racism" (Williams, LaVizzo-Mourey, and Warren, 1994:28).

History is, unfortunately, replete with examples of medical care and research founded on differentiation by race. For example, the integration of eugenics and racism within South Carolina's medical profession provoked objections to voluntary birth control programs:

> You have often heard the "nigger" as the great bugbear in the path of birth control. That they breed like rabbits, and [with] no desire for change.... That, with birth control [by whites] on one side of the hedge, and the negro on the other, spawning their millions, the Caucasian race will eventually be put out of business. (Dreher, 1931)

Ultimately, South Carolina addressed this issue through the adoption and implementation of a racially discriminatory sterilization program in its mental health hospital (Larson, 1995). The Nazi regime, distinguishing between the Aryan and the Jewish "races," progressively instituted measures to permit experimentation with and the extermination of members of the Jewish "race," which not only embodied " 'dangerous genes' in an individual medical sense [but also] 'racial poison' in a collective ethnic sense" (Lifton, 1986:77). The Jewish race, found by Nazi physicians to suffer from a higher incidence of certain metabolic and mental disorders than members of the Aryan race, became synonymous with disease: "There is a resemblance between Jews and tubercle bacilli: nearly everyone harbors tubercle bacilli and nearly every people of the earth harbors Jews; furthermore, an infection can only be cured with difficulty" (Peltret, 1935:565–566). The Tuskegee experiment involving syphilis and African-Americans in the rural South is perhaps one of the most infamous examples of race-based research in the United States and is discussed in greater detail in Chapter 6.

Despite the nebulous nature of "race" and the dangers inherent in our reliance on the concept, race continues to be used as a variable to explain health effects, often without any basis in reality. This is particularly true in the context of diseases associated with conduct that could be seen as immoral or uncautious (Gaines, 1994). Osborne and Feit (1992) note, for example, that the association of sexually transmitted diseases with race or ethnicity, absent a clear explanation of the hypotheses underlying the research, could lead the reader to believe that at least one of the following is true: (1) that members of a specified ethnic/racial group are more promiscuous than other Americans and that that promiscuity is inherited; (2) that promiscuity is not inherited, but that members of the specified group are more susceptible to sexually transmitted diseases than are others; (3) that members of the specified group are especially susceptible to the asexual transmission of sexually transmitted pathogens, which cannot differentiate potential hosts by race; (4) that members of the specified group do not contract sexually transmitted diseases either more frequently or in different ways than do other groups, but that they report these infections more often; or (5) that the apparent racial differences actually signify differences in socioeconomic status, education level, or lifestyle. Osborne and Feit (1992) propose an alternative conclusion: that the research reports indicating such differences are fraudulent, selective, or racially motivated. One must also consider, however, that such conclusions might be unthinking and uninformed, rather than fraudulent or malicious.

Ethnicity

Yinger (1994:3) has defined an ethnic group as

> a segment of a larger society whose members are thought, by themselves or others, to have a common origin and to share important segments of a common culture and who, in addition, participate in shared activities in which the common origin and culture are significant ingredients.

As such, three elements are critical to the formation of an ethnic group: (1) the perception by others in society of differences between the group members and others with respect to certain traits, such as language, religion, race, or homeland; (2) the perception of these same differences by the group members; and (3) the participation of group members in shared activities that are founded on their perceived common heritage or culture (Yinger, 1994).

By contrast, Montagu's (1964b:317) definition of ethnicity encompasses genetic differences and also recognizes the role of self-defined or self-imposed barriers:

> An ethnic group represents one of a number of populations, comprising the single species of *Homo sapiens*, which individually maintain their differences, physical and cultural, by means of isolating mechanisms such as geographic and social barriers. These differences will vary as the power of the geographic and social barriers acting upon the original genetic differences varies.

Race is often used as a criterion to define ethnicity, although its usage has varied over time and place (Yinger, 1994). The two terms have at times been used seemingly interchangeably. For example, in defining race, DuBois (1897:7) explained

> It is a vast family of human beings, generally of common blood and language, always of common history, traditions and impulses, who are both voluntarily and involuntarily striving together for the accomplishment of certain more or less vividly conceived ideals of life.

Similarly, *Dorland's Medical Dictionary* (Taylor, 1988) defined race as a function of ethnicity, genetics, and physical appearance:

> 1. an ethnic stock, or division of mankind; in a narrower sense, a national or tribal stock; in a still narrower sense, a genealogic line of descent; a class of persons of common lineage. In genetics, races are considered as populations having different distributions of gene frequencies. 2. a class or breed of animals; a group of individuals having certain characteristics in common, owing to a common inheritance; a subspecies.

Cooper (1994) also defines ethnicity with reference to race. Cooper first defines race as a biologic, rather than social, construct related to a single breeding population. The resulting racial classifications are based, in practice, on superficial phenotypic traits. Cooper defines ethnicity as "the relevant form of raciation among a species where cultural differentiation predominates." Ethnicity is produced through social evolution as the product of genes, culture, and social class.

van den Berghe (1967:9) explicit acknowledged the lack of demarcation between "race" and "ethnicity":

> In practice, the distinction between a racial and an ethnic group is sometimes blurred by several facts. Cultural traits are often regarded as genetic and inherited (e.g., body odor, which is a function of diet, cosmetics, and other cultural items); physical appearance can be culturally changed (by scarification, surgery, and cosmetics); and the sensory perception of physical differences is affected by cultural perceptions of race (e.g., a rich Negro may be seen as lighter than an equally dark poor Negro, as suggested by the Brazilian proverb: "Money bleaches").

It is this attention to race, however, that easily diverts our attention away from an examination of relevant cultural and ethnic differences. As an example, the African-American population of the United States is composed of individuals from diverse areas of the Caribbean and Africa, whose languages and histories are quite different (Williams *et al.*, 1994). The existence of such differences and their interaction with the larger environment may have important implications for our understanding of health status and disease prevention.

The Use of Race and Ethnicity in Health Research

Hahn and Stroup (1994) have identified numerous "challenges to public health surveillance" occasioned by the use of racial classifications:

1. There is a lack of scientific consensus regarding the conceptual validity of race and ethnicity.

2. Categories of race and ethnicity cannot be clearly delineated.
3. Racial and ethnic categories will change over time.
4. The scientific use of social categories may be wrongly interpreted as the endorsement of their validity. Consequently, reliance on racial and ethnic categories carries policy and ethical concerns.
5. Race and ethnicity are determinants of access to resources.
6. Biological characteristics should be measured appropriately in studies of disease. However, public health surveillance may rely on the assessment of race or ethnicity.

The first three issues have been addressed above; that discussion will not be repeated here. The three remaining premises are examined now in greater detail.

Our association of leprosy with various racial and ethnic groups provides an example of the broad-ranging social policy and political action that may ensue when we all too willingly accept our socially constructed ethnic classifications as reflective of immutable characteristics. The following statement by a physician exemplifies our willingness to equate group membership with disease:

> The questions as to whether the specific form of bacillus found in the lymphatics and sores of the leper can be transmitted through the medium of food, water and clothing, or by inoculation, may not be settled; but there are no doubt in the Chinese laundries of San Francisco, New Orleans, and New York, Asiatic men now at work who are in the early stages of the disease; and their practice of taking water in their mouths and spitting it out on the clothes they iron, is more than ever disgusting when considered in connection with the now possible transmission of disease by this means. (Jones, 1887:1245)

This association between the Chinese and leprosy fueled the belief in the superiority of the "Anglo-Saxon race," and ultimately led to the formulation and implementation of restrictions on Chinese immigration to the United States and the exclusion of individuals with leprosy (Gussow, 1989).

> At the present day Louisiana is threatened with an influx of Chinese and Malays, with filth, rice [sic] and leprous diseases. An inferior and barbarous race transferred from the burning heats of Africa has already been the occasion of the shedding of the blood of more than one million of the white inhabitants of the United States, and in the shock of arms and in the subsequent confusion and chaos attending the settlement of the question of African slavery, the liberties of the country have been well nigh destroyed, and it is but just that patriots should contemplate with dread the overflow of their country by the unprincipled, vicious and leprous bodies of Asia. The contact of a superior race with an inferior race must lead eventually to two results: The annihilation of one or the other, or the amalgamation of the two. The mixture of the blood of a noble race with that of one of the inferior mental and moral constitution may depress the former to the level of the latter, but can never endow the brain and heart of the African and Asiatic with the intelligence, independence, love of liberty, invention and moral worth of the Anglo-Saxon race. (Jones, 1887:1246–1247)

The politics of AIDS is also illustrative of the policy and ethical implications of reliance on racial and ethnic classifications, and provides a more recent example. The disease condition now known as AIDS (acquired immunodeficiency syndrome) was first labeled as such in 1982. The causative agent has since been identified as the human immunodeficiency virus (HIV), transmissible via the exchange of certain body fluids, such as blood, semen, and vaginal secretions. HIV/AIDS may be contracted through transfusion with contaminated blood or blood products or transplant with a contaminated organ; through unprotected sexual inter-course, possibly including oral intercourse; through the use of contaminated injection equip-ment; and through vertical transmission from mother to child. Transmission of the virus and progression of the disease may be facilitated by various cofactors; the rate of progression may, however, be altered through the use of various therapies (Abrams, 1997; Volberding, 1997). (For additional detail relating to HIV/AIDS, see Chapter 12).

Initial research into the etiology and epidemiology of AIDS focused on the identification of routes of transmission and risk factors for the disease. By 1982, within a year of identifying the first cases of what would come to be known as AIDS, the Centers for Disease Control and Prevention (CDC) had labeled Haitians a "risk group." This emphasis on group membership as a risk factor, rather than relevant behaviors, would ultimately result in the cultural and medical construction of "risk groups," whose members were often presumed to be at higher risk of contracting—and transmitting—HIV merely by virtue of their group membership: Haitians, homosexuals, heroin addicts, and hemophiliacs (Schiller, Crysteal, and Lewellen, 1994). These groups became known popularly as the "4-H club."

Haitians were ultimately seen not only as carriers of the disease, but its reservoir as well (Gilman, 1987). The labeling of Haitians as a risk group provided a scientific basis for the perpetuation of existing myths and stereotypes and the stigmatization of and discrimination against Haitians. One researcher noted:

> The link between AIDS and Haiti, strengthened in innumerable articles in the popular press, seemed to resonate with what might be termed a North American "folk model" of Haitians.... The press drew upon readily available images of squalor, voodoo, and boatloads of "disease-ridden" or "economic" refugees. One of the most persistently invoked asso-ciations related the occurrence of AIDS in Haitians to voodoo. Something that happened at those ritual fires, it was speculated, triggered AIDS in cult adherents, presumed to be the quasitotality of Haitians. (Farmer, 1990:416)

In addition, the characterization of AIDS transmission by risk group, rather than by behavior, may have engendered a false sense of security in individuals who did not identify themselves as members of these groups (Schiller et al., 1994).

Although differences in disease rates are often the result of differential access to re-sources, these differences have frequently been attributed to racial, or genetic, differences. For example, at one time Irish individuals were considered to be racially susceptible to rheumatic fever, which was linked to genes for red hair. Not surprisingly, as the Irish as a group became more prosperous, they experienced a decrease in the incidence of rheumatic fever, a disease associated with overcrowding and poverty (Paul, 1957). The incidence of the disease later increased among black migrants who had relocated from the South to urban areas (Newsholme, 1895).

Numerous studies have found an association between race and/or ethnicity and the differential utilization of health care resources. These differences have been attributed to sociocultural differences affecting physician and patient decision making (Eisenberg, 1979), patient treatment preferences (Maynard, Fisher, Passamani, and Pullum, 1986), patient–provider interactions (Franks, Clancy, and Naumberg, 1995), patient presentation style (Bird-well, Herbers, and Kroenke, 1993), patient familiarity with the procedures and patient educa-tion level (Wilson, May, and Kelly, 1994), differential access to specific types of hospitals (Blustein and Weitzman, 1995), variations in insurance coverage (Harris, Andrews, and Elixhauser, 1997), unmeasured environmental factors, and inadequately measured social indicators (Byrne *et al.*, 1994). Such conclusions, even when founded upon unmeasured variables and untested hypotheses, provide a disservice. As Morgenstern (1997:610) has noted, it is critical that we

> not attribute adjusted (residual) associations to the influence of specific unmeasured factors; rather, we should test our hypotheses by measuring those factors hypothesized to be responsible for health differences between groups.

Attribution of residual associations to unmeasured biological effects may lead to the spurious conclusion that, because the differences are biological, remedial action is of no use, thereby encouraging maintenance of the status quo. Similarly, to ascribe the differences to undefined, unexplained, and unmeasured cultural attributes may lead one to conclude that neither further examination nor action is necessary because such attributes remain firmly rooted. In either case, we fail to attend adequately to the needs of specific subpopulations. This uncritical explanation of differences may also transform minority communities into "mere statistical categories," reinforce existing stereotypes, "perpetuate the distortion of social reality," and help to create new stereotypes (Jones, LaVeist, and Lillie-Blanton, 1991; Schiller *et al.*, 1994; Sheldon and Parker, 1992:104; Williams, 1994:268). Also, in the context of health resource utilization, a finding of differential use fails to address whether one group is underutilizing care or another group is overutilizing procedures and treatments (Harris *et al.*, 1997).

Cooper (1994) has argued that ethnicity should replace race as the appropriate schema for public health surveillance due to the mutability of the classification scheme. However, it is not at all clear that racial or ethnic classifications as they are currently constructed are adequate for public health surveillance. Reliance on such constructs, without attention to the accurate measurement of variables such as socioeconomic characteristics, continues to allow the perpetuation of existing stereotypes and the development of policy founded on untested assumptions about a particular subgroup.

One must ask, then, whether there exists a legitimate use for the concept of race or ethnicity in health research. Numerous suggestions have been advanced. LaVeist (1994) has proposed that, since race refers to skin color rather than to culture, biology, or socioeconomic status, we measure skin color as a continuous variable. This approach fails, however, to delineate lines of demarcation along this continuum so, for example, it is unclear how light one's skin must be to be "very light" in comparison to "light," In addition, this scheme assumes (1) that it is the skin color itself that has relevance to the research question, and (2) that there is less variation in other factors of significance, which may be unconsidered or unmeasured, within each classification than there is across classifications.

Various researchers have persuasively argued that researchers (1) must justify the inclusion of a race/ethnicity variable in their analysis; (2) explicitly define race/ethnicity when they are used as variables; (3) report the manner in which race or ethnicity was assessed (e.g., self-report, direct observation, or record abstraction); and (4) attend to the social, economic, and political factors that affect health and health behaviors (Schulman, Rubenstein, Chesley, and Eisenberg, 1995; Williams, 1994).

Exercises

1. You are the chief epidemiologist for a department of public health in a large metropolitan area. You have been conducting a study to identify risk factors for low birth weight deliveries. The study, to date, has relied on birth certificates, medical records, and inter-

views with women recruited from publicly funded prenatal clinics, who are then followed through their deliveries. A proportion of the women have reported numerous events to you in the context of this study, including the use of illicit drugs, conduct toward other existing children that could be perceived as abusive or neglectful, and undocumented immigration status of some or all family members. Assume that you find an association between membership in a particular ethnic group, low birth weight upon delivery, and drug usage. What are the potential implications of these findings and how will you address them from both an ethical and scientific perspective?

2. The provisions of U.S. immigration law enacted in 1924 restricted the entry of certain groups due to their ostensible genetic inferiority: "Testimony before Congress by leaders of the American mental testing movement to the effect that Slavs, Jews, Italians and others were mentally dull and that their dullness was racial, or at least constitutional, gave scientific legitimacy to the [restrictive immigration] law" (Kamin, Lewontin, and Rose, 1984:27).

    a. What alternative explanations exist that could explain the perceived "dullness" of these groups' members?

    b. Ultimately, the immigration provisions were relaxed to permit the entry of limited numbers of individuals belonging to the enumerated groups. What, if any, long-term impact may have occurred on the health status or health access of these groups' members as a result of the initial attitudes and corresponding policies?

       i. *Design a study to assess the presence and extent of any such effects.*

       ii. *How might such attitudes and policies have impacted our approach to health research and our interpretation of research results, if they had any impact at all? Justify your response.*

3. If racial classification for the census is now based on self-identification, how can misreporting occur? What are the implications of such misreporting in the context of research?

References

Abrams, D.I. (1997). Alternative therapies for HIV. In M.A. Sande & P.A. Volberding (Eds.), *The Medical Management of AIDS* (5th ed., pp. 143–158). Philadelphia: W.B. Saunders Company.

Becker, E.L., & Landav, S.I. (1992). *Health Issues in the Black Community*. San Francisco: Jossey-Bass Publishers.

Birdwell, B.G., Herbers, J.E., & Kroenke, K. (1993). Evaluating chest pain. The patient's presentation style alters the physician's diagnostic approach. *Archives of Internal Medicine, 153*, 1991–1995.

Black, J. (1984). Afro-Caribbean and African families. *British Medical Journal, 290*, 984–988.

Blane, H.T. (1993). Ethnicity. In M. Galanter (Ed.), *Recent Developments in Alcoholism, Volume 11: Ten Years of Progress*. New York: Plenum Press.

Blustein, J., & Weitzman, B.C. (1995). Access to hospitals with high-technology cardiac services: How is race important? *American Journal of Public Health, 85*, 345–351.

Boas, F. (1940). *Race, Language and Culture*. New York: Free Press.

Byrne, C., Nedelman, J., & Luke, R.G. (1994). Race, socioeconomic status, and the development of end-stage renal disease. *American Journal of Kidney Diseases, 23*, 16–22.

Campbell, R.J. (1981). *Psychiatric Dictionary* (5th ed.). London: Oxford University Press.

Carlisle, D.M., Leake, B.D., & Shapiro, M.F. (1995). Racial and ethnic differences in the use of invasive cardiac procedures among cardiac patients in Los Angeles County, 1986 through 1988. *American Journal of Public Health, 85*, 352–356.

Cartwright, S. (1851). Diseases and peculiarities of the Negro race: Presented at the medical convention in Louisiana. *DeBow's Review, 11*, 64–69, 331–336.

Cooper, R.S. (1994). A case study in the use of race and ethnicity in public health surveillance. *Public Health Reports, 109*, 46–52.

Davis, J.F. (1991). *Who Is Black? One Nation's Definition*. University Park, PA: Pennsylvania State University Press.

Dreher, T.H. (1931). Birth control among the poor. *Journal of the South Carolina Medical Association, 27*, 331–332.

DuBois, W.E.B. (1897). The conservation of races. American Negro Academy, Occasional Paper, no. 2. Washington, DC: American Negro Academy.

Eisenberg, J.M. (1979). Sociological influences on medical decisionmaking by clinicians. *Annals of Internal Medicine, 90,* 957–964.

Farmer, P. (1990). The exotic and the mundane: Haitian immunodeficiency virus in Haiti. *Human Nature, 1,* 415–446.

Franks, P., Clancy, C.M., & Naumberg, E.H. (1995). Sex, access, and excess. *Annals of Internal Medicine, 123,* 548–550.

Gaines, A.D. (1994). Race and racism. In W. Reich (Ed.), *Encyclopedia of Bioethics.* New York: Macmillan.

Gilman, S. (1987). AIDS and syphilis: The iconography of the disease. In D. Crimp (Ed.), *AIDS: Cultural Analysis, Cultural Activism* (pp. 87–108). Cambridge, MA: MIT Press.

Gould, S.J. (1981). *The Mismeasure of Man.* New York: W.W. Norton.

Gray v. Ohio, 4 Ohio 353 (1831).

Gussow, Z. (1989). *Leprosy, Racism, and Public Health: Social Policy in Chronic Disease Control.* Boulder, CO: Westview Press.

Hahn, R.A. (1992). The state of federal health statistics on racial and ethnic groups. *JAMA, 267,* 268–271.

Hahn, R.A., Magder, L.S., Aral, S.O., Johnson, R.E., & Larsen, S.A. (1989). Race and the prevalence of syphilis seroreactivity in the United States population: A national sero-epidemiologic study. *American Journal of Public Health, 79,* 467–470.

Hahn, R.A., & Stroup, D.F. (1994). Race and ethnicity in public health surveillance: Criteria for the scientific use of social categories. *Public Health Reports, 109,* 7–15.

Harburg, E., Gleiberman, F., Ozgoren, F., Roeper, P., Schork, M.A., & Schull, W.J. (1978a). Skin color, ethnicity, and blood pressure. I: Detroit blacks. *American Journal of Public Health, 68,* 1177–1183.

Harburg, E., Gleiberman, F., Ozgoren, F., Roeper, P., Schork, M.A., & Schull, W.J. (1978b). Skin color, ethnicity, and blood pressure. II: Detroit whites. *American Journal of Public Health, 68,* 1184–1188.

Harris, D.R., Andrews, R., & Elixhauser, A. (1997). Racial and gender differences in the use of procedures for black and white hospitalized adults. *Ethnicity and Disease, 7,* 91–105.

Johnson, C.E., Jr. (1974). *Consistency of Reporting of Ethnic Origin in the Current Population Survey.* Washington, DC: Bureau of the Census [U.S. Department of Commerce Technical Paper No. 31].

Jones, J. (1887). *Medical and Surgical Memoirs ... 1855–1886* (Vol. 2). New Orleans. Quoted in Z. Gussow. (1989). *Leprosy, Racism, and Public Health: Social Policy in Chronic Disease Control.* Boulder, CO: Westview Press.

Jones, C.P., LaVeist, T.A., & Lillie-Blanton, M. (1991). "Race" in the epidemiologic literature: An examination of the *American Journal of Epidemiology, 1921–1990. American Journal of Epidemiology, 134,* 1079–1084.

Kamin, L., Lewontin, R., & Rose, S. (1984). *Not in Our Genes: Biology, Ideology, and Human Nature.* New York: Pantheon Books.

Kaufman, J.S., Cooper, R.S., & McGee, D.L. (1997). Socioeconomic status and health in blacks and whites: The problem of residual confounding and the resiliency of race. *Epidemiology, 8,* 621–628.

King, R.C., & Stansfield, W.D. (1990). *A Dictionary of Genetics.* London: Oxford University Press.

Klag, M.J., Whelton, P.K., Coresh, J., Grim, C.E., & Kuller, L.H. (1991). The association of skin color with blood pressure in US blacks with low socioeconomic status. *JAMA, 265,* 599–602.

Larson, E.J. (1995). *Sex, Race, and Science: Eugenics in the Deep South.* Baltimore, MD: Johns Hopkins University Press.

Lauderdale, D.S., & Goldberg, J. (1996). The expanded racial and ethnic codes in the Medicare data files: Their completeness of coverage and accuracy. *American Journal of Public Health, 86,* 712–716.

LaVeist, T.A. (1994). Beyond dummy variables and sample selection: What health services researchers ought to know about race as a variable. *Health Services Research, 29*(1), 1–16.

Lawrence, W. (1823). *Lectures on Physiology, Zoology, and the Natural History of Man, Delivered to the Royal College of Surgeons* [1819] (3rd ed.). London: South. Cited in R.J.C. Young. (1995). *Colonial Desire: Hybridity in Theory, Culture and Race.* London: Routledge.

Lee, N.C., Rubin, G.L., & Grimes, D.A. (1991). Measures of sexual behavior and the risk of pelvic inflammatory disease. *Obstetrics and Gynecology, 77,* 425–430.

Lifton, R.J. (1986). *The Nazi Doctors: Medical Killing and the Psychology of Genocide.* New York: Basic Books.

Massey, J. (1980). Using interviewer observed race and respondent reported race in the Health Interview Survey. *Proceedings of the American Statistical Association Meetings: Social statistics section* (pp. 425–428). Alexandria, VA: American Statistical Association.

Maynard, C., Fisher, L.D., Passamani, E.R., & Pullum, T. (1986). Blacks in the Coronary Artery Surgery Study (CASS): Race and clinical decision making. *American Journal of Public Health, 76,* 1446–1448.

McKenney, N.R., & Bennett, C.E. (1994). Issues regarding data on race and ethnicity: The Census Bureau experience. *Public Health Reports, 109,* 16–25.

Montagu, A. (1964a). *Man's Most Dangerous Myth: The Fallacy of Race* (4th ed. rev.). Cleveland, OH: World.

Montagu, A.M.F. (1964b). Discussion and criticism on the race concept. *Current Anthropology, 5,* 317.

Morgenstern, H. (1997). Defining and explaining race effects. *Epidemiology, 8,* 609–610.

Newsholme, A. (1895). Milroy lectures: Rheumatic fever. *Lancet, 1,* 589–596. Cited in R. Cooper. (1984). A note on the biologic concept of race and its application in epidemiologic research. *American Heart Journal, 108,* 715–723.

Nott, J.C. (1843). The mulatto a hybrid—Probable extermination of the two races if the whites and blacks are allowed to intermarry. *American Journal of the Medical Sciences, 6,* 252–256. Cited in R.J.C. Young. (1995). *Colonial Desire: Hybridity in Theory, Culture and Race.* London: Routledge.

Osborne, N.G., & Feit, F.D. (1992). The use of race in medical research. *JAMA, 267*(2), 275–279.

Paul, J.R. (1957). *The Epidemiology of Rheumatic Fever.* New York: American Heart Association.

Peltret —. (1935). Der Arzt als Fuhrer und Erzieher. *DA, 65,* 565–566. Cited in R.N. Proctor. (1988). *Racial Hygiene: Medicine Under the Nazis.* Cambridge, MA: Harvard University Press.

People v. Hall, 4 Cal. 399 (1854).

Peterson, E.D., Wright, S.M., Daley, J., & Thibault, G.E. (1994). Racial variation in cardiac procedure use and survival following acute myocardial infarction in the Department of Veterans Affairs. *JAMA, 271,* 1175–1180.

Qureshi, B. (1989). *Transcultural Medicine.* Dordrecht: Kluwer Academic.

Ryan, G.M., Abdella, T.N., McNeely, S.G., Baselski, V.S., & Drummond, D.E. (1990). *Chlamydia trachomatis* infection in pregnancy and effect of treatment on outcome. *American Journal of Obstetrics and Gynecology, 162,* 34–39.

Schiller, N.G., Crystal, S., & Lewellen, D. (1994). Risky business: The cultural construction of AIDS risk groups. *Social Science and Medicine, 38,* 1337–1346.

Schulman, K.A., Rubenstein, L.E., Chesley, F.D., & Eisenberg, J.M. (1995). The roles of race and socioeconomic factors in health services research. *Health Services Research, 30,* 179–195.

Segen, J.C. (1992). *The Dictionary of Modern Medicine.* Park Ridge, NJ: Parthenon Publishing Group.

Sheldon, T.A., & Parker, H. (1992). Race and ethnicity in health research. *Journal of Public Health Medicine, 14,* 104–110.

Siegel, J.S., & Passel, J.S. (1979). *Coverage of the Hispanic Population of the United States in the 1970 Census.* Washington, DC: Bureau of the Census. [Current Population Reports, United States Department of Commerce Publ. P23, No. 82].

Snipp, C.M. (1986). Who are American Indians? Some observations about the perils and pitfalls of data for race and ethnicity. *Population Research Policy Review, 5,* 237–252.

Taylor, E.J. (1988). *Dorland's Illustrated Medical Dictionary* (27th ed.). Philadelphia: W.S. Saunders Company.

van den Berghe, P.L. (1967). *Race and Racism: A Comparative Perspective.* New York: Wiley.

Volberding, P.A. (1997). Antiretroviral therapy. In M.A. Sande & P.A. Volberding (Eds.), *The Medical Management of AIDS* (5th ed., pp. 113–124). Philadelphia: W.B. Saunders Company.

Williams, D.R. (1994). The concept of race in *Health Services Research*: 1966 to 1990. *Health Services Research, 29,* 261–274.

Williams, D.R., LaVizzo-Mourey, R., & Warren, R.C. (1994). The concept of race and health status in America. *Public Health Reports, 109,* 26–41. Citing King, G., & Williams, D.R. (in press). Race and health: A multidimensional approach to African American health. In S. Levine, D.C. Walsh, B.C. Amick, & A.R. Tarlov (Eds.), *Society and Health: Foundation for a Nation.* New York: Oxford University Press.

Wilson, M.G., May, D.S., & Kelly, J.J. (1994). Racial differences in the use of total knee arthroplasty for osteoarthritis among older Americans. *Ethnicity and Disease, 4,* 57–67.

Yinger, J. (1994). *Ethnicity: Source of Strength? Source of Conflict?* Albany: State University of New York Press.

4

Sex, Gender, and Sexual Orientation

Introduction

It is generally assumed that sex and gender are sexually dimorphic, meaning that there exists a phylogenetically inherited structure of two types, male and female (Herdt, 1994). Lillie's (1939) thoughts represent an early explanation of such sexual dimorphism:

> What exists in nature is a dimorphism within species into male and female individuals, which differ with respect to contrasting characters, for each of which in any given species we recognize a male form and a female form, whether these characters be classed as of the biological, or psychological, or social orders. Sex is not a force that produces these contrasts; it is merely a name for our total impression of the differences.... In the strictly historical sense of these words, a male is to be defined as an individual that produces spermatozoa; a female one that produces ova; or individuals at least having the characters associated with these functions.

The identification of an individual as a biological male or female rests on an evaluation of one or more of the following elements: chromosomal sex, gonadal sex, morphological sex and secondary sex traits, and psychosocial sex or gender identity (Herdt, 1994). In general, it has been assumed that biological sex, determined by one or more of the first three elements, is inextricably linked with gender identity, as well as with gender role/social identity and sexual orientation (Bolin, 1994). This underlying assumption has been subject to ever-growing dispute in recent years. Each of these elements is discussed in greater detail here.

Biological Sex

This general overview of the development of biological sex presumes a basic knowledge of anatomy and human reproduction. Further details can be found in Moore and Persaud (1993).

The chromosomal sex of an embryo depends on whether the fertilization of the ovum occurs by an X-bearing or Y-bearing sperm. Fertilization by an X-bearing sperm results in an XX zygote, which will normally develop into a female. Fertilization by a Y-bearing sperm will produce an XY zygote, which normally develops into a male (Moore and Persaud, 1993).

However, the gonads of both males and females are identical in appearance prior to the seventh week of the embryo's development; during this period, they are referred to as indifferent or undifferentiated gonads.

Hermaphroditism or intersexuality occurs when there appears to be a discrepancy between the morphology of the gonads (testes or ovaries) and the appearance of the external genitalia. (For a discussion of the development of the testes and ovaries, see Moore and Persaud, 1993). True hermaphroditism is extremely rare and occurs only when both testicular and ovarian tissue are present. However, these tissues are generally nonfunctional (Krob, Braun, and Kuhnle, 1994; Moore and Persaud, 1993; Talerman *et al.*, 1990).

Gender Identity and Gender Role

Stoller (1968:viii–ix) distinguished between sex as a function of biology and gender as a function of culture:

> Dictionaries stress that the major connotation of sex is a biological one as, for example, in the phrases *sexual relations* or *the male sex....* It is for some of these psychological phenomena [behavior, feelings, thoughts, fantasies] that the term *gender* will be used: one can speak of the male sex or the female sex, but one can also talk about masculinity and femininity and not necessarily be implying anything about anatomy or physiology.

Gender has been defined as

> a multidimensional category of personhood encompassing a distinct pattern of social and cultural differences. Gender categories often draw on perceptions of anatomical and physiological differences between bodies, but those perceptions are always mediated by cultural categories and meanings.... Gender categories are not only "models of" difference ... but also "models for" difference. They convey gender-specific social expectations for behavior and temperament, sexuality, kinship and interpersonal roles, occupation, religious roles and other social patterns. Gender categories are "total social phenomena" ...; a wide range of institutions and beliefs find simultaneous expression through them, a characteristic that distinguishes gender from other social statuses. (Roscoe, 1994:341)

Despite this distinction, (biological) sex has often been considered synonymous with, or predictive of, gender (social role). The following excerpt illustrates how biological sex was determinative of social function:

> Thus it was claimed that women's low brain weights and deficient brain structures were analogous to those of lower races, and their inferior intellectualities explained on this basis. Woman, it was observed, shared with Negroes a narrow, childlike, and delicate skull, so different from the more robust and rounded heads characteristic of males of "superior" races. Similarly, women of higher races tended to have slightly protruding jaws, analogous to, if not as exaggerated as, the apelike jutting jaws of lower races. *Women and lower races were called innately impulsive, emotional, imitative rather than original, and incapable of the abstract reasoning found in white men.* (Stepan, 1990:39–40) (emphasis added)

Gender identity and gender role are distinct. Nanda's (1994:395–396) explanation is instructive:

> Gender identity has been defined as the private experience of gender role: the experience of one's sameness, unity and the persistence of one's individuality as male, female, or androgynous, expressed in both self-awareness and in behavior. Gender role is everything that a person says and does to indicate to others or to the self the degree to which one is either male, female or androgynous. Gender role would thus include public presentations of self in dress and verbal and nonverbal communication; the economic and family roles one plays; the sexual feelings (desires) one has and the persons to whom such feelings are directed; the sexual role one plays and emotions one experiences and displays; and the experiencing of one's body, as it is defined as masculine or feminine in any particular society. Gender identity and gender role are said to have a unity, like two sides of a coin.

Stoller's conceptualization of gender identity and gender role similarly distinguish between the private and the public experiences:

> I am using the word *identity* to mean one's own awareness (whether one is conscious of it or not) of one's existence or purpose in this world or, put a bit differently, the organization of those psychic components that are to preserve one's awareness of existing. (Stoller, 1968:x)

Gender identity is to be further distinguished from "core gender identity," a "person's unquestioning certainty that he belongs to one of only two sexes" (Stoller, 1968:39). Stoller elaborates as follows:

> This essentially unalterable core of gender identity [I am a male] is to be distinguished from the related but different belief, *I am manly* (or masculine). The latter attitude is a more subtle and complicated development. It emerges only after the child has learned how his parents expect him to express masculinity. (Stoller, 1968:40)

This, too, can be contrasted with gender role. "Core gender identity" signifies the feeling of "I am a male" or "I am a female," whereas gender role represents "a masculine or feminine way of behaving" (Walinder, 1967:4).

Gender identity is to be distinguished, as well, from sexual identity:

> The term "gender identity" [is] used … rather than various other terms which have been employed in this regard, such as the term "sexual identity." "Sexual identity" is ambiguous, since it may refer to one's sexual activities or fantasies, etc.… Thus, of a patient who says "I am not a very masculine man," it is possible to say that his gender identity is male although he recognizes his lack of so-called masculinity. (Stoller, 1964:220)

Sexual Orientation

We have come to equate the choice of one's sexual partner—male or female—with one's sexual orientation. It is clear, though, that homosexual behavior is not synonymous with homosexuality. For example, a recent study of male sexual behavior in the United States found that 2% of the respondents ages 20 to 39 reported having had any same sex sexual activity during the previous 10 years, but only 1% reported exclusively same-sex sexual activity for the same time period (Billy, Tanfer, Grady, and Keplinger, 1993). Identical sexual acts, including the choice of the sexual partner, may vary in meaning and significance, depending on their cultural and historical context (Vance, 1995). As illustrated by the following examples taken from both history and current events, we see that the biological sex of one's sexual partner may have as much or more to do with power, economic relations, and the availability of alternative partners as with sexual desire or orientation.

In a number of societies, sexual relations between younger and older men were structured by age (Greenberg, 1988). The older male often assumed the active role in the relationship, while the younger male assumed the passive role. The sexual act could include masturbation, anal intercourse, and/or fellatio. The motivation for these relationships varied depending on the culture, but could include the sexual transmission of special healing powers from the older male to the younger disciple; the belief that a boy must have semen implanted in his body by an adult in order to mature physically; a fear that heterosexual intercourse would deplete men's vitality; a scarcity of women; and a belief that heterosexual intercourse would harm men because of women's polluting qualities (Greenberg, 1988).

Homosexual behavior—as distinct from homosexuality—may also reflect a differential in power between the sexual partners. This includes, for example, the use of one's body rather than money to deter violence, a situation that may arise both on the street (Scacco, 1982), in prisons, and during war (Greenberg, 1988; Trexler, 1995).

The status of berdache and hijra both exemplify relations that might be termed homosexual based on only a superficial understanding of sexual behavior but, in fact, signify something quite different. Williams (1992:2) defined a berdache as "a morphological male who does not fit society's standard man's role, who has a nonmasculine character." Native Americans often referred to berdaches as "halfmen-halfwomen," although they were neither hermaphrodites nor transsexuals (Williams, 1992). Berdaches, who are now known as "two-spirit people" (Lang, 1996), existed within various Native American tribes, including the Cheyenne, Creek, Klamath, Mohave, Navaho, Pima, Sioux, and Zuni (Greenberg, 1988; Roscoe, 1991; Williams, 1992). Rather than being termed effeminate, two-spirit people are more accurately described as androgynous. They are not perceived as either men or women, but rather as an alternative gender. Often, two-spirit persons combined the behavior, social roles, and dress of both men and women. Although some assumed the passive role in a sexual relationship with another man, the sexual relationship was a secondary component of status as a berdache (Callender and Kochems, 1985; Williams, 1992). Homosexual behavior was not synonymous with status as a berdache (Williams, 1992). Similarly, some two-spirit *women* adopted some male roles and dress and had sexual relations with women (Schaeffer, 1965).

As a result of missionary efforts and U.S. government agents, the berdache tradition has declined. Younger Native Americans may have rejected the role of the berdache in favor of self-identity as a gay male (Williams, 1992).

The hijras of India have been characterized as "neither man nor woman and woman and man" (Nanda, 1990, 1994). Based on that status, hijras play a religious role, derived from Hinduism, by blessing newborn male children and performing at marriages (Nanda, 1990). Hijras are defined as such by their lack of desire for and sexual impotence with women, rather than by their sexual relations with men. Their impotence with women is attributed to a defective or absent male sexual organ, which is lacking due to an accident of birth or to intentional emasculation, the surgical removal of the male genitals (Nanda, 1990). In defining themselves, hijras collapse sex and gender into one category, defining themselves as "not men" because of their impotence with women and as "not women" because of their inability to bear children. They simultaneously incorporate aspects of the female role, such as dress, gendered erotic fantasies, desire for male sexual partners, and a gender identity of a woman or hijra, with those of a male role, such as coarse speech and the use of the hookah for smoking (Nanda, 1994). Clearly, despite their sexual relations with men, hijras are not defined and do not define themselves as homosexuals.

Homosexuality has been variously conceived of as an innate, relatively stable condition

(Murray, 1987); a congenital, but not hereditary condition (Heller, 1981); a form of congenital degeneracy (Gindorf, 1977); an earlier evolutionary form of the human race, that is, bisexual or hermaphroditic (Krafft-Ebing, 1965); a perverse and immature orientation resulting from family interactions during childhood development (Dynes, 1987; Freud, 1920); and the result of psychological processes similar to those that lead to heterosexuality, modifiable through various forms of therapy (Akers, 1977). It was not until 1973 that the American Psychiatric Association removed homosexuality as a mental illness from the *Diagnostic and Statistical Manual of Mental Disorders* (Greenberg, 1988).

Transsexuality and Transgenderism

Transsexuality

Transsexuals have been defined as "individuals with a cross-sex identity," regardless of their surgical status (Bolin, 1992:14), while transsexuality has been classified as a gender identity disorder resulting in "clinically significant distress or impairment in social, occupational, or other important areas of functioning" (Reid and Wise, 1995:241). Whether transsexuality *per se* constitutes a disorder, which then necessitates treatment, is subject to considerable dispute (Loue, 1996). Diagnosis rests on the presence of "a strong and persistent cross-gender identification" and "a persistent discomfort with one's sex or a sense of inappropriateness in the gender role of that sex" (Reid and Wise, 1995:241). Diagnosis requires that the condition be distinguished from hermaphroditism, from a desire to change sex in order to gain a cultural or social advantage, and from a desire to change sex due to nonconformity with prescribed sex roles (Reid and Wise, 1995:240).

Researchers have estimated that approximately 1 out of every 11,900 men (male to female) and approximately 1 out of every 30,400 women (female to male) are transsexuals (Bakker, van Kesteren, Gooren, and Bezemer, 1993). Estimates of the male-female sex ratio have varied widely, from 2.5:1 in the Netherlands to 5.5:1 in Poland (Bakker *et al.*, 1993; Godlewski, 1988; Pauley, 1968).

Treatment for transsexualism has included long-term hormonal therapy and sex change surgery. Genital reassignment surgery from female to male is complex and extensive and, consequently, must generally be performed in several stages (Hage, Bouman, de Graaf, and Bloem, 1993). Phalloplasty is used to construct a penis in a female-to-male transsexual (Hage, Bloem, and Suliman, 1993). In addition to the surgery, female-to-male transsexuals must often adhere to a long-term regimen of androgen administration (Sapino, Pietribiasi, Godano, and Bussolati, 1992). Potential adverse effects include necrosis, hernia, venous congestion, and phallic shaft fistulas (Hage, Bloem, and Suliman, 1993). Male-to-female transsexuals may also undergo extensive surgery (Eldh, 1993) and hormonal treatment (Valenta, Elias, and Domurat, 1992). Potential adverse effects include the lack of a sensate clitoris (Eldh, 1993), vaginal stenosis (Crichton, 1992; Stein, Tiefer, and Melman, 1990), and pain during sexual intercourse (Stein *et al.*, 1990). Many transsexuals may ultimately decide to forgo the surgery due to its high cost, the lack of health insurance coverage for the surgery (Gordon, 1991; Stein *et al.*, 1990), and the fear of an unsatisfactory surgical outcome (Crichton, 1992; Hage, Bout, Bloem, and Megens, 1993).

Transgenderism

The word "transgender" has several meanings. First, it can encompass all those who "challenge the boundaries of sex and gender" (Feinberg, 1996:x). Alternatively, it refers to those who reassign the sex they were labeled at birth, and those whose expressed gender is considered inappropriate for their apparent sex (Feinberg, 1996). A distinction is often made between transsexuals, who change or attempt to change the sex that they were assigned at birth, and transgender individuals, who "blur the boundar[ies] of the *gender expression*" traditionally associated with the biological sexes (Feinberg, 1996:x).

Such blurring may take the form of cross-dressing (Garber, 1992). Cross-dressing, or wearing the clothing that is most often associated with the opposite sex, may occur for various reasons and in numerous contexts. Women may assume an "imitation man look" in an attempt to be more successful in business (Molloy, 1977). Men, some homosexual and some heterosexual, may perform as female impersonators. Gay men may cross-dress as a means of self-assertion or activism (Garber, 1992). Cross-dressing has been central in theater (Baker, 1994; Heriot, 1975) and, to some degree, in religion (Barrett, 1931; Garber, 1992; Warner, 1982). It is important to recognize that not all of these behaviors are associated with being a transgendered individual.

Exercises

1. You are conducting a study to assess the unmet health care and social service needs of HIV-infected individuals in your state. The results of the study will be used as the basis of grant applications in your community for increased federal allocation and for grant applications by nonprofit organizations to private funding sources. The HIV-infected community is extremely diverse in terms of ethnicity, sex, sexual orientation, and gender role and identity.
   a. What issues may arise in the context of carrying out this study? Be as complete as possible in your response (e.g., ethical, personal issues, etc.).
   b. Explain how you will train your staff to be sensitive to the diverse concerns and sensitivities of the HIV-infected population.
   c. Design the demographic portion of the interview instrument. Make sure that it reflects both the diverse nature of the HIV-infected community and the potential concerns of those persons who will be interviewed.
2. Sexual behavior (age of initiation and number of sexual partners) has been hypothesized to be a potential risk factor for prostate cancer.
   a. Design a study that will test this hypothesized association. Include in your response a discussion of the study design, the study populations, and possible recruitment/ enrollment strategies.
   b. Discuss whether, and how, you will address sexual orientation in the context of this study.

References

Akers, R.L. (1977). *Deviant Behavior: A Social Learning Approach*. Belmont, CA: Wadsworth.

Baker, R. (1994). *Drag: A History of Female Impersonation in the Performing Arts*. New York: New York University Press.

Bakker, A., van Kesteren, F.J.M., Gooren, L.J.G., & Bezemer, P.D. (1993). The prevalence of transsexualism in the Netherlands. *Acta Psychiatrica Scandinavia, 87,* 237–238.

Barrett, W.P. (Trans.). (1931). *The Trial of Jeanne d'Arc*. London: Routledge.

Billy, J.O.G., Tanfer, K., Grady, W.R., & Klepinger, D.H. (1993). The sexual behavior of men in the United States. *Family Planning Perspectives, 25,* 52–60.

Bolin, A. (1992). Coming of age among transsexuals. In T.L. Whitehead & B.V. Reid (Eds.), *Gender Constructs and Social Issues* (pp. 13–39). Chicago: University of Chicago Press.

Bolin, A. (1994). Transcending and transgendering: Male-to-female transsexuals, dichotomy and diversity. In G. Herdt (Ed.), *Third Sex, Third Gender: Beyond Sexual Dimorphism in Culture and History* (pp. 447–485). New York: Zone Books.

Callender, C., & Kochems, L.M. (1985). Men and not-men: Male gender-mixing and homosexuality. *Journal of Homosexuality, 11*, 165–176.

Crichton, D. (1992). Gender reassignment surgery for male primary transsexuals. *South African Medical Journal, 83*, 347–349.

Dynes, W. (1987). *Homosexuality: A Research Guide*. New York: Garland.

Eldh, J. (1993). Construction of a neovagina with preservation of the glans penis as a clitoris in male transsexuals. *Plastic Reconstructive Surgery, 91*, 895–900.

Feinberg, L. (1996). *Transgender Warriors*. Boston: Beacon Press.

Freud, S. (1920). The psychogenesis of a case of homosexuality in a woman. In P. Rieff (Ed.). (1963). *Sexuality and the Psychology of Love* (pp. 133–159). New York: Collier.

Garber, M. (1992). *Vested Interests: Cross-Dressing and Cultural Anxiety*. New York: HarperCollins.

Gindorf, R. (1977). Wissenschaftliche Ideologien im Wandel: Die Angst von der Homosexualitat als intellektuelles Ereignis. In J.S. Hohmann (Ed.), *Der underdruckte Sexus* (pp. 129–144). Berlin: Andreas Achenbach Lollar. Cited in D.F. Greenberg. (1988). *The Construction of Homosexuality*. Chicago: University of Chicago Press.

Godlewski, J. (1988). Transsexualism and anatomic sex: Ratio reversal in Poland. *Archives of Sexual Behavior, 17*, 547–548.

Gordon, E.B. (1991). Transsexual healing: Medicaid funding of sex reassignment surgery. *Archives of Sexual Behavior, 20*, 61–79.

Greenberg, D.F. (1988). *The Construction of Homosexuality*. Chicago: University of Chicago Press.

Hage, J.J., Bloem, J.J.A.M., & Suliman, H.M. (1993). Review of the literature on techniques for phalloplasty with emphasis on the applicability in female-to-male transsexuals. *Journal of Urology, 150*, 1093–1098.

Hage, J.J., Bouman, F.G., de Graaf, F.H., & Bloem, J.J.A.M. (1993). Construction of the neophallus in female-to-male transsexuals: The Amsterdam experience. *Journal of Urology, 149*, 1463–1468.

Hage, J.J., Bout, C.A., Bloem, J.J.A.M., & Megens, J.A.J. (1993). Phalloplasty in female-to-male transsexuals: What do our patients ask for? *Annals of Plastic Surgery, 30*, 323–326.

Heller, P. (1981). A quarrel over bisexuality. In G. Chapple & H.H. Schulte (Eds.), *The Turn of the Century: German Literature and Art, 1890–1915* (pp. 87–115). Bonn: Bouvier Verlag Herbert Grundmann.

Herdt, G. (1994). Third sexes and third genders. In G. Herdt (Ed.), *Third Sex, Third Gender: Beyond Sexual Dimorphism in Culture and History* (pp. 21–81). New York: Zone Books.

Heriot A. (1975). *The Castrati in Opera*. New York: Da Capo Press.

Krafft-Ebing, R. V. (1965). *Psychopathia Sexualis: A Medico-Forensic Study* (H.E. Wedeck, Trans.). New York: G.P. Putnam's Sons. (Original work published 1886).

Krob, G., Braun, A., & Kuhnle, U. (1994). Hermaphroditism: Geographical distribution, clinical findings, chromosomes and gonadal histology. *European Journal of Pediatrics, 153*, 2–10.

Lang, S. (1996). There is more than just women and men: Gender variance in North American Indian cultures. In S.P. Ramet (Ed.), *Gender Reversals & Gender Cultures: Anthropological and Historical Perspectives* (pp. 183–196). London: Routledge.

Lillie, F. (1939). General biological introduction. In E. Allen (Ed.), *Sex and Internal Secretions: A Survey of Recent Research* (2nd ed.). Baltimore, MD: Williams and Wilkins.

Loue, S. (1996). Transsexualism in medicolegal limine: An examination and proposal for change. *Journal of Psychiatry and Law, Spring*, 27–51.

Molloy, J.T. (1977). *The Woman's Dress for Success Book*. New York: Warner Books.

Moore, K.L., & Persaud, T.V.N. (1993). *The Developing Human: Clinically Oriented Embryology* (5th ed.). Philadelphia: W.B. Saunders.

Murray, S.O. (1987). Homosexual acts and selves in early modern Europe. *Journal of Homosexuality, 15*, 421–439.

Nanda, S. (1990). *Neither Man Nor Woman: The Hijras of India*. Belmont, CA: Wadsworth Publishing Company.

Nanda, S. (1994). Hijras: An alternative sex and gender role in India. In G. Herdt (Ed.), *Third Sex, Third Gender: Beyond Sexual Dimorphism in Culture and History* (pp. 373–417). New York: Zone Books.

Pauley, I.B. (1968). The current status of the change of sex operation. *Journal of Nervous and Mental Disease, 147*, 460–471.

Reid, W.H., & Wise, M.G. (1995). *DSM-IV Training Guide*. New York: Brunner Manzel.

Roscoe, W. (1991). *The Zuni Man-Woman*. Albuquerque, NM: University of New Mexico Press.

Roscoe, W. (1994). How to become a berdache: Toward a unified analysis of gender diversity. In G. Herdt (Ed.), *Third Sex, Third Gender: Beyond Sexual Dimorphism in Culture and History* (pp. 329–372). New York: Zone Books.

Sapino, A., Pietribiasi, F., Godano, A., & Bussolati, G. (1992). Effect of long-term administration of androgens on breast tissues of female-to-male transsexuals. *Annals of the New York Academy of Science, 586*, 143–145.

Scacco, A. (Ed.). (1982). *Male Rape: A Casebook of Sexual Aggression*. New York: AMS Press.

Schaeffer, C.E. (1965). The Kutenai female berdache: Courier, guide, prophetess, and warrior. *Ethnohistory, 12,* 193–236.

Stein, M., Tiefer, L., & Melman, A. (1990). Followup observations of operated male-to-female transsexuals. *Journal of Urology, 143,* 1188–1192.

Stepan, N.L. (1990). Race and gender: The role of analogy in science. In D.T. Goldberg (Ed.), *Anatomy of Racism* (pp. 38–57) Minneapolis, MN: University of Minnesota Press.

Stoller, R.J. (1964). A contribution to the study of gender identity. *JAMA, 45,* 220–226.

Stoller, R.J. (1968). *Sex and Gender: On the Development of Masculinity and Femininity*. New York: Science House.

Talerman, A., Verp, M.S., Senekjian, E., Gilewski, T., & Vogelzang, N. (1990). True hermaphrodite with bilateral ovotestes, bilateral gonadoblastomas and the dysgerminomas, 46,XX/46,XY karotype, and a successful pregnancy. *Cancer, 66,* 2668–2671.

Trexler, R.C. (1995). *Sex and Conquest: Gendered Violence, Political Order, and the European Conquest of the Americas*. Ithaca, NY: Cornell University Press.

Valenta, L.J., Elias, A.N., & Domurat, E.S. (1992). Hormone pattern in pharmacologically feminized male transsexuals in the California state prison system. *JAMA, 84,* 241–250.

Vance, C.S. (1995). Social construction theory and sexuality. In M. Berger, B. Wallis, & S. Watson (Eds.), *Constructing Masculinity* (pp. 37–48). New York: Routledge.

Walinder, J. (1967). *Transsexualism: A Study of Forty-Three Cases*. (H. Fry, Trans.). Stockholm: Scandinavian University Books.

Warner, M. (1982). *Joan of Arc: The Image of Female Heroism*. New York: Vintage Books.

Williams, W.L. (1992). *The Spirit and the Flesh: Sexual Diversity in American Indian Culture*. Boston: Beacon Press.

5

Health Care Utilization and Access

As indicated in Chapter 3, race and ethnicity have often been associated with differential utilization of health care services and differences in access to care. This chapter explores the concepts of utilization and access, which might be the focus in a specific context, for example, utilization of cancer prevention strategies such as breast self-examination, mammograms, and Pap smears. The discussion focuses on health care access and utilization within the United States, but also encompasses non-U.S.-based research which may be relevant to some populations in the United States, given the diversity of the U.S. population. As the discussion in this chapter reveals, these concepts are both multidimensional and multifactoral and cannot be either measured or explained by a single variable.

Utilization in the Context of a Health System Model

Categorical Models

Wolinsky (1980) has summarized the various types of categorical models of health services utilization that have been used to explain why people do or do not use health care resources: (1) demographic models, relating utilization to such factors as age, sex, marital status, and family size; (2) social structural models, which tend to emphasize educational levels, occupation, and ethnicity; (3) social psychological models, which tend to focus on the perceived susceptibility to the illness, the perceived gravity of the illness, the anticipated benefits of action, and the existence of a cue to action; (4) family resource models, which examine variables of family income, health insurance, and the existence of a regular source of care; (5) community resource models, which are often economic supply models; and (6) organizational models, which often address the style of medical practice, the system for the delivery of care, the site at which services are provided, and the type of health workers who provide the care. None of these models has been adequate by itself to explain variations in utilization of treatments, procedures, or services. Health systems models are essentially a composite of these individual models.

Health Systems Models

Aday and Andersen (1974) have suggested a model for the examination of access to health care, health services utilization, and consumer satisfaction. This model consists of five major elements: health policy, the characteristics of the health delivery system, the characteristics of the population at risk, utilization of health care services, and consumer satisfaction. The system model of health care utilization can be analogized to the ecological model of disease, which considers the relationship and interaction between the host, the agent, and the entire environment (Janes, 1986; Dunn, 1984; Mechanic, 1972). Similarly, the Aday–Andersen model considers the relationship and interaction between the individual, the health care system, and the larger environment, including the policy context in which the interactions occur. Implicit in this model is the assumption that, as a system, its identifiable parts are mutually dependent on each other, that each part influences and is influenced by the others, and that the whole is a composite of not only its parts, but the interrelationships between its parts (Wellin, 1977). This model provides a structure for this discussion of health services utilization in general.

Aday and Andersen (1974) defined access to include not only the availability of financial and health systems resources in an area, but also the consumer's willingness to seek care. The level of consumer willingness is dependent on the individual's attitudes toward health care and his or her definition of illness (Mechanic, 1972).

Health policy essentially lays the foundation for access. The health care delivery system consists of two primary elements: (1) resources, such as labor, capital, personnel, and materials, and (2) organization, which refers to the process of entering the health care system and receiving treatment and to the structure of that system.

The characteristics of the population at risk encompass the enabling, predisposing, and need factors that constitute the individual determinants of utilization. The enabling component refers to the resources available to an individual for the use of services, such as income and insurance coverage. Predisposing factors include demographic characteristics of an individual, as well as his or her values related to health and illness. Need generally refers to the level of illness that the individual is experiencing. Individual determinants are discussed in greater detail below.

The utilization of health care services refers to the kind of service provided, the site of the service, the purpose of the service, the person or entity that provided the service, and the time interval for the service. Kinds of services include pharmacy services, surgical services, and nursing services. Services may be provided at an emergency department, a rehabilitation facility, a pharmacy, or other location. Care may be provided for preventive, curative, or custodial purposes. Various individuals may be involved in the provision of care, including a physician, nurse practitioner, pharmacist, or dentist.

Consumer satisfaction refers to the consumer's attitude toward the quantity and quality of care actually received. Both utilization and consumer satisfaction are outcome indicators of access.

Wolinsky (1976:225) proposed an expansion of the Aday–Andersen model to include "attitudes toward alternatives to the present health care delivery system." He hypothesized that these attitudes are directly influenced by the overall health policy.

Penchansky and Thomas (1981) have defined access as the degree of fit between the health care consumer and the health care system. As such, the elements of access—availability, accessibility, accommodation, affordability, and acceptability—are similar but not coterminous with Aday and Andersen's enabling factors. The concept of availability encompasses the adequacy of the supply of various providers and services in relation to the demand. Accessibility refers to the location of the services and of the consumers, in view of the consumers' resources and the requisite travel time. Accommodation relates to the organization of the services and the consumers' ability to work within that organization, such as office hours. Affordability considers the price of the services and the consumers' insurance, income, and ability to pay, as well as the consumers' perceptions of the value of the services. Finally, acceptability relates to consumers' attitudes about the providers' personal and professional characteristics and providers' attitudes about client characteristics.

Characteristics of the Population at Risk

Utilization of health services can be thought of either as the culmination of a process or the result of various individual determinants or predictors (Kroeger, 1983). Interestingly, although the process of health seeking could, itself, constitute one of the predictors of utilization, the literature has not identified it as such. Within the context of the Aday–Andersen model (1974), the health-seeking process pursued by an individual could be considered a predisposing component.

The Health Care-Seeking Process

Pathway Models for Seeking Care

A number of different pathway models have been proposed to explain the process of health seeking. Suchman (1965) developed a five-stage model of the disease process: (1) symptom experience, (2) assumption of the sick role, (3) medical care contact, (4) dependent patient, and (5) recovery or rehabilitation. Suchman further delineated five illness behavior patterns: (1) "shopping," or the process of searching for various sources of care; (2) fragmentation, whereby the patient receives care from several different medical providers at the same location; (3) procrastination, which refers to the patient's delay in seeking care following symptom recognition; (4) self-medication; and (5) discontinuity, which refers to the interruption of care.

Symptom experience consists of the experience of pain or discomfort, the recognition of this pain or discomfort as symptoms, and an emotional response to these symptoms. Assumption of the sick role refers to the patient's acknowledgement that he or she is ill and requires medical attention. According to Suchman, the individual is likely to seek support of family or friends during this stage in order to validate the illness and to be excused from his or her usual social obligations.

The third stage of medical care contact entails a decision to seek medical attention for the condition. Suchman hypothesized that the health care provider's initial diagnosis and proposed treatment play a significant role in the patient's future behavior.

The dependent-patient stage involves a transfer of control from the patient to the physician. This interaction, including the patient's acceptance of and adherence to the prescribed treatment regimen, may be tenuous due to the patient's and the provider's differing concepts of illness and treatment. The final stage in Suchman's model, that of recovery or rehabilitation, refers to the patient's relinquishment of the patient role as the result of either dismissal or withdrawal or the patient's assumption of a new role as a chronically ill individual.

Suchman (1965) further postulated that an individual's response to medical care is influenced by various group relationships at the community, social group, and family levels. A parochial group structure, characterized by close ties among family members and ethnic groups, was associated with low knowledge of disease, negativity toward medical care, and high dependency in illness. Community-level group structure referred to the extent to which individuals interacted with others of their own ethnic identity. Social group structure referred to the degree to which individuals participated in friendship groups of long duration. Family level was measured by the extent to which family authority and tradition played a part in an individual's life.

Fabrega (1972) has conceptualized disease as a six-stage process, consisting of (1) the labels of sick and normal, (2) relevant behaviors, (3) judgment of behaviors, (4) the consequences of judgments of behavior as sick, (5) the career of the sick person, and (6) the return to normality. Each of these steps comprises multiple elements. For example, the first step refers not only to the designation of an individual as sick or normal by himself/herself or others, but the process by which these labels are constructed and the status of an individual's adaptation to his or her environment. Unlike the Suchman model, Fabrega's framework was developed not so much as an explanation of the process in which the patient is engaged, but as a guide for an investigator's evaluation of health and illness.

Chrisman (1977), like Suchman, has also proposed a five-step model to explain this process: symptom definition, illness-related shifts in behavior, lay consultation and referral, treatment actions, and adherence. He emphasized, however, that all of these steps need not occur and that they need not be sequential in their occurrence.

Symptom definition "refers to the ways in which given symptoms are perceived, evaluated, and acted (or not acted) upon by different people" (Mechanic, 1968, 1969:191). This component encompasses a recognition of a deviation from what is considered normal, an evaluation of that deviation, an explanation of the deviation, and an assessment of the degree of threat that the deviation presents (Chrisman, 1977; Kasl and Cobb, 1966). (This evaluation of the degree of threat is akin to one element of the health belief model for behavior change, discussed here.) The degree of threat is reflected by the danger posed (i.e., the implications of the symptoms or the deviation) and the disability that the symptoms produce (i.e., the degree to which the symptoms affect on daily functioning). Much of this process of symptom definition is conducted on a solitary basis by the affected individual (Chrisman, 1977). In some instances, however, the symptoms may be recognized as such by others, rather than the individual experiencing them (Mechanic, 1968).

Role behavior shift occurs as the symptoms or deviation come to the attention of others, such as family members or friends. Chrisman (1977:357) explains how this shift occurs:

> Illness-related shifts in role behavior imply a "bargaining" process in which modified rights and obligations are established with others in the social environment.... Unambiguous acute symptoms place the individual in the strongest position for attaining the fullest extent of modifications in role behaviors and place upon him the strongest obligations to get well. On the other hand, ambiguous or chronic problems are not nearly so compelling.

Segall (1976) has identified two rights and two obligations that attend the recognition of the symptoms: (1) the right not to be held responsible for the condition, (2) the right to be exempted from one's usual social roles, (3) the obligation to try to become better, and (4) the obligation to seek help and to cooperate with that help, assuming that it is technically competent. Parsons (1951) views this role as permissible variations or modifications in one's usual role as a result of the sickness. Unlike Suchman, his view does not permit the formation of a new social identity with correlative rights and obligations. It is not at all clear that this "modification" model is appropriate in situations involving long-term, chronic, disabling conditions (Leventhal, Leventhal, and Nguyen, 1985; Minuchin, Rosman, and Baker, 1978).

Lay consultation and referral refers to the process by which an individual chooses among potential consultants and considers the substantive content of their appraisals in evaluating and validating the sickness and the shift in role(s) due to the sickness (Freidson, 1960). This process of lay consultation and referral also encompasses the decision of whether or not to consult a health care provider (Chrisman, 1977). Kleinman's (1980) hierarchy of resort notes that, not infrequently, evaluation and treatment of an illness is commenced at the level of the individual and then the family, prior to seeking care from a physician or other provider. Freidson (1970) has asserted that whether an individual ultimately visits a physician depends on the extent of congruence between the patient's beliefs and those of the physician and the degree of cohesiveness of the patient's social group.

Treatment actions refer to an individual's behaviors for the cure or amelioration of the perceived health problem. Chrisman's (1977) schema distinguishes between the type of treatment, such as traditional versus medical, and the source of the treatment, such as lay advisor versus physician. He further enumerates four categories of possible response to the sickness: (1) activity alterations, such as increased rest; (2) the application, ingestion, or injection of substances; (3) the use of ritual or verbal behaviors, such as prayer; and (4) reliance on other physical interventions, such as cupping.

Adherence refers to the extent to which an individual actually relies upon the advice that was given (Chrisman, 1977). Numerous determinants of adherence have been identified including, but not limited to, beliefs about the threat to one's health, knowledge and understanding of the treatment recommendation and its purpose, the availability of social support, illness symptoms, and the convenience, continuity, and sufficiency of the care provided (Kirscht and Rosenstock, 1979).

Igun (1979) proposed an 11-step model to describe the health-seeking process: (1) the experience of symptoms, (2) self-treatment, (3) communication to significant others, (4) assessment of the symptoms, (5) assumption of the sick role, (6) expression of concern, (7) assessment of the available sources of care and their appropriateness, (8) selection of a treatment plan, (9) treatment, (10) assessment of the treatment effects, and (11) recovery and rehabilitation. Progression through these stages is not inevitable; whether a particular individual moves from one stage to another depends on a number of factors.

The first stage of symptom experience, for example, consists of four components: the physical experience, the cue process, the cognitive aspect, and the emotional response. The individual must actually experience pain or discomfort or notice a change of appearance. A prompt, whether sudden or gradual, must bring the individual to an awareness that something is wrong with his or her health. The individual must then interpret the symptom experience, which may or may not be accompanied by a fear or anxiety response, depending on the meaning of the symptoms for the person. Whether the individual next moves into the self-treatment stage or the communication stage will depend on whether he or she understands the symptoms and can "label" them, and whether or not he or she believes that the symptoms are not serious and are amenable to self-treatment (Igun, 1979).

Models for Determining the Source of Care

Various researchers have explored the process by which help is sought following a determination to seek help. Kleinman (1980) identified three patterns of resort: simultaneous; hierarchical, exclusive type; and hierarchical, mixed type. Simultaneous resort refers to concurrent reliance on two or more sources of care in connection with a single illness episode: popular treatment, an allopathic practitioner, a homeopathic doctor or pharmacy, and sacred healers. Hierarchical resort of the exclusive type was more likely to occur in situations involving nonthreatening acute illness in adults. Individuals pursuing this pattern of care seek treatment sequentially from various types of practitioners, failing recovery through reliance on the initial treatment choice. Hierarchical resort of the mixed type was found to occur primarily in situations involving chronic or recurrent illness in an adult, and involves sequentially seeking out a variety of practitioners and simultaneous resort to these different sources of care, following the failure of the initial treatment.

Determinants of Health Care-Seeking Behavior

The Aday–Andersen Model

Extensive research has been conducted relating to individual determinants of health care utilization. According to Aday and Andersen's (1974) model, determinants can be classified as predisposing, enabling, or need factors. The alternative schema developed by the International Collaborative Study on Health Care (ICSHC) (Kohn and White, 1976) categorizes determinants instead as predisposing, enabling, or health services system factors. The ICSHC's designation of health services system factors is essentially equivalent to the health policy foundation of the Aday–Anderson model.

It is important, however, to view these individual determinants as parts of a whole, rather than focusing on a single factor in any given situation (Nichter and Nordstrom, 1989).

Predisposing Factors. Predisposing factors "describe the 'propensity' of individuals to use services" (Aday and Andersen, 1974:213). They include demographic characteristics, such as age and sex; social structure variables, such as occupation and ethnicity; and beliefs, which encompass values relating to health and illness, attitudes toward health services, and knowledge about disease (Andersen and Newman, 1973).

Age has been found to be a critical determinant in the decision to seek health care and the type of care sought. Wan and Soifer (1974), for example, found in their study of 2,168 households in five New York and Pennsylvania counties that age was an important predisposing factor.

Various differences in illness behavior have been noted between ethnic groups, indicating that illness behavior is, at least to some extent, culturally learned (Mechanic, 1972). Berkanovic and Telesky (1985) found few differences between black Americans, white Americans, and Mexican-Americans with respect to the frequency of illness reports, the extent of disability associated with reported illnesses, or the frequency with which they sought medical attention. Blacks, however, appeared less likely to define transitory physical sensations as illnesses. Berkanovic and Telesky further found that blacks, unlike whites and Mexicans, were more likely to consult a physician if it was easy to do so and if they felt particularly susceptible to illness. Unlike Mexicans and whites, the advice of others was not an important consideration in deciding whether or not to consult a physician. The researchers postulated that these differences might reflect an interactive effect between cultural differences, social networks, and cognitive orientations. Lawson, Kahn, and Heiman (1982) and Escobar, Randolph, and Hill (1986) reported less frequent utilization of inpatient mental health services by Hispanics, compared to other groups. Black women have been found to delay longer in seeking treatment for their own illness than for seeking care for others in the family (Jackson, 1981). (One must question, as always, the subgroup classifications as well as the meaning of the differences found.)

A comparison of the impact of social networks across studies is difficult due to the variations in definitions and measurements used between studies. McKinlay (1981:78) has offered one definition of social network: "that set of contacts with relatives, friends, neighbors, etc. through which individuals maintain a social identity and receive emotional support, material aid, services and information, and develop new social contacts." Social networks as such can be conceived of, then, as one component of Chrisman's (1977) lay consultation and referral process. Social networks can be characterized by their size, the strength of their ties, their density, their dispersion, the frequency of contact within the network, their directedness, and their reachability. McKinlay (1981) has distinguished between the network on which an individual relies during the pre-patient phase of his or her help-seeking activity and the formal or professional network that is activated once the individual passes into the patient phase of the help-seeking activity. The size and nature of an individual's social network has repeatedly been found to play a major role in the decision to seek care. Langlie (1977) found in her study of 383 urban adults that individuals were more likely to engage in preventive health behaviors if their social networks were characterized by high socioeconomic status and frequent interaction between non-kin.

The availability of support within a network may also be critical to the prevention or delay of illness (Dressler, 1990), perhaps reducing or obviating the need for health care services. Lower blood pressure has been found to be associated with membership in an extended family in rural settings (Scotch, 1963). Social support has also been found to protect against depression (Brown, Bhrolchain, and Harris, 1975) and to reduce psychological distress following the loss of employment (Gore, 1978). Berkman and Syme's (1979) study of 6,928 adults in Alameda County, California, demonstrated a relationship between absence of social ties and an increase in mortality. This association was independent of self-reported physical health status, socio-economic status, and a variety of health practices, including smoking, exercise, and alcohol consumption.

Health and illness beliefs are discussed here as predisposing factors. Although this discussion focuses on what are termed beliefs, we must bear in mind that these "beliefs" represent the reality of individuals' everyday experience and that what we refer to as "beliefs" of others constitutes, in their context, knowledge (Berger and Luckman, 1966).

This discussion uses the framework provided by the Aday–Andersen model of predisposing, enabling, and need characteristics. However, it is important to recognize that within the context of the pathway models, such as that of Chrisman, health and illness beliefs may play a critical role in the context of lay consultation and referral. Whether an individual chooses a particular consultant may depend on the congruence of his or her health and illness beliefs. Whether the patient and the provider are able to negotiate a mutual understanding of a particular illness episode can be thought of as an enabling variable (Kroeger, 1983), and is discussed here in that context. Models for the modification of health behaviors, which are often the product of health and illness beliefs, are discussed in a separate section.

First, health and illness beliefs may determine whether departures from the norm actually exist so as to be labeled "symptoms" and whether those symptoms warrant the label of "sickness" or "illness" (Scheff, 1966). This may occur on the societal level and/or the individual level. Transsexuality exemplifies this premise on a societal level. The *Diagnostic and Statistical Manual of Mental Disorders* refers to transsexualism as a "gender identity disorder" (Reid and Wise, 1995:241). However, the same behavior in another cultural context might not be seen as a deviation from the norm or, if it does constitute a departure from what is considered normal, it may not be seen as warranting attention (Loue, 1996). In such situations, the search for illness may be of greater harm to the individual than a failure to provide treatment (Scheff, 1963).

Variations in the classification of disease symptoms and illness categories may influence an individual's decision to seek care. As an example, an individual who believes that his or her symptoms are attributable to the inevitable process of aging may be less likely to seek care or to self-treat (Jackson, 1981). Health beliefs may also affect an individual's willingness to continue to seek treatment from that source and to adhere to a regimen of care (Harwood, 1981).

Beliefs about disease causation have direct implications for the methods that will be acceptable for the treatment of that disease (Lieban, 1977). For example, diseases due to magical manipulation of forces demand that sorcery or countersorcery be used in treating them (Rivers, cited in Wellin, 1977). Similarly, diseases believed to be the result of supernatural forces may require appeals to supernatural forces. Diseases that come about due to natural processes may require naturalistic treatment. The source of care may, in turn, be associated with different expectations and perceptions of recovery (Nichter and Nordstrom, 1989).

The presumed cause of the illness may affect the extent to which the illness can be discussed openly. This has clear implications for communication in the context of the treatment process. Also, beliefs regarding the interrelationship of various illnesses may promote a belief that these illnesses are amenable to similar treatments. For example, the classification of various discrete diseases as "weak lung" has been found to be a contributing factor to the development of a belief that certain medications are useful for all illnesses that weaken the lungs (Nichter, 1994).

In addition, health beliefs have implications for health behaviors, such as the appropriateness of particular actions; who is to follow these prescriptions; and whether, how, and by whom change in behavior is to be effected. For example, reliance on the hot–cold conceptual framework influences reasoning about health, susceptibility, and illness (Nichter, 1987). Such reasoning may lead to a rejection of "modern" medications, such as vaccines, based on the belief that they will have deleterious effects on the body (Nichter, 1987).

Young and Garro (1982), however, concluded from their study of two rural communities in Mexico, that accessibility, rather than the degree of conceptual consistency between ethnomedical theory and Western biomedical theory, explained individuals' decisions regarding the source of care. Kunstadter (1975) has also suggested that the decision-making process is more likely to be influenced by factors such as cost and accessibility rather than distinctions between health and illness beliefs.

Enabling Factors. Kleinman (1980) found in his study of patients, illness, and health care in Taiwan that various enabling factors played an important role in the decision to seek health care and the form of that care: the family's socioeconomic status, orientation to Western or traditional values, and past experiences with health care; the geographic nature (rural or urban) of the setting; and the patient's proximity to specific treatment resources.

The importance of financial assets and access has been documented in numerous other studies. Wan and Soifer (1974), for example, found that the two most critical enabling variables in the utilization of physician services were the average cost of a physician's visit and the availability of insurance coverage. Rosenstock (1969), in his review of various studies, found that there is a direct association between income level and efforts to find preventive or diagnostic health services in the absence of illness symptoms. Newacheck and Starfield (1988) reported that low-income children with health problems have fewer physician visits on an adjusted basis than do their counterparts with a higher income.

Interestingly, socioeconomic status may also be related to the type of care sought.

Kleinman's (1980) findings with respect to social class were particularly striking: only upper middle-class families treated all sickness episodes by resorting to care from Western-style physicians, and only lower-class families treated all sickness episodes at home without resorting to health care professionals or folk curers. Gesler (1979) and Heller, Chalfont, Quesada, and Rivera-Workey (1981) similarly found in their studies in Nigeria and Mexico, respectively, that higher socioeconomic status was related to greater reliance on Western-style health care. These findings relating socioeconomic status, social class, and the use of Western-style medicine have not, however, been consistent across all studies and locations. Garrison (1977) found that wealthier Puerto Ricans in New York were more likely to consult spiritualists for illness episodes than were poorer individuals.

Insurance status has been closely linked to individuals' ability to obtain care. Hayward, Shapiro, Freeman, and Corey (1988) found that insured, working-age adults had less access to medical care than the elderly, who were able to obtain care through the publicly funded Medicare program. Freeman and Corey (1993) concluded from their study of health insurance status and access to care among low-income persons 65 years of age and younger that the poor and the near-poor have limited access to care as a result of copayments and deductibles required by private health care insurance plans. Uninsured and publicly insured patients have been found less likely to undergo various high-cost or high-discretion medical procedures upon hospitalization (Hadley, Steinberg, and Feder, 1991; Wenneker, Weissman, and Epstein, 1990), are less likely to have contact with a medical care provider, and have fewer ambulatory visits when compared with privately insured patients (Agency for Health Care Policy and Research, 1991; Freeman, Aiken, Blendon, & Corey, 1990).

Whether an individual will seek treatment may depend "on the conceptual and emotional congruence between the ... healers and their patients" (Kroeger 1983). However, even when the patient and the provider have divergent beliefs regarding the etiology of an illness, it may be possible for them to successfully negotiate an illness episode. Snell (1967), for example, found in his study of 20 black individuals who believed that they had been "hexed," that they could be treated effectively by a psychiatrist using hypnosis, despite the physician's disbelief in "hexing." It would appear, then, that the quality of the patient–provider interaction would be a critical factor in health-seeking behavior (Nichter and Nordstrom, 1989).

Kleinman (1980) and Nichter (1981) have both emphasized the negotiation process in the development of a response to an illness episode. The interaction between the patient and the provider in this negotiation ultimately helps resolve five critical questions: (1) the etiology of the illness episode, (2) the time of symptoms, (3) the pathophysiology of the illness, (4) the course of the illness, and (5) the preferred treatment regimen (Kleinman, 1980). The construction of these explanatory models may also be critical in an understanding of behavior, as well as illness (Nichter, 1981).

Logically, patient–provider communication will be affected by what each brings to the situation. In this context, not only explanatory models, but also semantic illness networks, prototypes, and chain complexes become relevant to the communication process. Semantic illness networks refer to the networks "of words, situations, symptoms and feelings which are associated with an illness and give it meaning for the sufferer" (Good, 1977:40). Essentially, semantic illness networks are the composite of explanatory models made over time (Young, 1982). The patient's statements are more easily understood if interpreted in the context of this illness experience (Young, 1982), although few practitioners have either the time or the skill to explore these pathways with their patients.

Although prototypes and chain complexes may have some effect on patient–provider communication, neither is easily accessible to a provider for incorporation into the therapeutic or diagnostic process. Prototypes, consisting of a string of recalled events that are often related to earlier illness episodes, are limited to the patient or to a small circle of individuals, making their generalization difficult. Chain complexes result from a variety of experiences, sensations, and symptoms and exist only in the mind of the patient. To the extent that they are unconscious, their accessibility becomes even more unlikely (Young, 1982).

Communication in general and negotiation in particular may be affected, as well, by the differential in power between the patient and the physician. This differential manifests in a variety of ways, including the provider characterization of patients as "good" (not responsible for their illnesses, unquestioning, "compliant," and affirming the physician's self-image) or "bad" (unresponsive to treatment, demanding, questioning of authority, "noncompliant"); deserving or undeserving of care; or interesting or uninteresting "cases" (Lupton, 1994). A thorough exploration of the reasons for this differential has alternatively been viewed (1) as premised on legitimate authority and beneficial to the physician, the patients, and society as a whole (Parsons, 1987); (2) as a means by which physicians can reinforce capitalist ideologies by exercising control over their patients' behaviors (Waitzkin, 1984); and (3) as a form of social organization for the voluntary maintenance of social order and conformity (Silverman, 1987).

Mechanic (1972) found in his review of the literature that factors unrelated to the illness may determine whether an individual is recognized as ill and whether an individual receives assistance. In the context of mental illness, for example, individuals who are incontinent, suicidal, homicidal, delusional, or disoriented are more likely to be recognized and labeled by others as ill and to receive attention for that illness. Others who have displayed bizarre and difficult behavior, but who have not displayed these characteristics, are less likely to be brought into care.

Need Factors.   The variable of poor health has been found to be one of the strongest predictors of physician utilization (Wan and Soifer, 1974). How individuals define and perceive health and illness, then, may have a direct bearing on their need, which then affects on the decision to seek services (Mechanic, 1979).

The perceived seriousness of a particular symptom will often affect the likelihood that an individual will respond to it (Mechanic, 1968). A symptom may be defined as serious by either the individual experiencing it or those around him or her. A symptom is more likely to be characterized by others as serious if activities are disrupted as a result of that symptom. Similarly, the more frequent and persistent a symptom is, the more likely it is that both the individuals and those around him or her will perceive the symptom as serious (Lemert, 1951).

In their 1971 study of 3,880 families comprising 11,822 persons, Andersen, Krantz, and Andersen (1975) found that most of the variance in physician contact was explained by individuals' worry about health and their symptoms. The severity of the diagnosis, the nature of the symptoms, the individual's perceptions about his or her health, and the frequency of pain accounted for most of the variance in the volume of visits. A 1975 study of 7,787 persons found that the symptoms and the individual's perceived health explained the greatest proportion of the variance in service utilization (Andersen and Aday, 1978).

Urdaneta, Saldana, and Winkler (1995) examined the reasons underlying families' search for care for a mentally ill member. More than one third of the 103 Mexican-American respondents reported that inappropriate behavior on the part of the ill member precipitated the search. Almost one third identified violence as the single factor that forced them to seek help.

Alternative Models

Mechanic (1978) has identified ten individual determinants of illness behavior: (1) the visibility or recognizability of symptoms; (2) the extent to which the symptoms are perceived as serious; (3) the extent to which the symptoms are disruptive of the individual's everyday life; (4) the frequency and persistence of the symptoms; (5) the individual's level of tolerance; (6) the individual's level of knowledge, the availability of information, and the individual's underlying cultural assumptions; (7) the existence of basic needs that may lead the individual to deny the situation; (8) the individual's needs which are in competition with an illness response; (9) the existence of competing interpretations; and (10) the availability of treatment and related issues, such as monetary costs, or the proximity of the available treatment.

While many of Mechanic's variables could be grouped in the Aday–Andersen schema, Wolinsky (1980) has suggested instead that they be viewed as components of four basic categories of determinants: (1) perception of the symptoms, (2) nature of the symptoms, (3) individual needs and competing rationales, and (4) non-social-psychological factors. Wolinsky (1980:125) notes that these ten variables are ultimately joined together by a common theme: "that illness behavior is a culturally and socially learned response pattern."

The Role of Beliefs and Behavior: Models of Behavior Change

Numerous models of behavior change have been developed to explain why individuals do or do not participate in health programs or utilize services to detect, prevent, or treat illness and how participation can be enhanced. These models are reviewed here only briefly. Readings pertaining to these models can be found in the reference list at the end of this chapter.

Health Belief Model

The health belief model (HBM) was initially formulated to help explain why people did not participate in programs to detect or prevent disease (Rosenstock, 1960, 1966, 1974). Kirscht (1974) later extended the model to apply to people's responses to symptoms. Becker (1974) used the model to examine people's behavior in response to diagnosed illness.

The HBM has been characterized as a value-expectancy model because it encompasses the desire to get well or to avoid illness (value) and the belief that a specific action will help the person prevent or alleviate illness symptoms (expectation). The HBM originally consisted of four components: perceived severity, perceived benefits, perceived barriers, and cues to action. Bandura (1977) later introduced the concept of self-efficacy.

Perceived susceptibility refers to the individual's risk of contracting a particular condition. Perceived severity refers to an individual's feelings about the seriousness of contracting a condition or, if already diagnosed, of terminating or not adhering to treatment recommendations. An individual's perceptions of the benefits from following a particular course of action to reduce the risk of disease constitute the perceived benefits. "Perceived barriers" encompasses the negative aspects of a particular course of action, such as cost, unpleasantness, or time required. Cues to action consist of "triggers" that prompt an individual to respond. Self-efficacy has been defined as "the conviction that one can successfully execute the behavior required to produce the outcomes" (Bandura, 1977:79).

Social Cognitive Theory

Social cognitive theory posits that human functioning results from the reciprocal interaction of three elements: cognitive, biological, and affective factors; behavior; and environmental factors. Consequently, any program that aims to change behavior must address four areas: information; the development of social and self-regulatory skills required for preventive action; skill enhancement and self-efficacy; and the enlistment and creation of requisite social supports.

The informational component must not only provide information about the disease at issue, but must also instill a sense that the individual has the ability to alter his or her health habits and provide information on how to do so (Maddux and Rogers, 1983). The informational component must also attend to how this information will be diffused and must often look to social networks for information dissemination/diffusion (Watters *et al.*, 1990). Modeling, role playing, and corrective feedback techniques have been used as vehicles for the development of self-regulative behaviors (Schinke and Orlandi, 1990; Kelly, St. Lawrence, Hood, and Brasfield, 1989).

Social norms influence behavior because of the anticipated social consequences to particular courses of action. People also regulate their own conduct by conforming their behavior to internalized self-sanctions (Bandura, 1989). Strong involvement in a social network that is supportive of specific behaviors may increase individuals' knowledge about the disease at issue, reinforce beliefs about self-efficacy, and strengthen motivation to adopt more protective behaviors (McKusick *et al.*, 1990; Fisher, 1988).

Theory of Reasoned Action

The theory of reasoned action posits that beliefs and behavior are causally linked. The individual's beliefs that a certain behavior leads to particular outcomes and his or her evaluation of these outcomes constitutes his or her attitude toward the behavior. The individual's perceptions of the attitudes of others to performing or not performing the behavior constitute the subjective norm. The intention to perform a particular behavior is a function of the relative importance of the individual's attitude and the subjective norm. The intention then determines whether the behavior will be performed (Ajzen and Fishbein, 1980; Fishbein and Ajzen, 1975; Fishbein, 1967). This theory presupposes that most socially relevant behaviors are amenable to volitional control, which may be effectuated either attitudinally or normatively.

Diffusion Theory

Diffusion refers to the process by which innovation is communicated to members of a particular social system (Rogers, 1983). Diffusion encompasses four elements: (1) an idea or practice that is perceived as new; (2) communication channels through which the messages are exchanged; (3) time or process; and (4) a social system, or the structure and function of relations between individuals. The communication of a message may be rendered more complicated if (1) the content of the communication is considered taboo by the message's audience; (2) the adoption of the targeted behavior cannot guarantee that the intended outcome will occur; and (3) the target population is unique, that is, extremely homophilous individuals have bonded together as a result of the criticism and ostracism that they have experienced from the larger society (Dearing, Meyer, and Rogers, 1994). As such, this theory focuses on the culture of the target group (Friedman, Des Jarlais, and Ward, 1994).

Diffusion theory posits that communication among unique population groups occurs frequently and is characterized by a high level of trust. In the context of a unique population, community members are unlikely to act as opinion leaders in this communication process because of the high visibility that such a role would demand and the risk of being viewed negatively by other group members.

The classic diffusion model is based on the notion that communication is diffused from the top down through a one-way channel of communication. Decentralized diffusion systems, in contrast, are premised on a two-way channel of communication between the source of the innovation and the potential adopter. Decentralized systems are more appropriate when the innovation does not involve high-level technology and when the adopter group is heterogeneous.

Decentralized diffusion systems place a great deal of emphasis on the agent of change, from whom the group members learn about the innovation. Generally, successful change agents have a high degree of homophily with the target community and will be perceived by the target group as being knowledgeable about the innovation (competence credibility) and trustworthy (safety credibility) (Rogers, 1983).

Diffusion theory posits that five characteristics of the innovation will determine whether or not it is adopted by the target population: (1) the perceived relative advantage offered by the innovation; (2) the degree to which the innovation is consistent with existing values and needs and with past experiences (compatibility); (3) the degree to which the innovation can be tried on a limited basis (triability); (4) the degree to which the innovation is visible to others; and (5) the complexity of the innovation. The greater the degree of difficulty in using the innovation, the less likely it is that it will be adopted (Rogers, 1983).

Exercises

1. Socioeconomic status (SES) has been identified as an enabling factor in obtaining medical care. However, SES can be defined in a variety of ways, including each of the following: annual individual income, annual household income, annual family income, monthly individual income (low, average, or high), monthly household income (low, average, or high), and monthly family income (low, average, or high). Additionally, income may vary over time, even within a short period of time.
    a. In this context, how comparable or consistent are the findings across studies implicating SES as a factor?
    b. Should there be a standard measure of SES and, if so, what should it be?
    c. What does SES really signify, particularly in view of its close association with income, occupational status, and education?
2. You are employed by your local public health department to develop health programs. Your community has been experiencing increasing cancer-related mortality rates over the last 5 years. Your supervisor has asked you to develop an outreach program that will encourage individuals to present for cancer screening to their physicians. This would include, for instance, procedures related to breast and cervical cancer screening for women and prostate cancer screening for men (within recommended age guidelines). Because you want your outreach program to work, you have decided to conduct the necessary preliminary research before designing and implementing your program.
    a. What might be some of the existing barriers to access to such testing? How will you determine what the actual barriers are?
    b. How will you decide which behavior change model you will use as the theoretical framework for your outreach program?
        i. *Which one will you select and why?*
        ii. *How do the systemic barriers to access that you identified in (a), if any, affect your choice of behavior change model?*

    c. Explain how you will operationalize each component of the behavior change model that you selected in (b).

    d. How will you evaluate the effectiveness of your outreach program?

References

Aday, L.A., & Andersen, R. (1974). A framework for the study of access to medical care. *Health Services Research, 9*, 208–220.

Agency for Health Care Policy and Research, Center for General Health Services Intramural Research. (1991). *National Medical Expenditure Survey: Health Insurance, Use of Health Services, and Health Care Expenditures: Research Findings 12.* Rockville, MD: Department of Health and Human Services [AHCPR Publ. No. 92-0017].

Ajzen, I., & Fishbein, M. eds. (1980). *Understanding Attitudes and Predicting Social Behavior.* Englewood Cliffs, NJ: Prentice Hall.

Andersen, R., & Aday, L.A. (1978). Access to medical care in the U.S.: Realized and potential. *Medical Care, 16*, 533–546.

Andersen, R., Kravits, J., & Andersen O.W. (Eds.). (1975). *Equity in Health Services: Empirical Analyses in Social Policy.* Cambridge, MA: Ballinger.

Andersen, R., & Newman, J.F. (1973). Societal and individual determinants of medical care utilization in the United States. *Milbank Memorial Fund Quarterly, 51*, 95–124.

Bandura, A. (1977). *Social Learning Theory.* Englewood Cliffs, NJ: Prentice-Hall.

Bandura, A. (1989). Self-regulation of motivation and action through internal standards and goal systems. In L.A. Pervin (Ed.), *Goal Concepts in Personality and Social Psychology* (pp. 19–85). Hillsdale, NJ: Lawrence Erlbaum.

Becker, M.H. (Ed.). (1974). The health belief model and personal health behavior. *Health Education Monographs, 2*, 324–473.

Berger, P.L., & Luckman, T. (1966). *The Social Construction of Reality: A Treatise in the Sociology of Knowledge.* New York: Doubleday.

Berkanovic, E., & Telesky, C. (1985). Mexican-American, Black-American, and White-American differences in reporting illnesses, disability and physician visits for illnesses. *Social Science and Medicine, 20*, 567–577.

Berkman, L.F., & Syme, S.L. (1979). Social networks, host resistance, and mortality: A nine-year follow-up study of Alameda County residents. *American Journal of Epidemiology, 109*, 186–204.

Brown, G.W., Bhrolchain, M.N., & Harris T. (1975). Social class and psychiatric disturbance among women in an urban population. *Sociology, 9*, 225–254.

Chrisman, N.J. (1977). The health seeking process: an approach to the natural history of illness. *Culture, Medicine, and Psychiatry, 1*, 351–377.

Dearing, J.W., Meyer, G., & Rogers, E.M. (1994). Diffusion theory and HIV risk behavior change. In R.J. DiClemente & J.L. Peterson (Eds.), *Preventing AIDS: Theories and Methods of Behavioral Interventions* (pp. 79–93). New York: Plenum Publishing Company.

Dressler, W.W. (1990). Culture, stress, and disease. In T. Johnson & C. Sargent (Eds.), *Medical Anthropology: Contemporary Theory and Method* (pp. 248–267). New York: Praeger.

Dunn, F.L. (1984). Social Determinants in Tropical Disease. In K.S. Warren & A.A.F. Mahmoud (Eds.), *Tropical and Geographical Medicine*, New York: McGraw-Hill.

Escobar, J.I., Randolph, E.T., & Hill, M. (1986). Symptoms of schizophrenia in Hispanic and Anglo veterans. *Culture, Medicine and Psychiatry, 10*, 259–276.

Fabrega, H., Jr. (1972). The study of disease in relation to culture. *Behavioral Science, 17*, 183–203.

Fishbein, M. (1967). Attitude and the prediction of behavior. In M. Fishbein (Ed.), *Readings in Attitude Theory and Measurement* (pp. 477–492). New York: John Wiley.

Fishbein, M., & Ajzen, I. (1975). *Belief, Attitude, Intention and Behavior: An Introduction to Theory and Research.* Reading, MA: Addison-Wesley.

Fisher, J.D. (1988). Possible effects of reference group-based social influence on AIDS-risk behavior and AIDS prevention. *American Psychologist, 43*, 914–920.

Freeman, H.E., Aiken, L.H., Blendon, R.J., & Corey, C.R. (1990). Uninsured working-age adults. Characteristics and consequences. *Health Services Research, 24*, 811–823.

Freeman, H.E., & Corey, C.R. (1993). Insurance status and access to health services among poor persons. *Health Services Research, 28*, 531–541.

Freidson, E. (1960). Client control and medical practice. *American Journal of Sociology, 65*, 374–382.

Freidson, E. (1970). *The Profession of Medicine: A Study in the Sociology of Applied Knowledge*. New York: Dodd and Mead.

Friedman, S.R., Des Jarlais, D.C., & Ward, T.P. (1994). Social models for changing health-relevant behavior. In R.J. DiClemente & J.L. Peterson (Eds.), *Preventing AIDS: Theories and Methods of Behavioral Interventions* (pp. 95–116). New York: Plenum Publishing Company.

Garrison, V. (1977). Doctor, espiritista, or psychiatrist: Health seeking behaviour in a Puerto Rican neighborhood of New York City. *Medical Anthropology, 1*, 165–191.

Gesler, W.M. (1979). Measurement in household surveys in developing areas. *Social Science and Medicine, 13D*, 223–226.

Good, B.J. (1977). The heart of what's the matter: The semantics of illness in Iran. *Culture, Medicine and Psychiatry, 1*, 25–58.

Gore, S. (1978). The effect of social support in moderating the health consequences of unemployment. *Journal of Health and Social Behavior, 19*, 157–165.

Hadley, J., Steinberg, E.P., & Feder, J. (1991). Comparison of uninsured and privately insured hospital patients: Condition on admission, resource use, and outcome. *JAMA, 265*, 374–379.

Harwood, A. (Ed.). (1981). *Ethnicity and Medical Care*. Cambridge, MA: Harvard University Press.

Hayward, R.A., Shapiro, M.F., Freeman, H.E., & Corey, C.R. (1988). Inequities in health services among insured Americans: Do working-age adults have less access to medical care than the elderly? *New England Journal of Medicine, 318*, 1507–1512.

Heller, P.L., Chalfant, H.P., Quesada, G.M., & Rivera-Workey, C. (1981). Class, familism and utilization of health services in Durango, Mexico: A replication. *Social Science and Medicine, 15A*, 539–541.

Igun, U.A. (1979). Stages in health-seeking: A descriptive model. *Social Science and Medicine, 13A*, 445–456.

Jackson, J.J. (1981). Urban black Americans. In A. Harwood (Ed.), *Ethnicity and Medical Care* (pp. 37–129). Cambridge, MA: Harvard University Press.

Janes, C.R. (1986). Migration and hypertension: An ethnography of disease risk in an urban Samoan community. In C.R. Janes, R. Stall, & S.M. Gifford (Eds.), *Anthropology and Epidemiology* (pp. 175–211). Dordrecht, Holland: D. Reidel Publishing Company.

Kasl, S.U., & Cobb, S. (1966). Health behavior, illness behavior, and sick role behavior. *Archives of Environmental Health, 12*, 246–266.

Kelly, J.A., St. Lawrence, J.S., Hood, H.V., & Brasfield, T.L. (1989). Behavioral intervention to reduce AIDS risk activities. *Journal of Consulting and Clinical Psychology, 57*, 60–67.

Kirscht, J.P. (1974). The health belief model and illness behavior. *Health Education Monographs, 2*, 387–408.

Kirscht, J.P., & Rosenstock, I.M. (1979). Patients' problems in following recommendations of health experts. In G.C. Stone, F. Cohen, & E. Adler (Eds.), *Health Psychology—A Handbook*. San Francisco: Jossey-Bass.

Kleinman, A. (1980). *Patients and Healers in the Context of Culture: An Exploration of the Borderland Between Anthropology, Medicine, and Psychiatry*. Berkeley, CA: University of California Press.

Kohn, R., & White, K.L. (Eds.) (1976). *Health Care: An International Study*. London: Oxford University Press.

Kroeger, A. (1983). Anthropological and socio-medical health care research in developing countries. *Social Science and Medicine, 17*, 147–161.

Kunstadter, P. (1975). Do cultural differences make any difference? Choice points in medical systems available in northwestern Thailand. In A. Kleinman, P. Kunstadter, E. Alexander, & J. Gale (Eds.), *Medicine in Chinese Cultures: Comparative Studies of Health Care in Chinese and Other Societies*. Washington, DC: United States Department of Health, Education, and Welfare [DHEW Publ. No. (NIH) 75-653].

Langlie, J.K. (1977). Social networks, health beliefs, and preventive health behavior. *Journal of Health and Social Behavior, 18*, 244–260.

Lawson, H.H., Kahn, M.W., & Heiman, E.M. (1982). Psychopathology, treatment outcome and attitude toward mental illness in Mexican American and European patients. *International Journal of Social Psychiatry, 28*, 20–26.

Lemert, E. (1951). *Social Pathology*. New York: McGraw-Hill.

Leventhal, H., Leventhal, E.A., & Nguyen, T.V. (1985). Reactions of families to illness: Theoretical models and perspectives. In D.C. Turk & R. D. Kerns (Eds.), *Health, Illness, and Families: A Life-Span Perspective*. New York: Wiley.

Lieban, R.W. (1977). The field of medical anthropology. In D. Landy (Ed.), *Culture, Disease, and Healing: Studies in Medical Anthropology* (pp. 13–31). New York: Macmillan Publishing Co., Inc.

Loue, S. (1996). Transsexualism in medicolegal limine: An examination and a proposal for change. *Journal of Psychiatry and Law, 24*, 27–51.

Lupton, D. (1994). *Medicine As Culture: Illness, Disease, and the Body in Western Societies*. London: Sage Publications.

Maddux, J.E., & Rogers, J.W. (1983). Protection motivation and self-efficacy: A revised theory of fear appeals and attitude change. *Journal of Experimental Social Psychology, 19*, 469–479.

McKinlay, J.B. (1981). Social network influences on morbid episodes and the career of help seeking. In L. Eisenberg & A. Kleinman (Eds.), *The Relevance of Social Science for Medicine* (pp. 77–107). Dordrecht, Holland: D. Reidel.

McKusick, L., Coates, T.J., Morin, S.F., Pollack, L., & Hoff, C. (1990). Longitudinal predictors of reductions in unprotected anal intercourse among gay men in San Francisco: The AIDS behavioral research project. *American Journal of Public Health, 80*, 978–983.

Mechanic, D. (1968). *Medical Sociology: A Selective View*. New York: Free Press.

Mechanic, D. (1969). Illness and care. In J. Kosa, A. Antonovsky, & I. Zola (Eds.), *Poverty and Health: A Sociological Analysis* (pp. 191–214). Cambridge, MA: Harvard University Press.

Mechanic, D. (1972). *Public Expectations and Health Care: Essays on the Changing Organization of Health Services*. New York: John Wiley and Sons, Inc.

Mechanic, D. (1978). *Medical Sociology* (2nd ed.). New York: Free Press.

Mechanic, D. (1979). Correlates of physician utilization: Why do major multivariate studies of physician utilization find trivial psychosocial and organizational effects? *Journal of Health and Social Behavior, 20*, 387–396.

Minuchin, S., Rosman, B.L., & Baker, L. (1978). *Psychosomatic Families*. Cambridge, MA: Harvard University Press.

Newacheck, P.W. & Starfield, B. (1988). Morbidity and use of ambulatory care services among poor and nonpoor children. *American Journal of Public Health, 78*, 927–933.

Nichter, M. (1981). Negotiation of the illness experience: Ayurvedic therapy and the psychosocial dimension of illness. *Culture, Medicine, and Psychiatry, 5*, 5–24.

Nichter, M. (1987). Cultural dimensions of hot, cold and sema in Sinhalese health culture. *Social Science and Medicine, 25*, 377–387.

Nichter, M. (1994). Illness semantics and international health: The weak lungs/TB complex in the Philippines. *Social Science and Medicine, 38*, 649–663.

Nichter, M., & Nordstrom, C. (1989). A question of medicine answering: Health commodification and the social relations of healing in Sri Lanka. *Culture, Medicine and Psychiatry, 13*, 367–390.

Parsons, T. (1951). *The Social System*. Glencoe: Free Press.

Parsons, T. (1987). Illness and the role of the physicians: A sociological perspective. In J.D. Stoeckle (Ed.), *Encounters Between Patients and Doctors: An Anthology* (pp. 147–156). Cambridge, MA: MIT Press.

Penchansky, R., & Thomas, J.W. (1981). The concept of access: Definitions and relationship to consumer satisfaction. *Medical Care, 19*, 127–140.

Reid, W.H., & Wise, M.G. (1995). *DSM-IV Training Guide*. New York: Brunner/Mazel.

Rogers, E.M. (1983). *Diffusion of Innovations* (3rd ed.). New York: Free Press.

Rosenstock, I.M. (1960). What research in motivation suggests for public health. *American Journal of Public Health, 50*, 295–301.

Rosenstock, I.M. (1966). Why people use health services. *Milbank Memorial Fund Quarterly, 44*, 94–124.

Rosenstock, I.M. (1969). Prevention of illness and maintenance of health. In J. Kosa, A. Antonovsky, & I. Zola (Eds.), *Poverty and Health: A Sociological Analysis* (pp. 168–190). Cambridge, MA: Harvard University Press.

Rosenstock, I.M. (1974). Historical origins of the health belief model. *Health Education Monographs, 2*, 328–335.

Scheff, T.J. (1963). Decision rules, types of error and their consequences in medical diagnosis. *Behavioral Science, 8*, 97–107.

Scheff, T.J. (1966). Users and non-users of a student psychiatric clinic. *Journal of Health and Human Behavior, 7*, 114–121.

Schinke, S.P., & Orlandi, M.A. (1990). Skills-based, interactive computer interventions to prevent HIV infection among African American and Hispanic adolescents. *Computers in Human Behavior, 6*, 235–246.

Scotch, N.A. (1963). Sociocultural factors in the epidemiology of Zulu hypertension. *American Journal of Public Health, 52*, 1205–1213.

Segall, A. (1976). The sick role concept: Understanding illness behavior. *Journal of Health and Social Behavior, 17*, 163–170.

Silverman, D. (1987). *Communication and Medical Practice: Social Relations in the Clinic*. London: Sage Publications.

Snell, J.E. (1967). Hypnosis in the treatment of the "hexed" patient. *American Journal of Psychiatry, 124*, 311–316.

Suchman, E. (1965). Social patterns of illness and medical care. *Journal of Health and Human Behavior, 6*, 2–16.

Urdaneta, M.L., Saldana, D.H., & Winkler, A. (1995). Mexican-American perceptions of severe mental illness. *Human Organization, 54*, 70–77.

Waitzkin, H. (1984). The micropolitics of medicine: A contextual analysis. *International Journal of Health Services, 14*, 339–378.

Wan, T.H. & Soifer, S.S. (1974). Determinants of physician utilization: a causal analysis. *Journal of Health and Social Behavior, 15*, 100–108.

Watters, J.K., Downing, M., Case, P., Lorvick, J., Cheng, Y., & Fergusson, B. (1990). AIDS prevention for intravenous drug users in the community: Street-based education and risk behavior. *American Journal of Community Psychology, 18,* 587–596.

Wellin, E. (1977). Theoretical orientations in medical anthropology: Continuity and change over the past half-century. In D. Landy (Ed.), *Culture, Disease, and Healing: Studies in Medical Anthropology* (pp. 47–58). New York: Macmillan Publishing Co., Inc.

Wenneker, M.B., Weissman, J.S., & Epstein, A.M. (1990). The association of payer with utilization of cardiac procedures in Massachusetts. *JAMA, 264,* 1255–1260.

Wolinsky, F.D. (1976). Health service utilization and attitudes toward health maintenance organizations: A theoretical and methodological discussion. *Journal of Health and Social Behavior, 17,* 221–236.

Wolinsky, F.D. (1980). *The Sociology of Health* Boston: Little, Brown.

Young, A. (1982). The anthropologies of illness and sickness. *Annual Review of Anthropology, 11,* 257–285.

Young, J.C., & Garro, L.Y. (1982). Variation in the choice of treatment in two Mexican communities. *Social Science and Medicine, 16,* 1435–1465.

II

The Health of Communities

6

African-American Health

Introduction

Numerous disparities have been observed in the health of individuals classified as African-Americans compared to those classified as white. African-Americans have a higher prevalence of hypertension than whites and a higher risk of cardiovascular disease (Tyroler, 1990). For heart disease, cancer, stroke, accidents, and pneumonia, mortality rates are higher for U.S. blacks compared to whites, even after adjusting for age and sex (Cooper, 1984; Cooper and David, 1986; Cooper *et al.*, 1981). The infant mortality rate among African-Americans is twice the rate among white infants. The life expectancy for African-Americans is 6 years less than that for whites (Council on Ethical and Judicial Affairs, American Medical Association, 1990). Men in Bangladesh are more likely to reach the age of 65 than black men living in Harlem (McCord and Freeman, 1990).

The underlying reasons for such differences are unclear. Barriers in accessing care may play a critical role. For example, although African-American men experienced a rate of anterior myocardial infarction that was three-quarters that of whites, they were only half as likely to undergo angiography and only one-third as likely to undergo bypass surgery (Ford *et al.*, 1989). A study of patients discharged with a preliminary diagnosis of circulatory disease or chest pain found that although African-Americans and whites had similar rates of hospitalization, whites were one-third more likely to undergo coronary angiography and were more than twice as likely as African-Americans to undergo bypass surgery or angioplasty (Wenneker and Epstein, 1989). A study of patients diagnosed with pneumonia at 16 different hospitals concluded that nonwhite patients received fewer hospital services than would be expected based on their health status (Yergan, Flood, LoGerfo, and Diehr, 1987). An investigation of the use of eye surgery among whites and African-Americans found that the rate of surgery among blacks was twice that of whites, but blacks were four times more likely than whites to have glaucoma. Access to liver and renal transplantation appears to be significantly more limited for African-Americans compared to whites (Butkus, 1991; Butkus, Maydrech, and Raju, 1992; Gonwa *et al.*, 1991).

Similar findings with respect to the utilization of relevant procedures have been reported even after adjusting for severity of illness (Hannan *et al.*, 1991) and even when financial incentives, such as health insurance, are absent or adjusted for in the analysis (Carlisle, Leake, and Shapiro, 1995; Wenneker and Epstein, 1989; Whittle, Conigliaro, Good, and Lofgren,

1993). African-Americans were more likely to be classified as ward patients than white Americans, even when they had comparable insurance coverage (Perkoff and Anderson, 1970). Compared with white patients, African-Americans have been more likely to report that their physician did not inquire adequately about their pain, did not tell them how long it would be before their prescription medicine worked, did not explain the seriousness of their illness or injury, and did not discuss test and examination findings (Blendon, Aiken, Freemen, and Corey, 1989). Access issues for uninsured African-Americans may be even more critical. Uninsured African-Americans are more likely to feel that it is difficult to obtain needed medical care and that they need more care than they are receiving (Neighbors and Jackson, 1987).

Numerous other theories have been advanced, particularly in an attempt to explain the disparity between blacks and whites in the risk of premature birth, which has been found to be significantly higher among blacks (Klebanoff, Shiono, Berendez, and Rhoads, 1989; Klebanoff *et al.*, 1991). The first presupposes that certain environmental or social factors differ in quantity between whites and blacks, but have a qualitatively different effect. The second theory attributes disparities in health to genetic biological differences between blacks and whites. A third theory ascribes these disparities to social and environmental factors that affect only blacks, such as institutionalized racism and discrimination (David and Collins, 1991; Massey, 1990; Reed, 1990). Various other researchers have asserted that many of these disparities in health status arise specifically as a result of ill treatment during the years of slavery, resulting in a "slave health deficit" (Byrd and Clayton, 1992; Morais, 1967). An examination of the history of African-Americans in the health system provides some insight into the basis for the existing disparities.

Historical and Cultural Context

African-American Health during Slavery

Many physicians in the pre-Civil War South believed that significant medical differences existed between blacks and whites. Some physicians argued that blacks were immune from certain diseases that affected whites, such as malaria, but were especially susceptible to other conditions, such as frostbite (Savitt, 1985). One Northern physician observed of blacks that:

> God has adapted him, both in his physical and mental structure, to the tropics.... His head is protected from the rays of a vertical sun by a dense mat of woolly hair, wholly impervious to its fiercest heats, while his entire surface, studded with innumerable sebaceous glands, forming a complete excretory system, relieves him from all those climatic influences so fatal, under the same circumstances, to the sensitive and highly organized white man. Instead of seeking to shelter himself from the burning sun of the tropics, he courts it, enjoys it, delights in its fiercest heats. (Van Evrie, 1861:251, 256)

African-Americans suffered from several causes of mortality, including pulmonary tuberculosis and neonatal tetanus, more so than whites. One particular form of tuberculosis, characterized by difficulty in breathing, abdominal pain, progressive debility and emaciation, and ultimately death, was so common among blacks that it became known as Negro Consumption or *Struma Africana*. Various explanations have been offered in attempts to explain the impact of this form of tuberculosis on blacks, including lack of an immune response to the disease due to lack of exposure and an increased susceptibility to serious first attacks of tuberculosis due to various factors, including malnutrition and preexisting illness (Savitt, 1985).

Epidemics of cholera, yellow fever, and typhoid were of special concern among slaves. Slaves were often particularly vulnerable to cholera as a result of the increased consumption of water required by their strenuous work. The water, however, was often contaminated and the slaves often suffered from nutritional deficiencies that adversely affected their ability to recover from cholera (Lee and Lee, 1977).

The especial vulnerability to some diseases was used by some as an illustration of blacks' inferiority (Savitt, 1985). The harsh conditions to which black slaves were subjected were rarely mentioned as contributing to their susceptibility to specific diseases or to their poor health.

Male slaves were valued for their work, while the value of female slaves was determined not only by their capacity for work, but their capacity to reproduce and to increase the human property that formed the basis for the slave economy. Because female slaves were property, without any degree of autonomy, they were subject to their masters' sexual desires (Jacobs, 1988; Smith, 1988). Slaves were physically mutilated for real and imagined offenses (Hurmence, 1984; Jacobs, 1988). Lavinia Bell's treatment as a slave was all too common:

> After that time she was sent into the cotton field with the other field hands, where the treatment was cruelly severe. No clothes whatever were allowed them, their hair was cut off close to their head, and thus were exposed to the glare of a southern sun from early morn until late at night. Scarcely a day passed without their receiving fifty lashes, whether they worked or whether they did not. They were also compelled to go down on their knees, and harnessed to a plough, to plough up the land, with boys for riders, to whip them when they flagged in their work. At other times, they were compelled to walk on hackles, used for hackling flax. Her feet are now dotted over with scars, caused by their brutality.... Still later, for some disobedience on her part, they hoisted her into a tree, locked a chain round her neck, and hand-cuffed her wrists, the marks being yet visible. There she was left for two days and nights, without a morsel to eat, being taunted with such questions as to whether she was hungry and would like something to eat ... (Blassingame, 1977:342–343)

This failure to provide food for a slave was regarded as "the most aggravated development of meanness even among slaveholders" (Douglass, 1968:34).

Disagreement exists with respect to the medical treatment that slaves received. Accounts from slaves seem to indicate that, even as judged by the standards of the time, medical care was often poor. Midwives or doctors were rarely in attendance at the birth of a slave's child. At least one author, however, has argued that medical care of slaves was often superior to that received by their owners, if only because the slave represented a financial investment which could be threatened by ill health (Kolchin, 1993). Slaves not infrequently resorted to remedies at home rather than report their illness to the person in charge and be required to submit to the medical care provided at the behest of the owner. Consequently, a dual system of health care developed (Savitt, 1985).

Poor living conditions exacerbated existing health problems. Although slaves were provided with housing, they were rarely provided with toilets (Blassingame, 1977). The housing itself was often characterized by poor ventilation, lack of light, and damp, earthen floors (Semmes, 1996). There was little opportunity to bathe or to wash clothes, resulting in the promotion of bedbugs and body lice. The soil and water were often infested with worms and larvae, to which the slaves were particularly vulnerable due to the lack of shoes and the poor sanitation (Blassingame, 1979; Savitt, 1978). Roundworm, threadworm, tapeworm, and hookworm infestations plagued many slaves. The practice of eating soil (geophagy), which was continued from West Africa, further promoted infestation with worms (Savitt, 1978).

Poor diets and food shortages further contributed to the development of poor health. Slaveowners frequently provided the slaves with pork, which was the preferred source of protein for the owners. However, the slaveowners retained the leanest cuts for themselves, and passed on the fatty portions, together with cornmeal, to the slaves. On some plantations, slaves rarely had dairy products, fruits, or vegetables (Stampp, 1956). Not surprisingly, the slaves' poor diet often resulted in deficiencies in vitamins, including vitamins A, B, C, and D. These deficiencies, in turn, led to diseases such as scurvy, beriberi, and pellagra (Savitt, 1978).

Slaves were the unwilling subjects of scientific experimentation. When compensation was offered, it was provided to the slaveowner. For example, the physician J. Marion Sims reached an agreement with one slaveowner to maintain several of his female slaves at his expense in exchange for their use in experiments aimed designed to repair vesico-vaginal fistulas (Sims, 1894).

African-American Health during Reconstruction

Poor housing and poor sanitation continued into the period of Reconstruction (Blassingame, 1973; Morais, 1967). African-Americans suffered from pellagra and other nutritional deficiencies (Johnson, 1966), for which they were held responsible. One physician opined

> His [the Negro] diet is fatty; he revels in fat; every pore of his sleek, contented face wreaks with unctuousness. To him the force-producing quality of the fats has the seductive fascination that opium leaves about the Oriental ... (Tipton, 1886, quoted in Charatz-Litt, 1992:717)

The high rates of death among African-Americans was attributable primarily to heart disease, tuberculosis, influenza, nephritis, cancer, pellagra, and malaria (Johnson, 1966). In fact, New York Life's and Equitable's actuaries predicted that blacks would be extinct by the year 2000 as the result of the extremely high mortality rate (Haller, 1971). Congress responded to the high death rates among African-Americans with the passage of the Freedmen's legislation, which opened universities, hospitals, soup kitchens, and clinics in the South (Blassingame, 1973; Morais, 1967).

African-American Health during the 20th Century

The late 1800s and the beginning of the 1900s were characterized by significant migration of African-Americans from rural to urban areas. The Great Migration to northern urban areas, which began in 1915, was associated with pull factors in the North, such as employment opportunities, and push factors from the South, including a depressed demand for labor, low wages, floods, segregation, discrimination, lynching, and poor educational opportunities (Woodson, 1969).

African-Americans continued to suffer from serious health problems despite migration to urban areas. During the early 1920s, tuberculosis was responsible for three times as many deaths among blacks as among whites in New York City. Harlem's rate of infant mortality from 1923 to 1927 was 111 per 1,000, compared to a rate of 64.5 per 1,000 for the entire city of New York (Osofsky, 1966). Such disparities, particularly in the South, have been attributed in part to the actions of the white medical community (Charatz-Litt, 1992). White physicians often refused to treat black patients. Black physicians were rendered less effective in treating patients due to their inferior medical training and their exclusion from membership in many medical associations and societies, thereby precluding them from accessing new techniques (Byrd and Clayton, 1992; Charatz-Litt, 1992; Seham, 1964).

The National Hospital Association (NHA) was organized in 1923 as a member of the National Medical Association (NMA). Although the NMA's mission emphasized the education of its black physician members, the NHA focused on equality for blacks in the Southern health care system (Charatz-Litt, 1992). It was not until the mid-1960s, however, that the American Medical Association (AMA) reaffirmed its intent to cease racially discriminatory exclusion policies and practices (Anonymous, 1965). The movement toward recognition of black physicians was due in large measure to the passage of federal legislation, such as the Civil Rights Act, requiring cessation of discriminatory and exclusionary policies and practices (Byrd and Clayton, 1992).

Blacks were often solicited as subjects of medical experiments. M. Robert Hines obtained spinal fluid from 423 sick and healthy black infants at an Atlanta hospital, apparently without the consent of the children's parents or guardians. A number of children suffered trauma, including blood in the spinal fluid, as a result of the needle puncture (Roberts, 1925).

The Tuskegee syphilis study is perhaps the most notorious scientific experiment conducted with blacks as subjects of research. In 1929, the United States Public Health Service (USPHS) conducted a study to examine the prevalence of syphilis among blacks and possible mechanisms for treatment. The town of Tuskegee, located in Macon County in Alabama, was found to have the highest rate of syphilis among the six counties that had been included in the study (Gill, 1932; Jones, 1981). This study, funded by the Julius Rosenwald Fund, concluded that mass treatment of syphilis would be feasible. However, funding became inadequate for the continuation of the project and the implementation of the treatment due to the economic depression that commenced in 1929 and which devastated the Fund's financial resources (Thomas and Quinn, 1991).

The Tuskegee study was initiated in 1932 by the USPHS to follow the natural history of untreated, latent syphilis in black males. The impetus for the study derived in part from conflict between the prevailing scientific view in the United States of the progression of syphilis in blacks and the results of a study by Bruusgard in Norway. The U.S. view held that syphilis affected the neurological functioning in whites, but the cardiovascular system in blacks. Bruusgaard, however, had found from his retrospective study of white men with untreated syphilis that cardiovascular effects were common and neurological complications rare (Clark and Danbolt, 1955). However, even at the time that the Tuskegee study was initiated, there existed general consensus within the medical community that syphilis required treatment even in its latent stages, despite the toxic effects of treatment. Moore (1933:237), a venereologist, observed:

> Though it imposes a slight though measurable risk of its own, treatment markedly diminishes the risk from syphilis. In latent syphilis ... the probability of progression, relapse, or death is reduced from a probable 25–30 percent without treatment to about 5 percent with it; and the gravity of the relapse if it occurs, is markedly diminished.

Interest in other racial differences also provided impetus to continue with the study. Blacks were believed to possess an excessive sexual desire, a lack of morality (Hazen, 1914; Quillian, 1906), and an attraction to white women stemming from "racial instincts that are about as amenable to ethical culture as is the inherent odor of the race ..." (Howard, 1903:424).

The original Tuskegee study was to include black males between the ages of 25 and 60 who were infected with syphilis. The study required a physical examination, x-rays, and a spinal tap. The original design did not contemplate the provision of treatment to those enrolled in the study, despite existing consensus in the medical community regarding the necessity of treatment (Brandt, 1985). However, those recruited for the study were advised that they were ill with "bad blood," a term referring to syphilis, and would be provided with treatment. The mercurial ointment and neoarsphenamine provided to subjects as treatment were ineffective and intended to be ineffective. Similarly, the spinal tap which was administered for diagnostic purposes only was portrayed as a "special treatment" to encourage participation. A control group of healthy uninfected men was added to the study as controls in 1933, following USPHS approval to continue with the study (Brandt, 1985).

The researchers themselves noted the conditions that made this extended study possible: follow-up by a nurse who was known to the participants and who came from the community from which they were recruited; the provision to the subjects of the research burial assistance, which they might not have otherwise been able to afford; the provision of transportation to the subjects by the nurse; and government sponsorship of the "care" that the subjects believed, and had been led to believe, was being furnished to them (Rivers, Schuman, Simpson, and Olansky, 1953).

The Tuskegee study continued for 40 years, despite various events that should have signaled its termination. First, the USPHS had begun to administer penicillin to some syphilitic patients in various treatment clinics (Mahoney *et al.*, 1944). By at least 1945, it was clear in the professional literature that syphilis infections would respond to treatment with penicillin, even in cases that had been resistant to treatment with bismuth subsalicylate and mapharsen, a then-standard treatment (Noojin, Callaway, and Flower, 1945). Yet, subjects of the Tuskegee study were not only not offered penicillin treatment, but were also prevented from receiving care when they sought it out (Thomas and Quinn, 1991). Second, a series of articles had been published in professional journals indicating that the subjects were suffering to a much greater degree than the controls with increased morbidity and a reduction in life expectancy (Deibert and Bruyere, 1946; Heller and Bruyere, 1946; Pesare, Bauer, and Gleeson, 1950; Vonderlehr, Clark, Wenger, and Heller, 1936). Yet, defenders of the study asserted as late as 1974 that there was inadequate basis for treatment with either penicillin or other regimens during the course of the study and that it was the "*shibboleth* of informed consent ... born in court decisions in California (1957) and Kansas (1960)" that provoked the furor over the study (Kampmeier, 1974:1352). Clearly, the Nuremberg Code of 1949 was ignored.

It was not until 1972 that the then-existing Department of Health, Education, and Welfare convened an advisory panel in response to the criticism triggered by media coverage of the experiment (Brandt, 1985). The report of that committee focused on the failure to provide penicillin treatment and the failure to obtain informed consent. According to Brandt (1985), this emphasis obscured the historical facts regarding the availability of drug treatment for syphilis prior to the advent of penicillin and ignored the fact that the men believed that they were receiving clinical care and did not know that they were part of an experiment (Brandt, 1985).

The Tuskegee study has had a far-reaching impact. The study has, for many blacks, become a "symbol of their mistreatment by the medical establishment, a metaphor for deceit, conspiracy, malpractice, and neglect, if not outright racial genocide" (Jones, 1992:38). As a consequence, educational programs designed to combat HIV in black communities have been met with distrust and a belief that AIDS and AIDS prevention and care represent forms of racial genocide (Jones, 1992; Thomas and Quinn, 1991).

Health Status

Infectious Disease

African-Americans have been disproportionately affected by HIV. AIDS has become the leading cause of death among African-American women in New York and New Jersey (Chu, Buehler, and Berkelman, 1990). In California, as of June 30, 1992, it was estimated that 270 of every 100,000 African-Americans was infected with HIV. In a statewide blinded serosurvey of 150,000 childbearing women conducted in 1990, it was found that 1 out of every 205 African-American women was infected, compared to 1 out of every 2,389 Latinas and 1 out of every 2,959 women classified as white (Office of AIDS, 1992). A recent study of mortality resulting from AIDS in South Carolina found that African-Americans with AIDS were at increased risk of death at one year as compared to whites (Scott *et al.*, 1997).

Chronic Disease

Cancer

The incidence of breast cancer has been increasing at a rate faster among black women than among white women (Ries *et al.*, 1991). In fact, breast cancer is the leading cause of cancer mortality in black women (Ries *et al.*, 1991). The 5-year survival rate for breast cancer has been found to be lower for black women than for white women (United States Department of Health and Human Services, 1991). In addition, the death rate from breast cancer appears to be increasing among black women (National Cancer Institute, 1995). This difference in survival has been attributed to diagnosis at a later stage of disease among black women (Eley *et al.*, 1994; Satariano, Belle, and Swanson, 1986), possibly related to underuse of mammography and/or delay in obtaining care (Baquet, Horm, Gibbs, and Greenwald, 1991; Burack *et al.*, 1993; Chu, Smart, and Karone, 1988; Dawson and Thomson, 1989; Seidman *et al.*, 1987; Shapiro *et al.*, 1982; Whitman *et al.*, 1991). A recent study of 585 African-American women age 40 or older found that 90% of the women were not receiving regular mammograms, 36% had never had a mammogram, and 33% had never heard of mammography (Mickey, Durski, Worden, and Danigelis, 1995). Differences in utilization of screening or in seeking care may, in turn, be related to differences in the perception of symptoms, access to care or care seeking behavior, or variations in provider referral (Burack *et al.*, 1993; Harwood, 1981; Lieben, 1977; National Center for Health Statistics, 1990; Spector, 1979).

Few studies have examined risk factors for breast cancer specifically in African-American women. A recent study conducted through Howard University found an increased risk of breast cancer associated with induced abortions among women diagnosed after the age of 50 (Laing *et al.*, 1993).

Cardiovascular Disease

The use of smokeless tobacco has increased in recent years (Consensus Conference, 1986). The use of smokeless tobacco entails considerable exposure to nicotine (Benowitz, Porchet, Sheiner, and Jacob, 1988; Gritz *et al.*, 1981), and nicotine may increase the risk of atherosclerotic vascular disease (Benowitz, 1991). One recent study found that although the use of smokeless tobacco was more common among whites than blacks, it was also of concern among blacks, and its use appears to have a modest effect on cardiovascular risk factors among young healthy men (Siegel *et al.*, 1992).

Sickle Cell Anemia

Sickle cell anemia is a disorder that is associated with a reduced life span of the red blood cell and vaso-occlusive events. The disorder is caused by a mutation in the β-hemoglobin gene (Steinberg, 1995). Heterozygous carriers have been found to have a survival advantage with respect to *Plasmodium falciparum* malaria (Embury, Hebbel, Mohandas, and Steinberg, 1994). Manifestations of homozygous sickle cell disease include dactylitis in children, painful crisis, hip disease, osteomyelitis, splenomegaly, chronic hypersplenism, acute chest syndrome, bone marrow embolism, and stroke (Serjeant, 1993). Oral manifestations include neuropathic infarction of the mandible (Taylor, Nowak, Giller, and Casamassimo, 1995). Sickle cell disease is diagnosed through hemoglobin electrophoresis or, if done prenatally, amniocentesis or fetoscopy (Alter, 1979; Burdick, 1994).

Hypertension

African-Americans experience a higher incidence of hypertension than do individuals classified as white (Hypertension Detection and Follow-up Program Cooperative Group, 1977). African-Americans also suffer higher mortality rates from heart disease, stroke, and hypertension–related heart disease compared to whites (Jamerson and DeQuattro, 1996). Renal failure associated with hypertension is also more frequent in African-Americans than in whites (U.S. Renal Data System, 1989). These differences have been attributed, at least in part, to the influence of socioeconomic status and "John Henryism" (James *et al.*, 1992). John Henryism has been defined as

> a strong behavioral predisposition to cope in an active, effortful manner with the psycho-social stressors of everyday life.... Persons manifesting the John Henryism coping style believe that daily stressors ... can be effectively managed (and high levels of psychological stress thus avoided) if they work hard and are determined to succeed. (James *et al.*, 1992:59)

Additional risk factors include older age, greater body mass index, lower educational attainment (Adams-Campbell, Brambilla, and McKinlay, 1993; Gillum, 1996), dietary patterns, and exercise habits (Williams, 1992).

Gender and racial discrimination have also been implicated in the development of hypertension among African-Americans. A recent study found that black women are more likely than white women to respond to unfair treatment by remaining silent. Black women who adopted silence as a coping mechanism were more likely to develop high blood pressure than those black women who talked to others and took action in response to such treatment (Krieger, 1990).

The increased incidence of hypertension among African-Americans has also been attributed to the effects of slavery. This explanation actually takes three forms, all of which have been subject to dispute (Curtin, 1992):

> The first hypothesis, which concerns the ancestral experience in Africa, emphasizes the possible genetic consequences of a low-salt diet over many centuries. In the second, which concerns genetic changes caused by the trauma of the ocean passage from Africa to America during the slave trade, the case is made that individuals who were losing salt from sweat, diarrhetic stools, and vomit were more likely to survive if they already had an ability to conserve salt. This ability, which had survival value in the slave trade, would be passed on to their children and would later cause hypertension and death in the African American community. For the third hypothesis, which concerns the genetic consequences of life under

slavery, the argument is less precise, but it holds that bad conditions caused high death rates and hence genetic change among the survivors. (Curtin, 1992:1681–1682)

Adherence to treatment regimens for hypertension has been found to be poor. This lack of adherence may be due, at least in part, to varying explanatory models of illness. For example, some African-Americans have been found to distinguish between "hypertension," which is considered a blood disease caused by hereditary and dietary factors and treatable through antihypertensive drugs and dietary control, and "high pertension," which is believed to be a disease of the nerves whose course is often unpredictable and untreatable. Adherence to a treatment regimen has been found to be significantly greater where "hypertension," rather than "high pertension," is at issue (Heurtin-Roberts, 1993; Heurtin-Roberts and Reisin, 1992).

Intentional Injury

Intentional injury has become an issue of increasing concern in African-American communities (Schneider, Greenberg, and Choi, 1992). The murder rate among African-American adolescents between the ages of 16 and 19 is 54.3 per 100,000, compared with 8.7 per 100,000 among whites (Bureau of Justice Statistics, 1990). Homicide has become the leading cause of death for black males ages 15 through 19 and occurs at a significantly higher rate among young black males and females compared to whites of the same age group and sex (DuRant *et al.*, 1994). A study in Philadelphia of 46,260 injury events recorded through emergency department records for African-Americans during a 4-year period found that intentional interpersonal incidents accounted for 32.2% of the hospital admissions and 42.7% of the deaths (Schwarz *et al.*, 1994). In a survey of 246 inner-city youth, who were predominantly black, 44% of the respondents reported that they could obtain a gun within one day, 42% reported that they had seen someone shot or knifed, and 22% had seen someone killed (Schubiner, Scott, and Tzelepis, 1993). During the preceding three months, 18% of the students reported having carried a gun and 32% had been in a physical fight. Although one study found that African-American adults believe that guns are too easy to obtain and that there would be less crime and fewer in-home accidents if the sale of handguns were banned, it was also found that the majority of individuals surveyed believed that having a gun at home would protect them (Price *et al.*, 1994).

Numerous factors have been associated with the self-reported use of violence, including exposure to violence, personal victimization, hopelessness, depression, family conflict, previous corporal punishment, purpose in life, self-assessment of the probability of being alive at the age of 25 (DuRant *et al.*, 1994), older age, male sex, and weapon-carrying behavior (Cotten *et al.*, 1994). Drug trafficking has also been found to be associated with the use of or victimization by violence (Stanton and Galbraith, 1994). Exposure to violence and being victimized by violence have been associated with the development of posttraumatic stress disorder (PTSD) (Fitzpatrick and Boldizar, 1993; Weisman, 1993) in addition to physical injury (Bureau of Justice Statistics, 1986, 1991).

Exercises

1. It has often been stated that good science is incompatible with bad ethics. This statement is based on the premise that obviously immoral conduct cannot generate useful or valid scientific findings and, additionally, the research findings resulting from immoral conduct

should not be admitted into the body of scientific knowledge, such as that which occurs through publication in professional journals. Yet, the findings from the Tuskegee study continue to be cited in authoritative works pertaining to syphilis (Caplan, 1992). Discuss the ethical, scientific, and political implications of our continued reliance on the Tuskegee findings.

2. The "slave trade deficit" posits that African-Americans are experiencing lower levels of health than are other Americans due to the cumulative effects of the conditions that they experienced during and immediately following the era of the slave trade.

   a. Do you agree with this hypothesis? Substantiate your answer by exploring, in detail, how African-American susceptibility to a specific disease or excess rates of a specific disease supports/does not support this hypothesis. (You choose the disease.)

   b. Using the disease that you chose in (a) above, design a study to test the hypothesis that the slave experience is associated with excess rates/excess risk of the disease. Include in your response a discussion of the study design, the population to be sampled, inclusion and exclusion criteria, potential confounders and effect modifiers, and potential sources of bias, including measurement issues.

   c. As an expert in health, a federal legislator has consulted you for your opinion regarding a particular issue that has arisen among his constituents. Various African-American groups have asserted that the federal government should pay out sums to African-Americans as reparation for the time that their relatives in previous generations spent in slavery and for the resulting health effects that they and their communities are experiencing. What opinion do you have for the legislator, acting in your capacity as an epidemiologist? Support your response with specific examples.

References

Adams-Campbell, L.L., Brambilla, D.J., & McKinlay, S.M. (1993). Correlates of the prevalence of self-reported hypertension among African-American and white women. *Ethnicity and Disease, 3*, 119–125.

Alter, B.P. (1979). Prenatal diagnosis of hemoglobinopathies and other hematologic diseases. *Journal of Pediatrics, 95*, 501–513.

Anonymous. (1965). AMA reaffirms effort to end discrimination. *Journal of the National Medical Association, 57*, 105.

Baquet, C.R., Horm, J.W., Gibbs, T., & Greenwald, P. (1991). Socioeconomic factors and cancer incidence among blacks and whites. *Journal of the National Cancer Institute, 83*, 551–557.

Benowitz, N.L. (1991). Nicotine and cardiovascular disease. In F. Adlhofer & K. Thurau (Eds.), *Effects of Nicotine on Biological Systems* (pp. 579–596). Basel, Switzerland: Birkhauser Verlag.

Benowitz, N.L., Porchet, H., Sheiner, L., & Jacob, P. (1988). Nicotine absorption and cardiovascular effects with smokeless tobacco use: Comparison with cigarettes and nicotine gum. *Clinical Pharmacology and Therapy, 44*, 23–28.

Blassingame, J.W. (1973). *Black New Orleans, 1860–1880*. Chicago, IL: University of Chicago Press.

Blassingame, J.W. (Ed.). (1977). *Slave Testimony: Two Centuries of Letters, Speeches, Interviews, and Autobiographies*. Baton Rouge, LA: Louisiana State University Press.

Blassingame, J.W. (1979). *The Slave Community* (rev. ed.). New York: Oxford University Press.

Blendon, R.J., Aiken, L.H., Freeman, H.E., & Corey, C.R. (1989). Access to medical care for black and white Americans: A matter of continuing concern. *JAMA, 261*, 278–280.

Brandt, A.M. (1985). Racism and research: The case of the Tuskegee syphilis study. In J.W. Leavitt & R.L. Numbers (Eds.), *Sickness and Health in America: Readings in the History of Medicine and Public Health* (pp. 331–343). Madison, WI: University of Wisconsin Press.

Burack, R.C., Gimotty, P.A., Stengle, W., Warbasse, L., & Moncrease, A. (1993). Patterns of use of mammography among inner-city Detroit women: Contrasts between a health department, HMO, and private hospital. *Medical Care, 31*, 322–334.

Burdick, E. (1994). Sickle cell disease: Still a management challenge. *Postgraduate Medicine, 96*, 107–115.

Bureau of Justice Statistics. (1986). *Teenage Victims: A National Crime Survey Report*. Washington, DC: United States Department of Justice.

Bureau of Justice Statistics. (1990). *Black Victims*. Washington, DC: United States Department of Justice.

Bureau of Justice Statistics. (1991). *Criminal Victimization in the United States, 1989*. Washington, DC: United States Department of Justice.

Butkus, D.E. (1991). Primary renal cadaveric allograft survival in blacks—Is there still a significant difference? In P.J. Morris & N.L. Tilney (Eds.), *Transplantation Reviews*, (Vol. 5, pp. 91–99). Philadelphia: W.B. Saunders.

Butkus, D.E., Maydrech, E.F., & Raju, S.S. (1992). Racial differences in the survival of cadaveric renal allografts: Overriding effects of HLA matching and socioeconomic factors. *New England Journal of Medicine, 327*, 840–845.

Byrd, W.M., & Clayton L.A. (1992). An American health dilemma: A history of blacks in the health system. *Journal of the National Medical Association, 84*, 189–200.

Caplan, A.L. (1992). When evil intrudes. *Hastings Center Report, 22*, 29–32.

Carlisle, D.M., Leake, B.D., & Shapiro, M.F. (1995). Racial and ethnic differences in the use of invasive cardiac procedures among cardiac patients in Los Angeles County, 1986 through 1988. *American Journal of Public Health, 85*, 352–356.

Charatz-Litt, C. (1992). A chronicle of racism: The effects of the white medical community on black health. *Journal of the National Medical Association, 84*, 717–725.

Chu, J., Smart, C.R., & Karone, E. (1988). Analysis of breast cancer mortality and stage distribution by age (for the Health Insurance Plan Clinical Trial). *Journal of the National Cancer Institute, 80*, 1125–1132.

Chu, S., Buehler, J., & Berkelman, R. (1990). Impact of the human immunodeficiency virus epidemic on mortality in women of reproductive age, United States. *JAMA, 264*, 225–229.

Clark, E.G., & Danbolt, N. (1955). The Oslo study of the natural history of untreated syphilis. *Journal of Chronic Disease, 2*, 311–344.

Consensus Conference. (1986). Health applications of smokeless tobacco. *JAMA, 255*, 1045–1048.

Cooper, R.S. (1984). A note on the biologic concept of race and its application to epidemiologic research. *American Heart Journal, 108*, 715–723.

Cooper, R.S., & David, R.J. (1986). The biological concept of race and its application to public health and epidemiology. *Journal of Health, Politics, Policy, & Law, 11*, 97–116.

Cooper, R.S., Steinhauer, M., Miller, W., David, R., & Schatzkin, A. (1981). Racism, society, and disease: An exploration of the social and biological mechanisms of differential mortality. *International Journal of Health Services, 11*, 389–414.

Cotten, N.U., Resnick, J., Browne, D.C., Martin, S.L., McCarraher, D.R., & Woods, J. (1994). Aggression and fighting behavior among African-American adolescents: Individual and family factors. *American Journal of Public Health, 84*, 618–622.

Council on Ethical and Judicial Affairs, American Medical Association. Black-white disparities in health care. *JAMA, 263*, 2344–2346.

Curtin, P.D. (1992). The slavery hypothesis for hypertension among African Americans: The historical evidence. *American Journal of Public Health, 82*, 1681–1686.

David, R.J., & Collins, J.W., Jr. (1991). Bad outcomes in black babies: Race or racism? *Ethnicity and Disease, 1*, 236–244.

Dawson, D.A., & Thompson, G.B. (1989). Breast cancer risk factors and screening: United States, 1987. *Vital Health Statistics, 10*, 1–60.

Deibert, A.V., & Bruyere, M.C. (1946). Untreated syphilis in the male Negro. III. Evidence of cardiovascular abnormalities and other forms of morbidity. *Journal of Venereal Disease Information, 27*, 301–314.

Douglass, F. (1968). *Narrative of the Life of Frederick Douglass, An American Slave, Written by Himself*. New York: New American Library. (Original work published 1845)

DuRant, R.H., Cadenhead, C., Pendergrast, R.A., Slavens, G., & Linder, C.W. (1994). Factor associated with the use of violence among urban black adolescents. *American Journal of Public Health, 84*, 612–617.

Eley, J.W., Hill, H.A., Chen, V.W., Austin, D.F., Wesley, M.N., Muss, H.B., Greenberg, R.S., Coates, R.J., Correa, P., Redmond, C.K., Hunter, C.P., Herman, A.A., Kurman, R., Blacklow, R., Shapiro, S., & Edwards, B.K. (1994). Racial differences in survival from breast cancer: Results of the National Cancer Institute black/white cancer survival study. *JAMA, 272*, 947–954.

Embury, S.H., Hebbel, R.P., Mohandas, N., & Steinberg, M.H. (1994). *Sickle Cell Disease: Basic Principles and Clinical Practice*. New York: Raven Press.

Fitzpatrick, K.M., & Boldizar, J.P. (1993). The prevalence and consequences of exposure to violence among African-American youth. *Journal of the Academy of Child and Adolescent Psychiatry, 32*, 424–430.

Ford, E., Cooper, R., Castaner, A., Simmons, B., & Mar, M. (1989). Coronary arteriography and coronary bypass surgery among whites and other racial groups relative to hospital-based incidence rates for coronary artery disease: Findings from NHDS. *American Journal of Public Health, 79*, 347–440.

Gill, D.G. (1932). Syphilis in the rural Negro: Results of a study in Alabama. *Southern Medical Journal, 25*, 985–990.

Gillum, R.F. (1996). Epidemiology of hypertension in African American women. *American Heart Journal, 131*, 385–395.

Gonwa, T.A., Morris, C.A., Mai, M.L., Husberg, B.S., Goldstein, R.M., & Klintmalm, G.D. (1991). Race and liver transplantation. *Archives of Surgery, 12*, 1141–1143.

Gritz, E.R., Baer-Weiss, V., Benowitz, N.L., Van Vunakis, H., & Jarvik, M.E. (1981). Plasma nicotine and cotinine concentrations in habitual smokeless tobacco users. *Clinical Pharmacology and Therapy, 30*, 201–209.

Haller, J.S. (1971). *Outcasts from Evolution: Scientific Attitudes of Racial Inferiority*. New York: McGraw-Hill.

Hannan, E.L., Kilburn, H., O'Donnell, J.F., Lukacik, G., & Shields, E.P. (1991). Interracial access to selected cardiac procedures for patients hospitalized with coronary artery disease in New York State. *Medical Care, 29*, 430–441.

Harwood, A. (Ed.). (1981). *Ethnicity and Medical Care*. Cambridge, MA: Harvard University Press.

Hazen, H.H. (1914). Syphilis in the American Negro. *JAMA, 63*, 463–466.

Heller, J.R., Jr., & Bruyere, P.T. (1946). Untreated syphilis in the male Negro. II. Mortality during 12 years of observation. *Journal of Venereal Disease Information, 27*, 34–38.

Heurtin-Roberts, S. (1993). "High pertension"—The uses of a chronic folk illness for personal adaptation. *Social Science and Medicine, 37*, 285–294.

Heurtin-Roberts, S., & Reisin, E. (1992). The relation of culturally influenced lay models of hypertension to compliance with treatment. *American Journal of Hypertension, 5*, 787–792.

Howard, W.L. (1903). The Negro as a distinct ethnic factor in civilization. *Medicine (Detroit), 9*, 424.

Hurmence, B. (Ed.). (1984). *My Folks Don't Want Me to Talk About Slavery: Twenty-One Oral Histories of Former North Carolina Slaves*. Winston-Salem, NC: John F. Blair.

Hypertension Detection and Follow-up Program Cooperative Group. (1977). Race, education and prevalence of hypertension. *American Journal of Epidemiology, 106*, 351–361.

Jacobs, H. (1988). *Incidents in the Life of a Slave Girl*. New York: Oxford University Press.

Jamerson, K., & DeQuattro, V. (1996). The impact of ethnicity on response to antihypertensive therapy. *American Journal of Medicine, 101(suppl. 3A)*, 22S–32S.

James, S.A., Keenan, N.L., Strogatz, D.S., Browning, S.R., & Garrett, J.M. (1992). Socioeconomic status, John Henryism, and blood pressure in black adults: The Pitt County study. *American Journal of Epidemiology, 135*, 59–67.

Johnson, C.S. (1966). *Shadow of the Plantation*. Chicago: University of Chicago Press.

Jones, J. (1981). *Bad Blood: The Tuskegee Syphilis Experiment—A Tragedy of Race and Medicine*. New York: Free Press.

Jones, J.J. (1992). The Tuskegee legacy: AIDS and the black community. *Hastings Center Report, 22*, 38–40.

Kampmeier, R.H. (1974). Final report on the "Tuskegee syphilis study." *Southern Medical Journal, 67*, 1349–1353.

Klebanoff, M.A., Shiono, P.H., Berendez, H.W., & Rhoads, G.G. (1989). Facts and artifacts about anemia and preterm delivery. *JAMA, 262*, 511–515.

Klebanoff, M.A., Shiono, P.H., Shelby, J.V., Trachtenberg, A.I., & Graubard, B.I. (1991). Anemia and spontaneous preterm birth. *American Journal of Obstetrics and Gynecology, 164*, 59–63.

Kolchin, P. (1993). *American Slavery 1619–1877*. New York: Hill and Wang.

Krieger, N. (1990). Racial and gender discrimination: Risk factors for high blood pressure? *Social Science and Medicine, 30*, 1273–1281.

Laing, A.E., Demenais, F.M., Williams, R., Kissling, G., Chen, V.W., & Bonney, G.E. (1993). Breast cancer risk factors in African-American women: The Howard University tumor registry experience. *Journal of the National Medical Association, 85*, 931– 939.

Lee, A.S., & Lee, E.S. (1977). The health of slaves and the health of freedmen: A Savannah study. *Phylon, 38*, 170–180.

Lieben, R.W. (1977). The field of medical anthropology. In D. Lundy (Ed.), *Culture, Disease, and Healing* (pp. 13–31). New York: Macmillan Publishing Company.

Mahoney, J., Arnold, R.C., Sterner, B.L., Harris, A., & Zwally, M.R. (1944). Penicillin treatment of early syphilis. II. *JAMA, 126*, 63–67.

Massey, D.S. (1990). American apartheid: Segregation and the making of the underclass. *American Journal of Sociology, 96*, 329–357.

McCord, C., & Freeman, H.P. (1990). Excess mortality in Harlem. *New England Journal of Medicine, 322*, 173–177.

Mickey, R.M., Durski, J., Worden, J.K., & Danigelis, N.L. (1995). Breast cancer screening and associated factors for low-income African-American women. *Preventive Medicine, 24*, 467–476.

Moore, J.E. (1933). *The Modern Treatment of Syphilis*. Baltimore: Charles C. Thomas.

Morais, H.M. (1967). *The History of the Negro in Medicine* (2nd ed.). New York: Publishers Co., Inc.

National Cancer Institute. (1995, January) *Annual Cancer Statistics Review*. Bethesda, MD: United States Department of Health and Human Services.

National Center for Health Statistics. (1990). *Breast Cancer Risk Factors and Screening: United States, 1987* [Vital Health Statistics, Series 10, No. 172].

Neighbors, H.W., & Jackson, J.S. (1987). Barriers to medical care among adult blacks: What happens to the uninsured? *Journal of the National Medical Association, 79*, 489–493.

Noojin, R.O., Callaway, J.L., & Flower, A.H. (1945). Favorable response to penicillin therapy in a case of treatment-resistant syphilis. *North Carolina Medical Journal, January*, 34–37.

Office of AIDS, Department of Health Services. (1992, October) *Epidemiologic Overview of HIV/AIDS Among African-Americans in California*. Sacramento, CA: Author.

Osofsky, G. (1966). *Harlem: The Making of a Ghetto, Negro New York, 1890–1930*. New York: Harper and Row.

Perkoff, G.T., & Anderson, A. (1970). Relationship between demographic characteristics, patient's chief complaint, and medical destination in an emergency room. *Medical Care, 8*, 309–323.

Pesare, P.J., Bauer, T.J., & Gleeson, G.A. (1950). Untreated syphilis in the male Negro: Observation of abnormalities over sixteen years. *American Journal of Syphilis, Gonorrhea, and Venereal Diseases, 34*, 201–213.

Price, J.H., Kandakai, T.L., Casler, S., Everett, S., & Smith, D. (1994). African-American adults' perceptions of guns and violence. *Journal of the National Medical Association, 86*, 426–432.

Quillian, D.D. (1906). Racial peculiarities: A cause of the prevalence of syphilis in Negroes. *American Journal of Dermatology & Genito-Urinary Disease, 10*, 277–279.

Reed, W.L. (1990). Racism and health: The case of black infant mortality. In P. Conrad & R. Kern. (Eds.), *The Sociology of Health and Illness* (3rd ed., pp. 34–44). New York: St. Martin's Press.

Ries, L.A.G., Hanket, B.F., Miller, B.A., Hartman, A.M., & Edwards, B.K. (1991). *Cancer Statistics Review 1973–1988*. Bethesda, MD: National Cancer Institute [NIH Publ. No. 91-2789].

Rivers, E., Schuman, S.H., Simpson, L., & Olansky, S. (1953). Twenty years of followup experience in a long-range medical study. *Public Health Reports, 68*, 391–395.

Roberts, M.H. (1925). The spinal fluid in the newborn. JAMA, *85*, 500–503.

Satariano, W., Belle, S., & Swanson, M. (1986). The severity of breast cancer at diagnosis: A comparison of age and extent of disease in black and white women. *American Journal of Public Health, 76*, 779–782.

Savitt, T.L. (1978). *Medicine and Slavery: The Diseases and Health Care of Blacks in Antebellum Virginia*. Chicago: University of Illinois Press.

Savitt, T.L. (1985). Black health on the plantation: Masters, slaves, and physicians. In J.W. Leavitt & R.L. Numbers (Eds.), *Sickness and Health in America: Readings in the History of Medicine and Public Health* (2nd. ed. rev., pp. 313–330). Madison, WI: University of Wisconsin Press.

Schneider, D., Greenberg, M.R., & Choi, D. (1992). Violence as a public health priority for black Americans. *Journal of the National Medical Association, 84*, 843–848.

Schubiner, H., Scott, R., & Tzelepis, A. (1993). Exposure to violence among inner-city youth. *Journal of Adolescent Health, 14*, 214–219.

Schwartz, D.F., Grisso, J.A., Miles, C.G., Holmes, J.H., Wishner, A.R., & Sutton, R.L. (1994). A longitudinal study of injury morbidity in an African-American population. JAMA, *271*, 755–760.

Scott, W.K., Sy, F.S., Jackson, K.L., Macera, C.A., & Harris, N.S. (1997). Survival after AIDS diagnosis in South Carolina, 1982–1992. *The Journal of the South Carolina Medical Association, 93*, 5–12.

Seham, M. (1964). Discrimination against Negroes in hospitals. *New England Journal of Medicine, 271*, 940–943.

Seidman, H., Gelb, S.K., Silverberg, E., La Verda, N., & Lubera, J.A. (1987). Survival experience in the breast cancer detection demonstration project. *Cancer Journal for Clinicians, 37*, 258–290.

Semmes, C.E. (1996). *Racism, Health, and Post-Industrialism: A Theory of African-American Health*. Westport, CT: Praeger.

Serjeant, G.R. (1993). The clinical features of sickle cell disease. *Bailliere's Clinical Haematology, 6*, 93–115.

Shapiro, S., Venet, W., Strax, P., Venet, L., & Roeser, R. (1982). Prospects for eliminating racial differences in breast cancer survival rates. *American Journal of Public Health, 72*, 1142–1145.

Siegel, D., Benowitz, N., Ernster, V., Grady, D.G., & Hauck, W.W. (1992). Smokeless tobacco, cardiovascular risk factors, and nicotine and cotinine levels in professional baseball players. *American Journal of Public Health, 82*, 417–421.

Sims, J.M. (1894). *The Story of My Life*. New York: D. Appleton.

Smith, V. (1988). Introduction. In H. Jacobs, *Incidents in the Life of a Slave Girl* (pp. xxvii–xl). New York: Oxford University Press.

Spector, R.E. (1979). *Cultural Diversity in Health and Illness*. New York: Appleton-Century Crafts.

Stampp, M. (1956). *The Peculiar Institution: Slavery in the Ante-Bellum South*. New York: Vintage Books.

Stanton, B., & Galbraith, J. (1994). Drug trafficking among African-American early adolescents: Prevalence, consequences, and associated behaviors and beliefs. *Pediatrics, 1993,* 1039–1043.

Steinberg, M.H. (1995). Genetic modulation of sickle cell anemia. *Proceedings of the Society for Experimental Biology and Medicine, 209,* 1–13.

Taylor, L.B., Nowak, A.J., Giller, R.H., & Casamassimo, P.S. (1995). Sickle cell anemia: A review of the dental concerns and a retrospective study of dental and bony changes. *Special Care in Dentistry, 15,* 38–42.

Thomas, S.B., & Quinn, S.C. (1991). The Tuskegee syphilis study, 1932 to 1972: Implications for HIV education and AIDS risk education programs in the black community. *American Journal of Public Health, 81,* 1498–1504.

Tipton, F. (1886). The Negro problem from a medical standpoint. *The New York Medical Journal,* 569–572. Cited in C. Charatz-Litt. (1992). A chronicle of racism: The effects of the white medical community on black health. *Journal of the National Medical Association, 84,* 717–725.

Tyroler, H.A. (1990). Socioeconomic status, age, and sex in the prevalence and prognosis of hypertension in blacks. In J.H. Laragh & B.M. Brenner (Eds.), *Hypertension: Pathophysiology, Diagnosis and Management* (pp. 159–174). New York: Raven Press.

United States Department of Health and Human Services. (1991). *Health, United States, 1991.* Hyattsville, MD: Author [Publ. No. PHS 92-1237].

U.S. Renal Data System. (1989). *USRDS 1989 Annual Report.* Bethesda, MD: National Institutes of Health.

Van Evrie, J.H. (1861). *Negroes and Negro "Slavery,"* New York.

Vonderlehr, R.A., Clark, T., Wenger, O.C., & Heller, J.R., Jr. (1936). Untreated syphilis in the male Negro. A comparative study of treated and untreated cases. *Venereal Disease Information, 17,* 260–265.

Weisman, G.K. (1993). Adolescent PTSD and developmental consequences of crack dealing. *American Journal of Orthopsychiatry, 63,* 553–561.

Wenneker, M.B., & Epstein, A.M. (1989). Racial inequalities in the use of procedures for patients with ischemic heart disease in Massachusetts. *JAMA, 261,* 253–257.

Whitman, S., Ansell, D., Lacey, L., Chen, E.H., Ebie, N., Dell, J., & Phillips, C.W. (1991). Patterns of breast and cervical cancer screening at three public health centers in an inner-city urban area. *American Journal of Public Health, 81,* 1651–1653.

Whittle, J., Conigliaro, J., Good, C.B., & Lofgren, R.P. (1993). Racial differences in the use of invasive cardiovascular procedures in the Department of Veterans Affairs medical system. *New England Journal of Medicine, 329,* 621–627.

Williams, D.R. (1992). Black–white differences in blood pressure: The role of social factors. *Ethnicity and Disease, 2,* 126–141.

Yergan J., Flood, A.B., LoGerfo, J.P., & Diehr, P. (1987). Relationship between patient race and the intensity of hospital services. *Medical Care, 25,* 592–602.

Woodson, C.G. (1969). *A Century of Negro Migration.* New York: Russell and Russell.

7

Asian and Pacific Islander Health

Introduction

Although Asians and Pacific Islanders, as defined by the U.S. census, constitute only 3% of the U.S. population, they are the fastest-growing minority group in the United States (1990 Census in Lum, 1995; Takaki, 1989). This growth is due to several factors, including the passage and implementation of the Immigration Act of 1965, which removed provisions excluding Asians from entry into the United States, and the influx of refugees from Southeast Asia beginning in 1975 (Burr and Mutchler, 1993; Lin-Fu, 1988; McKenney and Bennett, 1994; Takaki, 1989).

The Asian and Pacific Islander population of the United States is extremely diverse, encompassing at last count 29 different Asian groups and 20 different Pacific Islander groups, which together speak more than 100 languages (Loue, Lloyd, and Loh, 1996). According to the 1980 census, six subgroups accounted for more than 95% of the Asian Pacific Islander population: Chinese, Filipino, Japanese, Asian Indian, Korean, and Vietnamese (Lin-Fu, 1988).

The Asian and Pacific Islander population is equally diverse with respect to socio-economic status, migration patterns, access to health care, and risk for specific diseases; these factors are interrelated. For example, as a group, Japanese-Americans tend to be more highly acculturated and of higher socioeconomic status. This is not surprising, in view of their migration to the United States since the late 19th century. In contrast, recent arrivals from Southeast Asia tend to be poor and less acculturated, and face increased barriers to health care, such as language (Takada, Ford, and Lloyd, 1998). Southeast Asian refugees may have also suffered higher levels of stress and trauma in migration, which may, in turn, affect their health.

As a group, Asians and Pacific Islanders appear to have few health problems and to be well insured for health care (Mayeno and Hirota, 1994; Smith and Ryan, 1987). Unfortunately, these aggregated data mask the large variation within the Asian and Pacific Islander population. The 1980 census, for example, indicated that 7.5% of all Asian-Americans have an annual family income over $50,000 (Mayeno and Hirota, 1994). However, Asian-Americans also had the highest proportion of unrelated persons (individuals not living in the same household) with yearly incomes below $2,000 (Mayeno and Hirota, 1994). A San Diego survey of Asian Americans found that 75.8% lived below the poverty level, while 53% of the Vietnamese in a San Francisco Bay area survey reported incomes below the federal poverty level (Mayeno and Hirota, 1994).

Many Asians and Pacific Islanders work in low-wage jobs, such as factory and service industry positions, which often do not provide either employer-sponsored health insurance or sufficient resources to permit the employees to purchase health insurance. A recent study in Boston's Chinatown found that 61% of the employed uninsured earned less than $10,000 per year (Mayeno and Hirota, 1994). Studies conducted in California and Chicago have similarly found that high proportions of some Asian-American groups lacked health insurance (Mayeno and Hirota, 1994).

Cultural and Historical Context

Language and Acculturation

Language may constitute a significant barrier to care. Limited reading skills in both one's native language and in English may reduce one's ability to read and understand signs in health care facilities, paperwork and informational materials, as well as provider instructions (Mayeno and Hirota, 1994). A study conducted in San Diego in 1988 found that 60% of the individuals surveyed attributed difficulty in obtaining health care to language (Mayeno and Hirota, 1994).

Levels of acculturation differ not only between individuals but across groups as well. Individuals who acculturate better to U.S. society tend to rely to a greater degree on Western medicine. Groups and individuals who do not acculturate are more likely to rely on alternative explanatory models of health and illness and, consequently, more traditional methods of care. For example, many Southeast Asians view health as a state of equilibrium or balance with disease and illness resulting from disequilibrium or an imbalance of specific forces or elements (Jenkins, Le, McPhee, and Stewart, 1996; Miller, 1995; Shimada, Jackson, Goldstein, and Buchwald, 1995; Uba, 1992), often treatable with herbal medicines (Jenkins *et al.*, 1996). The lack of health professionals who understand the cultural context of Asians and Pacific Islanders may interact with the difficulties in communication due to language differences to further compound the problems faced in accessing care (Takada, Ford, and Lloyd, 1998).

Explanatory Models of Health and Illness

An understanding of culture-specific explanatory models for health and illness is critical to understanding how individuals interpret and respond to illness episodes. These conceptualizations of health and illness, which differ from the Western medical perspective, may influence individuals' willingness to seek care and to adhere to the medical recommendations that they receive.

Numerous studies of health beliefs among Southeast Asians have often failed to distinguish between these cultural groups (e.g., Thai, Lao, Cambodian, etc.). Not infrequently, researchers have failed to specify which Southeast Asian groups are being discussed, making cross-study comparisons difficult.

Mattson (1995) has identified three categories of illness causation common to many Southeast Asians: (1) physical causes, such as accidents or spoiled food; (2) metaphysical causes, such as an imbalance of *yin* and *yang*, of hot and cold energy, of diet, or of emotions; and (3) supernatural causes, such as evil spirits or soul loss. Disease results from imbalance and disharmony, and illness is attributed to deficiencies or excesses of physical, spiritual, or natural elements. These beliefs affect individuals' health-seeking behaviors and utilization of services.

For instance, Mattson (1995) notes that many Southeast Asian women will avoid pelvic examinations because they believe that dilation of the vagina with a speculum will expose the woman to wind and result in the loss of heat and the influx of cold. In situations in which an illness is believed to have been brought about by an imbalance of *yin* and *yang*, individuals are more likely to self-medicate with herbs than to seek out a traditional or religious healer or Western health care provider (Uba, 1992).

The Mien, a Southeast Asian hill people, originally migrated from China to various parts of Southeast Asia in the 13th century. Although they have continued to live predominantly in Thailand and in Laos, Mien began emigrating to various countries in the mid-1970s (Moore and Boehnlein, 1991). The Mien believe that illness may result from environmental exposures, such as dampness, inadequate food, or germs. Such illnesses can be cured by using herbal remedies or by modifying the environmental factors. An illness that does not respond to such treatment is thought to be a disorder of the spirit world, such as soul loss, requiring treatment by a shaman. Regardless of the postulated cause of the illness, emotional distress tends to be expressed through the verbalization of somatic symptoms (Moore and Boehnlein, 1991). This manner of expressing emotional distress has been noted among other Asian groups as well.

The Hmong, another hill tribe of Southeast Asia, emigrated from China into Vietnam, Laos, Thailand, and Myanmar (Quincy, 1988). The Central Intelligence Agency (CIA) of the United States began recruiting Hmong assistance for the "secret army" beginning in 1962. This effort and the subsequent series of events resulted in Hmong resettlement in the United States. Capps (1994) has examined the impact of migration to the United States on the Hmong traditional health and illness beliefs, one of the few studies to concern itself with modifications to health beliefs following migration from a developing to a developed nation.

Capps found that many Hmong converted to Christianity and abandoned animistic practices following relocation to Kansas City. Although Hmong individuals frequently continued to attribute illness to a "traditional" cause, such as sorcery or ancestral spirits' removal of their protection of individuals in response to improper behavior, individuals refused to consult a shaman for healing because of fear that they would be ostracized from the now-converted Hmong community. Interestingly, consultation with a shaman has been replaced by prayer.

Fright illness (*ceeb*) continues to be a common illness among Hmong immigrants. This syndrome results from immersion in cold water, a car accident, or other unexpected and similarly startling events. *Ceeb* is believed to tighten the veins, resulting in a reduced flow of blood and cold extremities. The Kansas City Hmong no longer treat *ceeb* with soul-calling rituals, but rely instead on massage and prayer (Capps, 1994).

Koucharang, believed by Cambodians to be the result of turbulent emotions or of "thinking too much," is characterized by intrusive thoughts, headaches, and suicidal ideation. It is not, however, perceived to be a kind of mental illness. The syndrome has most often been noted among Cambodians exposed to severe violence in their home countries and has been documented among Cambodian refugees in California and Massachusetts (Frye and D'Avanzo, 1994b). Because it is not perceived as a mental disorder, individuals suffering from *koucharang* are unlikely to seek out either counseling or medical services.

Chinese, including Chinese in the United States, have been found to have five basic explanations for disease causation: wind, which is thought to enter the body when it is in an especially vulnerable state; an imbalance of hot and cold; poison; blockages of *ch'i*, the energy force; and fright. Gould-Martin and Ngin (1981) have found that Chinese Americans are often able to reconcile the popular Chinese explanation for specific illnesses with the popular Western explanation, such as wind as a cause of illness (Chinese) and wind-borne dust as a cause of illness (Western).

Many East Indians subscribe to the precepts of Ayurvedic medicine. A detailed review of Ayurvedic principles is beyond the scope of this chapter. Briefly, Ayurveda enumerates five elements in the universe: water, fire, earth, wind, and ether. Fire, water, and wind constitute the three humors found in the body as bile, phlegm, and wind, respectively. An imbalance in these humors results in illness, whereas homeostasis maintains health. Humoral equilibrium can be lost due to the consumption of foods that are inappropriately "hot" or "cold," that is, the nature of the food is such that it increases or decreases the heat in the body (Ramakrishna and Weiss, 1992). This emphasis on diet may affect patient expectations of the patient–provider relationship in that patients may expect physicians to conduct not only a complete examination and history, but also a complete dietary history (Ramakrishna and Weiss, 1992).

Expectations and values are not governed by tradition alone; they are also subject to other influences. Many patients may believe, for example, that capsules are stronger than tablets and that injections are superior to all other forms of treatment (Ramakrishna and Weiss, 1992). Such beliefs affect patients' willingness to seek out care, the acceptability of the care received, and willingness to adhere to medical recommendations (Shimada *et al.*, 1995).

Historical Context

The migration experience of Asians and Pacific Islanders clearly differs between individuals and between specific groups; broad generalizations are, therefore, suspect. Also, the large number of subgroups classified as Asian and Pacific Islander renders impossible an examination of the migration experience and historical context of each group. This section presents a brief overview of three Asian and Pacific Islander subgroups. We must ask ourselves whether and how the migration experience of these populations relates to their current health and health care and the potential implications for health research.

Chinese Americans

Early Chinese migrants to the United States often came as laborers, intending to work temporarily in this country and to return home with their earnings. During the latter half of the 19th century, approximately 46,000 Chinese migrated to Hawaii, and 380,000 migrated to the U.S. mainland between 1849 and 1930 (Takaki, 1989). Many of these individuals sought refuge from ongoing conflict, including the British Opium Wars (1839–1842, 1856–1864) and peasant rebellions such as the Red Turban Rebellion (1854–1864), and from harsh economic conditions. The typical immigrant of this period was male, married, and generally unaccompanied by his wife and family due to the expense and, in the mainland United States, to legislation restricting the entry of Chinese women (Osumi, 1982; Peffer, 1986; Wu, 1972).

The Chinese lived predominantly in rural areas for several decades, many of them settling in California and other areas in the West (Takaki, 1989). Gradually, the Chinese became an urban population, representing a wide range of socioeconomic statuses (Cao and Novas, 1996).

Initially, Chinese were employed in California as workers in the gold fields, in railroad construction, and in manufacturing (Cao and Novas, 1996). By the late 1860s, Chinese workers in San Francisco constituted almost half of those employed in four major occupations: boots and shoe manufacturing, woolens, tobacco farming, and sewing (Takaki, 1989). The Chinese population also became increasingly active in agriculture, primarily as laborers (Cao and Novas, 1996). However, the growing "ethnic antagonism" (Takaki, 1989:92) that confronted the Chinese in mines, fields, and factories ultimately propelled them into self-employment situations, often in laundry, retail, or restaurants.

In the South, Chinese laborers were seen as role models for black workers due to their hard work and sense of economy. In the Northeast, the Chinese population often worked in factories. Women were often employed as housekeepers, servants, cooks, miners, seamstresses, and laundresses. And, in a world dominated by men, many women were employed as prostitutes. Many of these women were treated as slaves and not infrequently became addicted to opium (Takaki, 1989).

Despite the growing reliance on the Chinese workforce in the late 1800s and early 1900s, the Chinese remained an "internal colony" (Takaki, 1989:99), excluded from full participation in what was perceived to be a homogeneous white society. This exclusion was premised on the perception of the Chinese as inferior, undesirable, and a threat to the survival of American society as a result of myriad potent and incurable diseases that they brought with them to the United States ("yellow peril") (Gussow, 1989). Their subordinate position was reinforced through various legal and political mechanisms, including court decisions disregarding the testimony of Chinese witnesses (Heizer and Almquist, 1971), the Chinese Exclusion Act of 1882 (Takaki, 1989), the Geary Act of 1892, which required the registration of all Chinese persons in the United States (Cao and Novas, 1996), the establishment of segregated schools, and political rhetoric (Lyman, 1971).

Although the Chinese were often perceived by others as temporary settlers, many immigrants formed Chinatowns and *fongs*, groupings of village associations. Recreation often took the form of Chinese theater and festivals. Viewed from the outside, Chinatowns were ghettos. In San Francisco's Chinatown in 1934, an average of 20.4 persons shared each bathroom and an average of 12.3 persons shared each kitchen. Over three quarters of Chinatown dwellings were found to be substandard, compared to one fifth of the dwellings in other parts of the city. The rate of tuberculosis was three times higher in Chinatown than in San Francisco's other residential areas (Lee, 1938).

One of the major issues remained the separation of China-born and U.S.-born Chinese from each other. Even as late as 1930, 80% of the U.S. Chinese population was male (Takaki, 1989). Under then-existing immigration laws, those Chinese born in the United States could bring in their overseas-born children, but could not bring in their China-born wives. Some such children came as "paper sons," claiming U.S. citizenship based on forged or purchased identity papers.

Education was seen as a bridge for second-generation Chinese Americans to improve their situation. Second-generation Chinese were often caught between two worlds, uncomfortable with the Chinese language, but denied social and economic opportunities because of their appearance. Second-generation Chinese often found themselves confined to a low-skill job market (Takaki, 1989).

The situation changed significantly with the advent of World War II and the development of animosities between the United States and Germany and Japan. Chinese became friends. Employment opportunities became available to Chinese in the armed services and in the defense industries. The exclusion laws that had been in place to prevent the entry of Chinese into the United States were repealed, and Chinese immigrants were, for the first time, eligible to apply for naturalization as citizens of the United States (Takaki, 1989).

Japanese Americans

At the time the Chinese Exclusion Act of 1882 came into effect, there were just over 2,000 Japanese on the U.S. mainland. Within 40 years, the population reached an estimated 138,834 (Takaki, 1989). By 1930, approximately half of the Japanese population consisted of first-generation immigrants (*Issei*), while the other half comprised second-generation Japanese (*Nisei*). Almost half of the Japanese population resided in California. Many of the immigrants were farmers, merchants, and students, and many were quite well-educated (Spickard, 1996). Many, including the farm laborers and cannery workers, worked under harsh conditions characterized by long hours. Their poor diets not infrequently led to malnutrition and night blindness (Takaki, 1989).

The U.S. Japanese urban economy expanded greatly during the early 1900s. Enterprises, which included barber shops, poolrooms, laundries, hotels, and stores, provided the Japanese community with employment. Other Japanese entered farming on a large scale, obtaining land to farm through contracts, sharing, leasing, or ownership (Spickard, 1996).

The Japanese were often the target of both verbal and physical discrimination. Japanese were seen as competitors and a menace to American labor, so much that labor organizations called for the expansion of the Chinese Exclusion Act to include the Japanese. The California legislature in 1913 passed legislation denying land ownership to "aliens ineligible to citizenship," which included the Japanese (California Statutes, 1913). A 1920 law prohibited these individuals from leasing agricultural land or acquiring it under the names of U.S.-born minor children, a strategy that had been used earlier to avoid the impact of the 1913 land ownership law (Takaki, 1989). The 1921 "Ladies' Agreement" barred the immigration of picture brides and sharply curtailed Japanese immigration to the United States (Kanzaki, 1921). The 1924 general immigration law specifically excluded from entry aliens ineligible to citizenship (i.e., the Japanese).

Numerous other, more personal objections were voiced against the *Issei*. The Japanese were seen as incapable of being good Americans, as "unassimilable ... with great pride of race, [having] no idea of assimilating in the sense of amalgamation" (McClatchy, quoted in Daniels, 1962:99). The Japanese were characterized as filthy individuals whose "nests pollute the communities like the running sores of leprosy" (*American Defender*, quoted in Ogawa, 1971: 13). Japanese men were perceived as sexually aggressive, lusting after white women (*Los Angeles Times*, quoted in Ogawa, 1971:15) and represented new, devious attempts by Japan to take over American territory (Spickard, 1996).

As with the Chinese, education was seen as a way out, a bridge to something better. Despite efforts to acquire higher education, however, *Nisei* were often trapped in the ethnic labor market, often due to racism and discrimination (Spickard, 1996). Numerous strategies were developed in an attempt to overcome these barriers, including the promotion of U.S. nationalism within the Japanese-American community, and the cultivation of an "American" lifestyle (Takaki, 1989).

The Japanese attack on Pearl Harbor during World War II fueled fears of the Japanese and ultimately resulted in the mass internment of Japanese Americans on the mainland United States, but not Hawaii. Japanese, many of them native-born American citizens, were ordered to report to evacuation centers, from which they were transported to one of ten internment camps and housed in barracks and stalls that were often filthy and congested (Commission on Wartime Relocation and Internment of Civilians, 1997; Spickard, 1996; Takaki, 1989). Adults worked as wage earners for the government. It has been estimated that those who were interned suffered approximately $370 million in direct property losses, equivalent to between $1 billion and $3 billion in 1983 dollars, not including lost income and lost opportunities (Taylor, 1986). Despite their treatment by the U.S. government, about 33,000 *Nisei* served in the Armed Forces during the Second World War. It was not until 1988, though, that the U.S. government acknowledged the wrong committed by the internment (Reagan, 1988).

The Filipino Community

Unlike the Chinese and Japanese migrants to the United States, Filipino migrants came to Hawaii and to the mainland United States from what was a U.S. territory. By the mid-1930s, approximately 110,000 Filipinos had migrated to Hawaii; approximately 40,000 had arrived on the mainland. Most were poor and uneducated men, who saw themselves as temporary sojourners (Takaki, 1989).

On the mainland, most Filipinos worked in agriculture, with the remainder employed as service workers or in the Alaska salmon fisheries. Work in the fields entailed long hours, low pay, and often unsatisfactory conditions. Workers were often housed in crowded, flimsy bunkhouses that lacked insulation and sewage disposal. Continuing poor conditions ultimately prompted the Filipino workers in some areas to organize, demonstrate, and win concessions from the growers (Takaki, 1989).

Despite their status as "little brown brothers" in the Philippines, Filipinos encountered intense racial discrimination in the United States. They were often segregated or refused service altogether, prohibited from living in certain areas, and were ineligible to apply for citizenship. The passage of the Tydings McDuffie Act of 1934 granted commonwealth status to the protectorate of the Philippines, and all Filipinos were subsequently reclassified as aliens, rather than nationals, laying the foundation for efforts to deport and repatriate them to their original home (Cao and Novas, 1996). Fears of Filipino sexuality and the resulting threat to white racial purity sparked and fueled racial violence (Takaki, 1989). Anti-miscegenation laws in many states prohibited intermarriage between Filipinos and whites. Those who intermarried often experienced social ostracism (Takaki, 1989).

World War II appears to have been somewhat of a watershed in Americans' perceptions of Filipinos. Filipino loyalty and patriotism prompted revisions to states' land laws that had prohibited the sale or leasing of land to Filipinos, the expansion of immigration provisions to permit the entry of Filipinos, and the revision of the citizenship laws to allow for the eligibility of Filipinos (Takaki, 1989).

Health Status

Infectious Disease

Acquired Immunodeficiency Syndrome

Initially, little attention was focused on HIV/AIDS in the Asian and Pacific Islander populations, due to both the relatively few cases that had been reported in this population and the erroneous belief that Asians and Pacific Islanders might be genetically immune to the infection (Gock, 1994; Lee and Fong, 1990). As of December 1997, a total of 4,589 AIDS cases among Asians and Pacific Islanders had been reported to the Centers for Disease Control and Prevention (CDC). For 1997, Asians and Pacific Islanders had the lowest rate of AIDS cases among all ethnic groups, 4.5 per 100,000 (CDC, 1997). These data mask, however, an alarming increase in the rate of reported AIDS cases among Asians and Pacific Islanders which, for the years 1987 through 1990, was similar to all other ethnic groups combined (Gock, 1994). Additionally, in large metropolitan areas with large Asian and Pacific Islander populations, the Asian and Pacific Islander communities have experienced the highest rate of increase in reported AIDS cases of any ethnic group (Toleran, 1991).

Numerous factors may contribute to the increase in HIV transmission among Asians and Pacific Islanders, including persistent stereotypes regarding immunity to the infection (Gock, 1994), low levels of knowledge about HIV and its transmission and prevention (Albrecht *et al.*, 1989; DiClemente, Zorn, and Temoshok, 1986; Siegel *et al.*, 1991; Strunin, 1991), risky sexual behaviors (Cochran, Mays, and Leung, 1991), and a belief in the inability to prevent infection stemming from a belief in karmic destiny (Loue *et al.*, 1996). Prevention efforts are rendered more challenging due to the cultural and linguistic diversity of the Asian and Pacific Islander communities (Brown, 1992; Gock, 1994; Loue *et al.*, 1996), cultural taboos related to sex communication (Brown, 1992; Loue *et al.*, 1996), and the need to develop specific strategies for those engaging in higher-risk behaviors within the broader Asian and Pacific Islander communities (Brown, 1992).

Hepatitis B

The great majority of the 200 million individuals chronically infected with hepatitis B virus (HBV) worldwide are in Asia (Hann, 1994), so it is not surprising that hepatitis B infection is more common among Asian-Americans than among other U.S. ethnic groups. Untreated, HBV may lead to hepatocellular carcinoma, chronic active hepatitis, and chronic liver disease (Hann, 1994; Mayeno and Hirota, 1994). HBV chronic carrier rates ranging from 5% to 15% have been reported in various Asian and Pacific Islander subpopulations (Franks *et al.*, 1989; Hann, London, McGlynn, and Blumberg, 1987; London, 1990; McGlynn, London, Hann, and Sharrar, 1986; Szmuness *et al.*, 1978). Several studies have indicated that the death rate among Chinese-American males suffering from hepatocellular carcinoma is significantly higher than the rate among whites (Fraumeni and Mason, 1974; Szmuness *et al.*, 1978).

HBV is often transmitted in the Asian and Pacific population perinatally. Data indicate that the risk of perinatal transmission is 16 times greater among Asians and Pacific Islanders than it is for the entire U.S. population (Mayeno and Hirota, 1994). Barriers to the prevention of transmission include lack of knowledge about HBV and/or the relationship between HBV and liver disease (Jackson, Rhodes, Inui, and Buchwald, 1997; Jenkins *et al.*, 1996; Sworts and Riccitelli, 1997), and lack of immunization (Jenkins, McPhee, Bird, and Bonilla, 1990).

Tuberculosis

Asian-Americans are also disproportionately affected by tuberculosis. The incidence rate among Asians and Pacific Islanders is more than six times that of the U.S. population as a whole, due in part to the high prevalence of tuberculosis in the countries of origin (Mayeno and Hirota, 1994).

Chronic Disease

Cancer

Chinese, Japanese, and Filipinos appear to have lower cancer incidence rates than whites for all anatomic sites combined (Jenkins and Kagawa-Singer, 1994). However, Chinese-Americans have been found to be at relatively high risk for cancer of the nasopharynx, liver, and esophagus (Barringer, Gardner, and Levin, 1993; Lum, 1995), while Japanese-Americans are at higher risk of stomach cancer (Barringer *et al.*, 1993) and are experiencing an increasing rate of colorectal and breast cancer (Barringer *et al.*, 1993; Lin-Fu, 1988; Lum, 1995). Native Hawaiians have higher cancer incidence rates than do whites for all anatomic sites combined (Heckler, 1985) and, in particular, experience an increased incidence in breast, cervical, esophageal, lung, pancreatic, and stomach cancers (Jenkins and Kagawa-Singer, 1994). Despite the lower overall cancer incidence rates experienced by Chinese, Japanese, and Filipinos, their survival experience is generally poorer than whites (Jenkins and Kagawa-Singer, 1994).

In general, migration studies seem to indicate that incidence rates of cancer among immigrant groups approach those of the U.S. population over time. For example, Thomas (1979) found that the incidence rates of breast, prostate, colon, rectal, and pancreatic cancer increased among Chinese and Japanese after immigration to the United States from their countries of origin. Similar increases in incidence rates have been noted for prostate cancer among Chinese men (Yu et al., 1991), breast cancer among Chinese women (Yu et al., 1991), and breast cancer among Japanese women (Shimizu et al., 1991). Decreases in the incidence rates of liver, stomach, cervical, and esophageal cancers have been noted among Chinese and Japanese following immigration to the United States (Thomas, 1979). These changes in incidence rates have been attributed, depending on the particular site of the cancer, to dietary changes, differences in food handling techniques and preservation methods, and improved screening (Jenkins and Kagawa-Singer, 1994).

The chewing of betel quid, which consist of areca nut (betel nut), betel leaf, lime paste, and leaf tobacco, may represent a culture-specific risk factor for oral cancer, oral leukoplakia, and mucosal lesions ("betel chewer's mucosa") (Reichart, Schmidtberg, and Scheifele, 1996). A mixture of these ingredients is placed between the gum and the cheek for long periods of time, gradually causing the permanent staining of the teeth and mouth (Pickwell, Schimelpfening, and Palinkas, 1994). Use of betel quid appears to be declining due to dislike of the residual staining (Reichart et al., 1996).

Asians and Pacific Islanders as a group have been found less likely to undergo screening procedures for various cancers, including mammograms (Centers for Disease Control, 1992a), Pap smears (Centers for Disease Control, 1992b; Han et al., 1989), and rectal examinations and stool occult blood tests (Jenkins et al., 1990). Numerous barriers to preventive screening have been identified, including lack of knowledge (Tash, Chung, and Yasunobou, 1988; Wirthlin Group, 1992), embarrassment over the physical examination and/or being touched by a stranger, the belief that cancer is untreatable, and fear of the equipment (Bailey et al., 1996; Kelly et al., 1996; Yi and Prows, 1996). Culture-sensitive interventions include reliance on female physicians to conduct women's examinations, detailed explanations related to the purpose of screening and the use of equipment, and explanations of the results (Bailey et al., 1996; Kelly et al., 1996).

Cardiovascular Disease

Hypertension. The various risk factors that have been identified for hypertension among Asians and Pacific Islanders have been classified as either biological or sociocultural (Tamir and Cachola, 1994). Biological variables include increased body mass and alcohol consumption. Sociocultural risk factors include educational level, ethnicity, and level of knowledge and awareness (Tamir and Cachola, 1994).

Increased age has been found to be associated with increased blood pressure levels among Japanese-Americans (American Heart Association, 1991), Chinese immigrants in Boston (Choi et al., 1990), and Southeast Asians (Bates, Hill, and Barrett-Connor, 1989). Stavig, Igra, and Leonard (1984) found an association between elevated body mass and increased prevalence of hypertension among Filipinos and other Asian and Pacific Islander groups. Several studies have detected a positive association between increased alcohol consumption and increased prevalence of hypertension among Filipinos (Angel, Armstrong, and Klatsky, 1989; Stavig *et al.*, 1984).

In comparison with the general population, Asians and Pacific Islanders have been found to be less knowledgeable about hypertension, with fewer visits to their physicians and less frequent measure of their blood pressure (Stavig, Igra, and Leonard, 1988). Education has been found to be negatively associated with hypertension among Asians and Pacific Islanders in general (Stavig *et al.*, 1984). However, education is positively correlated with hypertension among Filipino men specifically (Angel *et al.*, 1989). Although Filipinos are more likely to be aware of the implications of high blood pressure in comparison with other Asian and Pacific Islander groups, they also experience the highest rates of hypertension among Asian and Pacific Islander groups (Stavig *et al.*, 1988). Culturally and linguistically appropriate health education interventions have been found to be effective in addressing this lack of knowledge (Chen *et al.*, 1994).

Coronary Heart Disease.   In general, mortality rates due to heart disease among Asians-Americans are lower than those among U.S. whites but in excess of the rates in the countries of origin (Barringer *et al.*, 1993; Syme *et al.*, 1975). These differences have been attributed to a U.S. diet that is higher in animal fat, dairy, and simple carbohydrates, as well as a sedentary lifestyle (Nichaman *et al.*, 1975).

Smoking constitutes one of the major risk factors for coronary heart disease (Tamir and Cachola, 1994). Numerous studies have found high rates of smoking among specific Asian Pacific Islander populations, among men in general (Moeschberger *et al.*, 1997; Zane, Takeuchi, and Young, 1994), and among Cambodian and Lao men in particular (Moeschberger *et al.*, 1997). Chinese men and women have been found less likely to smoke than other Asian and Pacific Islander groups (Klatsky and Armstrong, 1991). The prevalence of smoking among Filipinos has been found to vary across studies, ranging from 20% (Asian and Pacific Islander Health Forum, 1991) to 32.9% (Klatsky and Armstrong, 1991) among men and from 6 to 7% among women (Asian and Pacific Islander Health Forum, 1991). A number of factors appear to be positively associated with the prevalence of smoking in specific subgroups, including alcohol consumption, marriage (Klatsky and Armstrong, 1991), and employment status (Moeschberger *et al.*, 1997). High levels of education appear to be negatively correlated with smoking and positively correlated with levels of acculturation (U.S. Department of Health and Human Services, 1990).

Mental Health and Illness

Diagnosis of mental or emotional disorders among Asians and Pacific Islanders is often complex, due to language differences, difficulties in the application of Western diagnostic criteria to the presenting symptoms, and a lack of understanding by mental health professionals of the cultural context of the presenting symptoms (Ong, 1995). Moreover, many Asians and Pacific Islanders may be reluctant to use Western mental health services, often due to differing concepts of mental health and illness and the appropriate treatment for such disorders. For example, many Asians and Pacific Islanders may express depression and anxiety somatically, perhaps due to the stigma associated with mental illness (Cheung and Dobkin de Rios, 1982; Flaskerud and Soldevilla, 1986; Kim and Rew, 1994). Typical presenting symptoms include anxiety, dizziness, fatigue, irritability, and lack of appetite (Flaskerud and Soldevilla, 1986; Kim and Rew, 1994). These symptoms may be attributed to karma, the actions of ancestral spirits (Ong, 1995), possession by evil spirits (Flaskerud and Soldevilla, 1986), character weakness, or misdeeds (Flaskerud and Soldevilla, 1986; Kim and Renfrew, 1994). Treatment may consist of praying to ancestors, avoiding "thinking too much," and reliance on traditional techniques to restore balance in the body and in the environment (Flaskerud and Soldevilla, 1986; Frye and D'Avanzo, 1994a; Kim and Rew, 1994; Ong, 1995).

Mental health problems most commonly reported among Asians and Pacific Islanders are depression, schizophrenia, and problems associated with family discord, loss of status, and loss of self-esteem (Agbayani-Siewert, 1994; Flaskerud and Soldevilla, 1986; Kim and Rew, 1994; Kuo, 1984; Ying, 1990). The experience of immigration itself, isolation from peers, poverty, and alienation from younger family members have been identified as risk factors for mental illness among Asians and Pacific Islanders (Lum, 1995). Southeast Asians, in particular, have been found to have high rates of anxiety, depression, and PTSD, often in response to their escape experiences or the events that occurred during their resettlement in refugee camps (Carlson and Rosser-Hogan, 1993; Clarke, Sack, & Goff, 1993; Lin-Fu, 1988; Palinkas and Pickwell, 1995; Sack *et al.*, 1993; Tran, 1993). Racism has also been identified as a potential risk factor for impaired mental health and a barrier to the receipt of appropriate mental health services (Cheung and Dobkin de Rios, 1982).

Health care providers may not associate their patients' varied somatic complaints with a mental health disorder. Chronic headache has been found to be associated with depression among a sample of Cambodians (Handelman and Yeo, 1996). "Extreme sadness" and "thinking too much" are culture-bound syndromes among Cambodians that are associated with PTSD (Frye and D'Avanzo, 1994a; Moore and Boehnlein, 1991). "Thinking too much" is characterized by headache, chest pain, palpitations, shortness of breath, excess sleeping, and withdrawal. Alcohol and drugs may be used to cope with "thinking too much," although suicide may also be viewed as an option (Frye and D'Avanzo, 1994a).

Exercises

1. The *Diagnostic and Statistical Manual IV* (American Psychiatric Association, 1994:424) defines posttraumatic stress disorder as

> the development of characteristic symptoms following exposure to an extreme traumatic stressor involving direct personal experience of an event that involves actual or threatened death or serious injury, or other threat to one's physical integrity; or witnessing an event that involves death, injury, or a threat to the physical integrity of another person; or learning about unexpected or violent death, serious harm, or threat of death or injury experienced by a family member or other close associate.

Symptoms include persistent re-experiencing of the traumatic event, persistent avoidance of stimuli associated with the trauma, numbing of general responsiveness, and symptoms of increased arousal, such as difficulty concentrating or falling asleep, hypervigilance, and an exaggerated startle response. It is clear, however, that all individuals who undergo such experiences do not present with these symptoms. As a health researcher, you are interested in identifying those factors that may predispose individuals who undergo this type of experience to develop PTSD. Assume that your community has a large number of refugees, particularly from Southeast Asia.
   a. What are the ethical concerns related to a study seeking to identify predisposing factors for PTSD in a refugee population? If there are no concerns, indicate that. Explain your response with reference to any relevant international and/or national documents.
   b. Assume for the purpose of this question only that you are able to overcome any ethical

issues that you may have identified. Design a study that will enable you to identify predisposing factors for PTSD. Include in your response a discussion of the strengths and weaknesses of the proposed design.

    c. Assume that a proportion of the prospective participants in your study were tortured prior to their arrival in the United States. Assuming further that you are able to overcome any ethical concerns associated with your study, how might these experiences affect your ability to recruit participants? How will you address these issues?

2. You are interested in examining high-risk behaviors for HIV transmission within the Asian and Pacific Islander populations of your community, due to the increasing rate of new cases of AIDS. Your findings will be used as the basis for the development of culturally sensitive intervention efforts.

    a. There is great diversity of culture, national origin, and language among the various subgroups now classified as Asian and Pacific Islander. How does an individual who, for example, is a U.S.-born Chinese male in his early 20s come to identify with a female Filipino immigrant in her 40s and to self-classify as Asian and Pacific Islander?

    b. One potential consequence to your study is the stigmatization of individuals and/or specific subgroups in the community. How will you reduce or eliminate this risk?

    c. In view of the great diversity among Asians and Pacific Islanders, how will you design (i) your study and (ii) your intervention to be "culturally sensitive"?

References

Agbayani-Siewert, P. (1994). Filipino American culture and family: Guidelines for practitioners. *Journal of Contemporary Human Services, September*, 429–438.

Albrecht, G.L., Levy, J.A., Sugrue, N.M., Prohaska, T.R., & Ostrow, D.G. (1989). Who hasn't heard about AIDS? *AIDS Education and Prevention, 1*, 261–267.

American Heart Association. (1991). Cardiovascular diseases and stroke in African Americans and other racial minorities in the United States: Special report. *Circulation, 83*, 1463–1480.

American Psychiatric Association. (1994). *Diagnostic and Statistical Manual of Mental Disorders* (4th ed.). Washington, DC: Author.

Angel, A., Armstrong, M.A., & Klatsky, A.L. (1989). Blood pressure among Asian Americans living in Northern California. *American Journal of Cardiology, 64*, 237–240.

Asian and Pacific Islander Health Forum. (1991). Asian and Pacific Islander American Health Forum national agenda for Asian and Pacific Islander health. In *Proceedings of the Second Asian and Pacific Islander American Health Forum*. Cited in A. Tamir & S. Cachola. (1994). Hypertension and other cardiovascular risk factors. In N.W.S. Zane, D.T. Takeuchi, & K.N.J. Young (Eds.), *Confronting Critical Health Issues of Asian and Pacific Islander Americans* (pp. 209–246). Thousand Oaks, CA: Sage Publications.

Bailey, S., Bennett, P., Hicks, J., Kemp, C., & Warren, S.H. (1996). Cancer detection activities coordinated by nursing students in community health. *Cancer Nursing, 19*, 348–352.

Barringer, H.R., Gardner, R.W., & Levin, M.J. (1993). *Asians and Pacific Islanders in the United States*. New York: Russell Sage Foundation.

Bates, S.R., Hill, L., & Barrett-Connor, E. (1989). Cardiovascular disease risk factors in an Indochinese population. *American Journal of Preventive Medicine, 5*, 15–25.

Brown, W.J. (1992). Culture and AIDS education: Reaching high-risk heterosexuals in Asian-American communities. *Journal of Applied Communication Research, August*, 275–291.

Burr, J.A., & Mutchler, J.E. (1993). Nativity, acculturation, and economic status: Explanations of Asian American living arrangements in later life. *Journal of Gerontology, 48*, S55–S63.

California Statutes (1940). Cited in R. Takaki (1989). *Strangers from a Different Shore*. New York: Penguin Books.

Cao, L., & Novas, H. (1996). *Everything You Need to Know About Asian-American History*. New York: Penguin Books.

Capps, L.L. (1994). Change and continuity in the medical culture of the Hmong in Kansas City. *Medical Anthropology Quarterly, 8*, 161–177.

Carlson, E.B., & Rosser-Hogan, R. (1993). Mental health status of Cambodian refugees ten years after leaving their homes. *American Journal of Orthopsychiatry, 63,* 223–231.

Centers for Disease Control. (1992a). Behavioral risk factor survey of Chinese: California, 1989. *Morbidity and Mortality Weekly Report, 41,* 266–270.

Centers for Disease Control. (1992b). Behavioral risk factor survey of Vietnamese: California, 1992. *Morbidity and Mortality Weekly Report, 41,* 69–72.

Centers for Disease Control and Prevention. (1997). *HIV/AIDS Surveillance Report, 9,* 1–43.

Chen, M.S., Jr., Anderson, J., Moeschberger, M., Guthrie, R., Kuun, P., & Zaharlick, A. (1994). An evaluation of heart health education for Southeast Asians. *American Journal of Preventive Medicine, 10,* 205–208.

Cheung, F., & Dobkin de Rios, M.F. (1982). Recent trends in the study of mental health of Chinese immigrants to the United States. *Research in Race Relations, 3,* 145–163.

Choi, E.S.K., McGandy, R.B., Dallal, G.E., Russell, R.M., Jacob, R., Schaefer, E.J., & Sadowski, J.A. (1990). The prevalence of cardiovascular risk factors among elderly Chinese Americans. *Archives of Internal Medicine, 150,* 1167–1174.

Clarke, G., Sack, W.H., & Goff, B. (1993). Three forms of stress in Cambodian adolescent refugees. *Journal of Abnormal Child Psychology, 21,* 65–77.

Cochran, S.D., Mays, V.M., & Leung, L. (1991). Sexual practices of heterosexual Asian-American young adults: Implications for risk of HIV infection. *Archives of Sexual Behavior, 20,* 381–391.

Commission on Wartime Relocation and Internment of Civilians. (1997). *Personal Justice Denied.* Washington, DC: Civil Liberties Public Education Fund.

Daniels, R. (1962). *The Politics of Prejudice.* Berkeley, CA: University of California Press.

DiClemente, R.J., Zorn, J., & Temoshok, L. (1986). Adolescents and AIDS: A survey of knowledge, beliefs, and attitudes about AIDS in San Francisco. *Journal of Public Health, 76,* 1443–1445.

Flaskerud, J.H., & Soldevilla, E.Q. (1986). Filipino and Vietnamese clients: Utilizing an Asian mental health center. *Journal of Psychosocial Nursing, 24,* 32–36.

Franks, A.L., Berg, C.J., Kane, M.A., Browne, B.B., Sikes, R.K., Elsea, W.R., & Burton, A. (1989). Hepatitis B virus infection among children born in the United States to Southeast Asian refugees. *New England Journal of Medicine, 321,* 1301–1305.

Fraumeni, J.F., Jr., & Mason, T.J. (1974). Cancer mortality among Chinese-Americans, 1950–1969. *Journal of the National Cancer Institute, 52,* 659–665.

Frye, B.A., & D'Avanzo, C.D. (1994a). Cultural themes in family stress and violence among Cambodian refugee women in the inner city. *Advances in Nursing Science, 16,* 64–77.

Frye, B.A., & D'Avanzo, C. (1994b). Themes in managing culturally defined illness in the Cambodian refugee family. *Journal of Community Health Nursing, 11,* 89–98.

Gock, T.S. (1994). Acquired immunodeficiency syndrome. In N.W.S. Zane, D.T. Takeuchi, & K.N.J. Young (Eds.), *Confronting Critical Health Issues of Asian and Pacific Islander Americans* (pp. 247–265). Thousand Oaks, CA: Sage Publications.

Gould-Martin, K., & Ngin, C. (1981). Chinese-Americans. In A. Harwood (Ed.), *Ethnicity and Medical Care* (pp. 130–171). Cambridge, MA: Harvard University Press.

Gussow, Z. (1989). *Leprosy, Racism, and Public Health: Social Policy in Chronic Disease Control.* Boulder, CO: Westview Press.

Han, E.E.S., Kim, S.H., Lee, M.S., Miller, J. S.K., Rhee, S., Song, H., & Yu, E.Y. (1989). Korean Health Survey: A Preliminary Report: Los Angeles Health Education, Information and Referral Center. Cited in C.N.H. Jenkins & M. Kagawa-Singer. (1994). Cancer. In N.W.S. Zane, D.T. Takeuchi, & K.N.J. Young (Eds.), *Confronting Critical Health Issues of Asian and Pacific Islander Americans* (pp. 105–147). Thousand Oaks, CA: Sage Publications.

Handelman, L., & Yeo, G. (1996). Using explanatory models to understand chronic symptoms of Cambodian refugees. *Clinical Research and Methods, 28,* 271–276.

Hann, H.W.L. (1994). Hepatitis B. In N.W.S. Zane, D.T. Takeuchi, & K.N.J. Young (Eds.), *Confronting Critical Health Issues of Asian and Pacific Islander Americans* (pp. 148–173). Thousand Oaks, CA: Sage Publications.

Heckler, M.M. (1985). *Report of the Secretary's Task Force on Black and Minority Health* (Vol. I: Executive Summary). Washington, DC: U.S. Department of Health and Human Services.

Heizer, R.F., & Almquist, A.F. (1971). *The Other Californians.* Berkeley, CA: University of California Press.

Jackson, J.C., Rhodes, L.A., Inui, T.S., & Buchwald, D. (1997). Hepatitis B among the Khmer: Issues of translation and concepts of illness. *Journal of General Internal Medicine, 12,* 292–298.

Jenkins, C.N.H., & Kagawa-Singer, M. (1994). Cancer. In N.W.S. Zane, D.T. Takeuchi, & K.N.J. Young (Eds.), *Confronting Critical Health Issues of Asian and Pacific Islander Americans* (pp. 105–147). Thousand Oaks, CA: Sage Publications.

Jenkins, C.N.H, Le, T., McPhee, S.J., & Stewart, S. (1996). Health care access and preventive care among Vietnamese immigrants: Do traditional beliefs and practices pose barriers? *Social Science and Medicine, 43,* 1049–1056.

Jenkins, C.N.H., McPhee, S.J., Bird, J.A., & Bonilla, N.T.H. (1990). Cancer risks and prevention practices among Vietnamese refugees. *Western Journal of Medicine, 153,* 34–39.

Kanzaki, K. (1921). Is the Japanese menace in America a reality? *Annals of the American Academy of Political and Social Sciences,* 96–97.

Kelly, A.W., Chacori, M.D.M.F., Wollan, P.C., Trapp, M.A., Weaver, A.L., Barrier, P.A., Franz III, W.B., & Kittke, T.E. (1996). A program to increase breast cancer screening for Cambodian women in a Midwestern community. *Mayo Clinic Proceedings, 71,* 437–444.

Kim, S., & Rew, W. (1994). Ethnic identity, role integration, quality of life, and depression in Korean-American women. *Archives of Psychiatric Nursing, 8,* 348–356.

Klatsky, A.I., & Armstrong, M.A. (1991). Cardiovascular risk factors among Asian Americans living in Northern California. *American Journal of Public Health, 81,* 1423–1428.

Kuo, W.H. (1984). Prevalence of depression among Asian-Americans. *Journal of Nervous and Mental Disease, 172,* 449–457.

Lee, D.A., & Fong, K. (1990, February/March). HIV/AIDS and the Asian and Pacific Islander community. *SIECUS Report,* 16–22.

Lee, L.P. (1938). The need for better housing in Chinatown. *Chinese Digest.*

Lin-Fu, J.S. (1988). Population characteristics and health care needs of Asian Pacific Americans. *Public Health Reports, 103,* 18–27.

London, W.T. (1990). Prevention of hepatitis B and hepatocellular carcinoma in Asian residents in the United States. *Asian Journal of Clinical Science Monograms: Hepatitis B Virus Infections, 11,* 49–57.

Loue, S., Lloyd, L., & Loh, L. (1996). HIV prevention in U.S. Asian Pacific Islander communities: An innovative approach. *Journal of Health Care for the Poor and Underserved, 7,* 364–376.

Lum, O. (1995). Health status of Asians and Pacific Islanders. *Clinics in Geriatric Medicine, 11,* 53–67.

Lyman, S. (1971). Strangers in the city: The Chinese in the urban frontier. In F. Odo (Ed.), *Roots: An Asian American Reader.* Los Angeles: Continental Graphics.

Mattson, S. (1995). Culturally sensitive prenatal care for Southeast Asians. *JOGNN, 24,* 335–341.

Mayeno, L., & Hirota, S.M. (1994). Access to health care. In N.W.S. Zane, D.T. Takeuchi, & K.N.J. Young (Eds.), *Confronting Critical Health Issues of Asian and Pacific Islander Americans* (pp. 347–375). Thousand Oaks, CA: Sage Publications.

McGlynn, K., London, W.T., Hann, H.W., & Sharrar, R.G. (1986). Prevention of primary hepatocellular carcinoma in Asian populations in the Delaware Valley. *Advances in Cancer Control: Health Care Planning and Research* (pp. 237–246). New York: Alan R. Liss.

McKenney, N.R., & Bennett, C.E. (1994). Issues regarding data on race and ethnicity: The Census Bureau experience. *Public Health Reports, 109,* 16–25.

Miller, J.A. (1995). Caring for Cambodian refugees in the emergency department. *Journal of Emergency Nursing, 21,* 498–502.

Moeschberger, M.L., Anderson, M.A.S., Kuo, Y.F., Chen, M.S., Jr., Wewers, M.E., & Guthrie, R. (1997). Multivariate profile of smoking in Southeast Asian men: A biochemically verified analysis. *Preventive Medicine, 26,* 53–58.

Moore, L.J., & Boehnlein, J.K. (1991). Treating psychiatric disorders among Mien refugees from highland Laos. *Social Science and Medicine, 32,* 1029–1036.

Nichaman, M.Z., Hamilton, E.B., Kagan, A., Grier, T., Sacks, S.T., & Syme, S.L. (1975). Epidemiologic studies of CHD and stroke in Japanese men living in Japan, Hawaii and California: Distribution of biochemical risk factors. *American Journal of Epidemiology, 102,* 491–501.

Ogawa, D.M. (1971). *From Japs to Japanese: The Evolution of Japanese-American Stereotypes.* Berkeley, CA: McCutchan.

Ong, A. (1951). Making the biopolitical subject: Cambodian immigrants, refugee medicine, and cultural citizenship in California. *Social Science and Medicine, 40,* 1243–1257.

Osumi, M.D. (1982). Asians and California's anti-miscegenation laws. In N. Tsuchida (Ed.), *Asian and Pacific Islander Experiences: Women's Perspectives.* Minneapolis, MN: Asian/Pacific American Learning Resource Center and General College, University of Minnesota.

Palinkas, L.A., & Pickwell, S.M. (1995). Acculturation as a risk factor for chronic disease among Cambodian refugees in the United States. *Social Science and Medicine, 40,* 1643–1653.

Peffer, G.A. (1986). Forbidden families: Emigration experiences of Chinese women under the Page Law, 1875–1882. *Journal of American Ethnic History, 6,* 28–46.

Pickwell, S.M., Schimelpfening, S., & Palinkas, L.A. (1994). "Betelmania": Betel quid chewing by Cambodian women in the United States and its potential health effects. *Western Journal of Medicine, 160,* 326–330.

Quincy, K. (1988). *Hmong: History of a People*. Cheny, WA: East Washington University Press.

Ramakrishna, J., & Weiss, M.G. (1992). Health, illness, and immigration: East Indians in the United States. *Western Journal of Medicine*, *157*, 265–270.

Reagan, R. (1988). Text of Reagan's remarks. Reprinted in *Pacific Citizen*, August 19–26, 5.

Reichert, P.A., Schmidtberg, W., & Scheifele, C. (1996). Betel chewer's mucosa in elderly Cambodian women. *Journal of Oral Pathology and Medicine*, *25*, 367–370.

Sack, W.A., Clarke, G., Him, C., Dickason, D., Goff, B., Lanham, K., & Kinzie, J.D. (1993). A 6-year follow-up study of Cambodian refugee adolescents traumatized as children. *Journal of American Academy of Child and Adolescent Psychiatry*, *32*, 431–437.

Shimada, J., Jackson, J.C., Goldstein, E., & Buchwald, D. (1995). "Strong medicine": Cambodian views of medicine and medical compliance. *Journal of General Internal Medicine*, *10*, 369–374.

Shimizu, H., Ross, R.K., Bernstein, L., Yatani, R., Henderson, B.E., & Mack, T.M. (1991). Cancers of the prostate and breast among Japanese and white immigrants in Los Angeles County. *British Journal of Cancer*, *63*, 963–966.

Siegel, D., Lazarus, N., Krasnovsky, F., Dubin, M., & Chesney, M. (1991). AIDS knowledge, attitudes and behavior among inner city, junior high school students. *Journal of School Health*, *61*, 160–165.

Smith, M.J., & Ryan, A.S. (1987). Chinese-American families of children with developmental disabilities: An exploratory study of reactions to service providers. *Mental Retardation*, *25*, 345–350.

Spickard, P.R. (1996). *Japanese Americans: The Formation and Transformation of an Ethnic Group*. New York: Twayne Publishers.

Stavig, G.R., Igra, A., & Leonard, A.R. (1984). Hypertension among Asians and Pacific Islanders in California. *American Journal of Epidemiology*, *119*, 677–691.

Stavig, G.R., Igra, A., & Leonard, A.R. (1988). Hypertension and related health issues among Asians and Pacific Islanders in California. *Public Health Reports*, *103*, 28–37.

Strunin, L. (1991). Adolescents' perceptions of risk for HIV infection: Implications for future research. *Social Science and Medicine*, *32*, 221–228.

Sworts, V.D., & Riccitelli, C.N. (1997). Health education lessons learned: The H.A.P.I. kids program. *Journal of School Health*, *67*, 283–285.

Syme, S.L., Marmot, M.G., Kagan, A., Kato, H., & Rhoads, G. (1975). Epidemiologic studies of CHD and stroke in Japanese men living in Japan, Hawaii, and California: Introduction. *American Journal of Epidemiology*, *102*, 477–480.

Szmuness, W., Stevens, C.E., Ikram, H., Much, M.J., Harley, E.J., & Hollinger, B. (1978). Prevalence of hepatitis B infection and hepatocellular carcinoma in Chinese-Americans. *Journal of Infectious Diseases*, *137*, 822–829.

Takada, E., Ford, J., & Lloyd, L.S. (1998). Asian Pacific Islander health. In S. Loue (Ed.), *Handbook of Immigrant Health* (pp. 303–327). New York: Plenum Press.

Takaki, R. (1989). *Strangers from a Different Shore*. New York: Penguin Books.

Tamir, A., & Cachola, S. (1994). Hypertension and other cardiovascular risk factors. In N.W.S. Zane, D.T. Takeuchi, & K.N.J. Young (Eds.), *Confronting Critical Health Issues of Asian and Pacific Islander Americans* (pp. 209–246). Thousand Oaks, CA: Sage Publications.

Tash, E., Chung, C.S., & Yasunobu, C. (1988). *Hawaii's Health Risk Behaviors, 1987*. Honolulu, HI: Hawaii State Department of Health, Health Promotion and Education Branch.

Taylor, S.C. (1986). Evacuation and economic loss. In R. Daniels, S.C. Taylor, & H.H.L. Kitano (Eds.), *Japanese Americans: From Relocation to Redress* (pp. 163–167). Salt Lake City, UT: University of Utah Press.

Thomas, D.B. (1979). Epidemiologic studies of cancer in minority groups in the Western United States. *National Cancer Institute Monographs*, *53*, 103–113.

Toleran, D.E. (1991). Pakikisama: Reaching the Filipino community with AIDS prevention. *MIRA*, *5*, 1, 8–10.

Tran, T.V. (1993). Psychological traumas and depression in a sample of Vietnamese people in the United States. *Health and Social Work*, *18*, 184–194.

Uba, L. (1992). Cultural barriers to health care for Southeast Asian refugees. *Public Health Reports*, *107*, 544–548.

United States Department of Health and Human Services, Public Health Service. (1990). *Healthy People 2000: National Health Promotion and Disease Prevention Objectives*. Washington, DC: Government Printing Office [DHHS Publ. No. PHS 91-50212].

Wirthlin Group. (1992, Jan.). Breast Cancer Survey for the American Cancer Society. Paper presented at the National Breast Summit. Cited in C.N.H. Jenkins & M. Kagawa-Singer. (1994). Cancer. In N.W.S. Zane, D.T. Takeuchi, & K.N.J. Young (Eds.), *Confronting Critical Health Issues of Asian and Pacific Islander Americans* (pp. 105–147). Thousand Oaks, CA: Sage Publications.

Wu, C.T. (1972). *Chink! A Documentary History of Anti-Chinese Prejudice in America*. New York: World.

Yi, J.K., & Prows, S.L. (1996). Breast cancer screening practices among Cambodian women in Houston, Texas. *Journal of Cancer Education*, *11*, 221–225.

Ying, Y-W. (1990). Explanatory models of major depression and implications for help-seeking among immigrant Chinese-American women. *Culture, Medicine, and Psychiatry, 14*, 393–408.

Yu, H.E., Randall, E.H., Gao, Y.-T., Gao, R., & Wynder, E.L. (1991). Comparative epidemiology of cancers of the colon, rectum, prostate and breast in Shanghai, China versus the United States. *International Journal of Epidemiology, 20*, 76–81.

Zane, N.W.S., Takeuchi, D.T., & Young, K.N.J. (Eds.). (1994). *Confronting Critical Health Issues of Asian and Pacific Islander Americans*. Thousand Oaks, CA: Sage Publications.

8

Hispanic Health

Introduction

According to the 1990 census, the Hispanic population was estimated to be over 22 million, or approximately 9% of the U.S. population (U.S. Bureau of the Census, 1992, 1993). The classification "Hispanic" obscures the diversity of this population. Individuals of Mexican heritage account for 64.3% of all Hispanics, while Puerto Ricans (10.6%), Cubans (4.7%), Central and South Americans (13.4%), and others (7%) comprise the remainder (Furino, 1992). Two-thirds of the Hispanic population lives in urban areas (U.S. Bureau of the Census, 1990). The various subgroups have tended to settle in different geographic areas, with Mexicans living predominantly in California and Texas, Puerto Ricans in New York, and Cubans in Florida (Furino, 1992; Mendoza, 1994; U.S. Bureau of the Census, 1988).

The U.S. Department of Commerce, Bureau of the Census, refers to all individuals with an ethnic origin from Spanish-speaking countries as "Hispanic." This includes Spain, Puerto Rico, Cuba, and Central and South American countries. "Hispanic" is a more general term than "Latino," which is usually used to refer to persons whose ethnic origin is from a Spanish-speaking country in Latin America (Mendoza, 1994).

In comparison with other groups, Hispanics have a higher fertility rate, give birth to children at a younger age, and have more children (U.S. Bureau of the Census, 1993). Although Mexican and Cuban families are likely to be headed by two parents, over 60% of children of parents of Puerto Rican descent are in single-parent households, a situation strongly associated with poverty (Commonwealth Fund, 1995, cited in Guendelman, 1998). A recent study of mortality patterns among adult Hispanics suggests that older Hispanics experience lower overall mortality in comparison with non-Hispanic whites, but mortality among young and middle-aged Hispanics is similar to that of non-Hispanic whites (Liao *et al.*, 1998).

Of all Hispanic families, one third live below the U.S. poverty level (U.S. Bureau of the Census, 1993). Cuban-Americans are the least likely of Hispanic groups to be living in poverty, while Puerto Ricans are the most likely to be poor (U.S. Bureau of the Census, 1990). Hispanics are more likely to be employed in service, agricultural, or blue-collar jobs, where employers are less likely to provide health insurance benefits (Trevino, Moyer, Burciaga, Valdez, and Stroup-Benham, 1991; U.S. Bureau of the Census, 1990), sick leave, parental leave, disability benefits, or retirement benefits (Bassford, 1995). A recent study found that among uninsured Hispanics, 60% of Cuban-Americans, 53% of Mexican-Americans and 46% of Puerto Ricans were employed (Trevino *et al.*, 1991). Mexican-Americans are more likely to be employed than are Puerto Ricans, but are less likely to have health insurance, due to lack of employer-sponsored insurance and inability to afford private insurance premiums (Council on Scientific Affairs, 1991; Valdez *et al.*, 1993). Cuban-Americans are more likely to have higher education and income levels and private health insurance. Puerto Ricans, however, who tend to have lower levels of both income and employment, are most likely to be insured by Medicaid (Lipton and Katz, 1989; Trevino and Moss, 1983). The less favorable occupational status and lower incomes are reflective of the lower educational levels among Hispanics. For example, only 50% of young adult Hispanics have a high school diploma (U.S. Bureau of the Census, 1993) and over 10% have less than 5 years of school (U.S. Bureau of the Census, 1988).

Cultural and Historical Context

Language and Acculturation

As with Asians and Pacific Islanders, language may constitute a significant barrier to care. Research has demonstrated that Hispanic patients who speak English are more likely to have a regular source of care than those who speak only Spanish (Hu and Covell, 1986) and may be more willing to utilize available services (Trevino, Bruhn, and Bunce, 1979). Yet, English literacy is low in the Hispanic population in general. Less than half of the Hispanic elderly are estimated to be fully literate in either English or Spanish (Cuellar, 1990).

Acculturation levels may vary across and within groups. Lower levels of acculturation have been associated with reduced likelihood of utilizing inpatient and outpatient care (Wells *et al.*, 1989), poorer oral health outcomes (Marcell, 1994), and more favorable prenatal health behaviors, including abstinence from alcohol, drug, and cigarette use during pregnancy (Moore and Devitt, 1989; Marin, Perez-Stables, and Marin, 1989; U.S. Department of Health and Human Services, 1996). Higher levels of acculturation have been associated with an increased likelihood of unplanned pregnancies, pregnancy complications, and delivery of pre-term and low birth weight infants (Guendelman and English, 1995), as well as increased prenatal stress, less social support during pregnancy, higher medical risk, and greater drug and alcohol use (Zambrana, Scrimshaw, Collins, and Dunkel-Schetter, 1997). The relative lack of health providers who understand the cultural context of their Hispanic patients may exacerbate the provider–patient communication difficulties arising from differences in language (Council on Scientific Affairs, 1991).

Explanatory Models of Health

Hispanic individuals may interpret and respond to illness episodes using culture-specific explanatory models. These models have often been referred to as "folk illnesses" or "culture-bound syndromes," treatable through "folk practices" (Council on Scientific Affairs, 1991). These explanatory models are important because they may influence individuals' decisions to seek care or to utilize a specific form of care.

Numerous explanatory models have been documented. These illnesses have been classified into three categories, based on the presumed underlying causative mechanisms. The first, "natural" illnesses, includes *aigre* or *mal aire* (bad air), *empacho* (intestinal obstruction), and *mollera caida* (fallen fontanelle). Magical diseases encompass *encono* (the festering of wounds), *mal ojo* (evil eye), and *maleficio* (witchcraft). *Melarchico* (melancholy), *susto* (fright), and *ataque de nervios* ("nervous attack") comprise the third category relating to psychological and interpersonal etiology (Scheper Hughes and Stewart, 1983). The symptoms, causes, and recommended treatment for each are described in Table 8.1. The complaints of symptoms may, in fact, be biologically based and require accurate diagnosis and treatment (DeLaCancela, Guarnaccia, and Carrillo, 1986; Hispanic Health Alliance, 1990; Trotter, 1985).

Many illnesses have been attributed to an imbalance of hot–cold in food or in climate. The vast literature addressing hot–cold syndromes and therapeutics can only be touched on here. Messer (1981:133) has explained this paradigm:

> [H]ot-cold syndromes ... view health as a balance of opposing or complementary (hot–cold) qualities and illness as an imbalance or alteration in one quality. Where such terms are used, all body conditions, foods and medicines can be potentially classified as some degree of hot–cold.... The general rule for health maintenance is avoidance of extremes of any one quality. In the event of imbalance (illness) the procedure is treatment by the principle of opposites. The particular body condition is analyzed to be one or the other quality and is brought back into balance by introduction of quantities of the opposite quality.

The entrance of cold into the body has been said to cause the following syndromes: chest cramps, earaches, headaches, paralysis, pains due to sprains, stomach cramps, rheumatism, teething, and tuberculosis. An excess of heat is responsible for *algodoncillo* (whitening of the lips, tongue, and gums), *dispela* (outbreak of red spots on the extremities), dysentery, sore eyes, *fogazo* (red spots in the mouth and on the tongue), kidney ailments, *postemilla* (abscess in tooth), sore throats, warts, and rashes. Diarrhea, enteritis, and toothache can result from extremes of either hot or cold (Currier, 1966).

Treatment for maladies brought on by humoral imbalance includes the ingestion of teas (Kay and Yoder, 1987), herbal preparations (Foster, 1988), specific food preparations, or a combination of these remedies (Mathews, 1983). Illness can be prevented through the avoidance of exposures to heat or cold insults (Foster, 1984). In the case of unfamiliar maladies, the choice of a specific remedy often depends on preceding episodes of similar illness and a remembrance of the illness–remedy–outcome link (Mathews, 1983).

Reliance on humoral theory serves to (1) explain what has happened; (2) provide a prescription for what is to be done; and (3) afford individuals a degree of control over and an understanding of their own health (Foster, 1984). Additionally, the hot–cold paradigm provides a framework in which individuals can deal with anxieties and desires that cannot be addressed directly. Burgess and Dean (1962:68) have said of the hot–cold framework:

> Other ways of attempting to deal with the internal stress of threats to life or to emotional security are to over-estimate external dangers, or to attribute internal threats almost entirely to external influences of various kinds; and, with this, to attempt magically to evade or appease an apparently external threat, or to balance one type of threat against another. The practice of giving "heating" or "cooling" foods in particular kinds of clinical conditions may be a form of this kind of balancing technique for evading what are regarded as threatening influences—not of a nutritional kind.

Humoral medicine, however, remains a subject of controversy. Despite the apparent widespread reliance on the hot–cold dichotomy, as evidenced by the studies noted above, various investigations have found that a significant proportion of the population under study was unaware of the classifications (Kay, 1977); that the categorization of terms often varies between urban and rural populations within the same area (Weller, 1983); and that the

Table 8.1. Illness Categories, Symptoms, and Treatments among Hispanic Patients[a]

Illness	Cause	Symptoms	Treatment	Source
Aigre/mal aire	"Bad air"; caused by exposure to drafts and night air	Nausea, vomiting, headaches, dizziness, earaches, facial paralysis		Curandero/a, physician
Ataque de nervios	Acute stress	Seizure-like responses; dissociation, including visual or auditory hallucinations; intense fear, anger, or anxiety		Curandero/a, physician
Empacho	Food adherence to the intestinal wall	Intestinal obstruction, abdominal pain, loss of appetite or bloating	Small dose of mercury administered on spine; pinching spine	Curandero/a, sobradora
Mollera caida	A fall or an abrupt withdrawal of the nipple while feeding; fallen fontanelle of the parietal bone of the cranium; diagnosed only in infants. Acutally due to dehydration	Depression of the fontanelle	Pushing the palate; shaking infant upside down, dipping infant's head into water, putting egg on fontanelle	Mother, curandero/a, physician
Encono	"Festering of wounds"; infection of open wound or scar caused by exposure to individual who intentionally or unintentionally caused the wound to fester			Curandero/a

Mal ojo	"Evil eye"; sudden reversal of emotional or physical well-being due to "evil eye"	General malaise, sleepiness, severe headache	Herb tea; sweeping victim with broom; finding person who has cast mal ojo and having him caress patient	Curandero/a, physician
Maleficio	Witchcraft of a malevolent witch (bruja)	Unexplained physical or emotional disorder		Abolario
Melarchico	"Melancholy"; caused by change in environment or loss of or separation from loved one	Depression; loss of appetite, insomnia		
Susto/mal de espanto	1. Infection caused by intestinal parasites 2. Traumatic effect of emotional event; loss or reduction of vital force	Restlessness during sleep; listlessness; loss of appetite; disinterest in dress and personal hygiene; loss of strength; depression	1. Herbs, massage, antihelminthic treatment 2. Offering to spirits; spraying with cold liquor from mouth of healer; placing bed over burning coals in order to sweat; sweeping the patient with a broom to brush out illness	Curandero/a, physician

[a]Sources: Ortiz de Montellano (1987); Martin et al. (1985); Scheper-Hughes and Stewart (1983); Signorini (1982); Schreiber and Homiak (1981); Edgerton, Karno, and Fernandez (1970); Nall and Spielberg (1967); Rubel (1964).

interpretation and the application of the hot–cold distinction differs between groups (Browner, 1985). Logan (1977:95), commenting on the deficiencies of humor-related research, stated:

> Most ethnographic accounts of humoral medicine are descriptive, in that no specific hypotheses or sets of relationships are central to the given research. It is of limited use simply to report that a given people classify certain items or conditions as hot and others as cold. For without explanation, that is, without relating the data to some fact of the group's culture, ecology, or biological adaptations, the data tell us little more than certain items and conditions are judged, by some informants, to be hot or cold.

Use or nonuse of traditional healing practices is closely related to health and illness beliefs; the beliefs may indicate the appropriateness of a particular source of care or form of treatment. The extent to which individuals adhere to cultural practices necessarily affects the extent to which they engage in self-diagnosis and self-prescription and the extent to which they are willing to consult with traditional healers or Western-style health care providers (Ludman *et al.*, 1989).

Brandon (1991) found in his New York/New Jersey-based study of santeria that many of the Hispanics interviewed used home-grown plants to treat minor illnesses, such as inflammations, skin eruptions, muscle pains, and fevers. Healing rites, such as *rogacion de cabeza* (rogation of the head), were used to treat more serious maladies, such as depression, mental confusion, and high blood pressure. The cure requires that the patient recite a series of prayers and that the santero place a plant or animal preparation on the patient's head, to be worn for 24 hours. Unfortunately, Brandon did not explore how or why individuals chose between care from a santero or care from a medical provider.

Hispanic patients may seek assistance from traditional healers for a variety of conditions, including *aigre, empacho, mollera caida, encono, mal ojo, maleficio, melarchico,* or *susto* (see Table 8.1). Treatment may consist of herbal preparations, prayers, burning incense, or massages, depending on the nature of the malady and the expertise of the healer (Martinez and Martin, 1966). Treatment may be sought from a folk healer (*curandero/a*), a masseuse/ bonesetter (*sobadora*), or an herbalist (*albolario*), depending on the nature of the symptoms (Scheper Hughes and Stewart, 1983; Creson *et al.*, 1969) (see Table 8.2).

The selection of the medicinal substance to be used for healing is based on its metaphoric hot or cold quality (Foster, 1985; Browner, 1985). Once selected, these substances must be prepared for use, which often entails compounding multiple ingredients into the treatment,

Table 8.2. Traditional Health Practitioners Serving Hispanic Communities[a]

Type of healer	Illness treated	Methods used
Sobrador (bonesetter/ masseur)	Musculoskeletal pains and stiffness; cuts and bruises	Massage; joint manipulation; stretching mobilization (repetitive small amplitude movements applied rhythmically to the joints)
Albolario	Illness caused by witchcraft	Herbs
Curandero(a)		Laying on the hands; prayer; rituals; herbs; teas
Partera (midwife)	"Female disorders"	

[a]Sources: Mayers (1989); Anderson (1987); Scheper Hughes and Stewart (1983); Baca (1969).

such as an ointment or infusion. The method of treatment administration depends not only on the symptoms or illness, but also on the humoral goals of the treatment. As an example, the extraction of heat may be accomplished through reliance on *emplastos*, a poultice consisting of grape leaves applied to the temples and cheeks with saliva. The expulsion of heat can be accomplished by purges or induced vomiting, brought about by a compound of cold ingredients such as salt, rose leaves and petals, and ash leaves (Foster, 1985).

Historical Context

It is beyond the scope of this chapter to provide a summary of the historical context of each Hispanic group in the United States. Accordingly, a brief review is provided of the history of Mexicans and Puerto Ricans, the two largest Hispanic communities in the United States.

The Mexican American Context

The United States–Mexico border extends from the mouth of the Rio Grande River to the Pacific Ocean, a distance of almost 2,000 miles. The border was established as the result of the 1848 Treaty of Guadalupe Hidalgo, which ended the Mexican War, as it is referred to in the United States, or the American Intervention, as it is known in Mexico (Ehrlich, Bilderback, and Ehrlich, 1979). Tension from a variety of sources over time has characterized the border area and continues to do so: Mexican opposition to slavery in Texas and assistance to escaping slaves during the 1850s; the authorized incursion of U.S. troops into Mexico during the 1870s; the massacre of Americans at Santa Ysabel in 1916; the influx of American investors into Mexico in the 1920s; the expropriation of American-owned oil companies in Mexico by the Mexican government during the late 1930s; the introduction of U.S. agribusiness in Mexican farming throughout the 1940s, 1950s, and 1960s, with disastrous economic consequences; the establishment and subsequent termination of the U.S. Bracero Program; the establishment of *maquiladoras* in border areas; and U.S. immigration policy (Ehrlich *et al.*, 1979; Samora, 1971).

Mexican immigration to the United States gradually increased until the onset of the Great Depression. During the period from 1900 through 1904, Mexicans represented only .07% of the total immigrant influx to the United States. However, that proportion had grown to 15.7% during the 1925–1929 period. Immigration decreased dramatically following the passage of the Deportation Act of March 4, 1929, which rendered some aliens deportable, and the May 4, 1929 law, which made it a felony for deported aliens to re-enter the U.S. illegally. The advent of the Great Depression further dampened Mexican immigration (Samora, 1971).

The need for agricultural labor during World War II, due in part to the forced relocation of Japanese-Americans from the West Coast, prompted the establishment of the Bracero Program in 1942. This program was intended to provide agricultural labor to the United States in shortage areas. The desire of growers to obtain cheap labor after World War II led to the maintenance of the program until the early 1960s. Numerous researchers have traced the beginnings of the "illegal immigration problem" to the initiation of the Bracero Program and the growers' encouragement of migration—legal and illegal—to the United States (Ehrlich *et al.*, 1979; Samora, 1971).

The Puerto Rican Experience

Puerto Rico's population increased significantly during the 19th century, primarily due to the influx of Spanish royalists (Wagenheim and Jimenez de Wagenheim, 1994). Unlike other locales of the Caribbean, the lighter-skinned population of Puerto Rico outnumbered those of darker skin color, and slaves constituted a very small proportion of the total population. Despite the relatively small number of slaves, the abolition of the slave system was an integral part of Puerto Rico's struggle for autonomy.

That autonomy was to be short-lived. Spain granted Puerto Rico a charter in 1897, permitting a substantial degree of home rule. The new Puerto Rico government convened for the first time on February 11, 1898, only to be surrendered by Spain to the invading Americans on October 18, 1898, as compensation for the losses brought about by war. The Americans viewed Puerto Rico as a real-estate venture even then, suitable as a naval base and for a winter vacation (Wagenheim and Jimenez de Wagenheim, 1994). U.S. military rule lasted only briefly, ending on April 12, 1900, with the appointment of a civilian governor by the president of the United States.

The American invasion brought with it economic changes as well as political ones. Prior to the invasion, Puerto Rico had had a diversified subsistence economy with four basic export crops: tobacco, cattle, coffee, and sugar. That economy was essentially converted to a sugar crop economy, of which 60% was owned by absentee U.S. investors (Gonzalez, 1966; Steward, 1965).

The first rebellion against American rule occurred in 1909. Since that time, independence from the United States has remained an ongoing issue. Attempts to increase home rule during the early 1900s were generally met with little sympathy, even as militant anti-American forces began to emerge in response to the high rates of starvation and disease occasioned by the later decline of the sugar cane-based economy and the control of the economy by absentee U.S. investors (Wagenheim and Jimenez de Wagenheim, 1994).

The Great Depression in the United States was felt in Puerto Rico. For example, a 1933 study of the offshore municipality of Vieques Island found that the total population of 11,000 persons earned a total income of $500 per week, or less than 7 cents per person per day.

During the years following World War II, the sagging Puerto Rico economy was boosted through the implementation of Operation Bootstrap, which promoted private investment instead of government development of industry. Liberal tax benefits and low wages were used to lure foreign investors (Rodriguez, 1994; Wagenheim and Jimenez de Wagenheim, 1994). However, these industries failed to provide sufficient employment and, as a result, surplus labor migrated to the mainland United States (Bonilla and Campos, 1981; Morales, 1986). Various benefits made possible through these ties with the mainland, such as citizenship, accessible air travel, and education systems, encouraged further migration (Rodriguez, 1994).

The first phase of Puerto Rican migration occurred between 1900 and 1945 (Stevens-Arroyo and Diaz-Stevens, 1982). As of 1910, there were only 1,513 Puerto Ricans living throughout 39 states. By 1920, the mainland Puerto Rican community had increased to 11,811 in 45 states (Wagenheim and Jimenez de Wagenheim, 1994). The majority, however, settled in New York City (Rodriguez, 1994). Many of these immigrants were employed in working-class occupations (Chenault, 1970; Handlin, 1959).

The "great migration" occurred during the years from 1946 through 1964. Although the great majority of migrants settled in New York, communities were also established in Connecticut, New Jersey, Chicago, and other areas (Stevens-Arroyo and Diaz-Stevens, 1982). Many of these migrants encountered intense racial prejudice in their new settlements, for which they were ill-prepared despite the efforts of the island government. Unable to pass as Americans, many Puerto Ricans attempted to dissociate themselves from the media-labeled "Puerto Rican problem" by calling themselves Hispanos or Latinos (Wagenheim and Jimenez de Wagenheim, 1994).

The migration period from 1965 through the present has been labeled "revolving door migration," reflecting the fluctuating in- and outmigration (Stevens-Arroyo and Diaz-Stevens, 1982). Although New York City continues to attract the majority of the migrants, approximately 40% of those arriving from the island now settle outside of New York (Wagenheim and Jimenez de Wagenheim, 1994). The term "Neo-Rican" is now used to describe the "hybrid person" who speaks and thinks in both English and Spanish but feels a stranger in both cultures (Wagenheim and Jimenez de Wagenheim, 1994:276).

Health Status

Infectious Disease

Acquired Immunodeficiency Syndrome

Although Hispanics comprise approximately 9% of the total U.S. population (U.S. Bureau of the Census, 1992, 1993), they account for 18% of all reported AIDS cases (Maldonado, 1998). Almost two thirds of reported AIDS cases among men born in Central and South America, Cuba, and Mexico are attributed to male-to-male sex, while almost two thirds of AIDS cases among Puerto Ricans are associated with injection drug use (Diaz, Buehler, Castro, and Ward, 1993; Selik, Castro, Pappaioanou, and Buehler, 1989). Although Hispanic children account for only 13% of all U.S. children, 24% of childhood AIDS cases occur among Hispanic children. Perinatal transmission accounts for 88% of Hispanic pediatric AIDS cases (Diaz, 1992). Limited knowledge of the transmission and prevention, as well as cultural norms that proscribe condom use, contribute to the transmission (Council on Scientific Affairs, 1991).

Tuberculosis

Recent research has revealed a decrease in the rate of tuberculosis for U.S.-born persons and an increase in the rates among the foreign-born (Anonymous, 1996; Cantell, Snider, Cauthen, and Onorato, 1995). The rate of tuberculosis among Hispanics is 22.4 per 100,000, compared to 4 per 100,000 among whites (Cantell *et al.*, 1995). The incidence of tuberculosis is substantially higher among Hispanics living in large urban areas, such as New York and Los Angeles, compared to those living elsewhere (Centers for Disease Control, 1987).

Parasitic Infections

Migrant farm worker communities and recent immigrants from Central America and U.S.–Mexico border areas may be at risk of soil-transmitted parasites, including roundworm, whipworm, and hookworm (Arfaa, 1981). Over one third of 124 children screened in a Massachusetts community clinic were found to have pathogenic parasites, with the highest rates among Brazilian and Central American children (Bass, Mehta, and Eppes, 1992).

Chronic Disease

Cancer

In general, Hispanics appear to have a lower overall rate of cancer compared to non-Hispanic whites (National Cancer Institute, 1985). However, Hispanics have been found to have an excess incidence of cancer of the stomach, esophagus, pancreas, and cervix (De-LaRosa, 1989; Secretary's Task Force on Black and Minority Health, 1986a). Mortality due to stomach cancer is twice as high in Hispanics compared to whites (Public Health Service, 1987; Secretary's Task Force on Black and Minority Health, 1986b). These differences in cancer incidence are believed to be related to dietary factors. The traditional diet among Hispanic groups is high in fiber and vegetable sources of protein, potentially accounting, in part, for the lower rates of colon and breast cancer (Garcia-Palmieri *et al.*, 1980).

Many Hispanics may delay cancer screening (Marks, Garcia, and Solis, 1990; National Cancer Institute, 1985) and often lack the knowledge necessary to recognize the early warning signs of cancer (National Cancer Institute, 1989; Clark, Matire and Bartholomew Inc., 1985; Shai, 1986; Villar and Menck, 1994). Ultimately, this may contribute to lower cancer survival rates (Marks *et al.*, 1990; National Cancer Institute, 1985). For example, Hispanic women are less likely to undergo mammograms and other forms of breast cancer screening (Fulton, Rakowski, and Jones, 1995; Kirkman-Liff and Jacobs Kronenfeld, 1992; Marks *et al.*, 1987; Saint-Germain and Longman, 1993) and are also less likely to perceive themselves as susceptible to breast cancer (Fulton *et al.*, 1995). Hispanic women often present with breast cancer at a later stage of the disease and with a larger tumor, which may contribute to a poorer outcome (Samet, Hunt, and Goodwin, 1990). This is particularly true of Mexican-American women, who tend to have worse outcomes than either Puerto Ricans or Cuban-Americans (Villar and Menck, 1994). Hispanics have been found less likely than non-Hispanic whites to undergo a digital rectal examination, a fecal occult blood test, and a sigmoidoscopy (Perez-Stable *et al.* 1994).

Cardiovascular Disease

Cardiovascular mortality among Hispanics appears to be lower than that among non-Hispanic whites and African-Americans (Diehl and Stern, 1989; Gillum, 1997; Los Angeles County Department of Health Services, 1993; National Center for Health Statistics, 1989; Secretary's Task Force on Black and Minority Health, 1986b). However, cardiovascular disease remains the leading cause of death among Hispanics (National Center for Health Statistics, 1995).

Hypertension is often unrecognized and untreated among Hispanics (Barrios *et al.*, 1987; Kumanyika *et al.*, 1989). For example, in the Hispanic Health and Nutrition Examination Survey (HHANES), almost one half of the Puerto Ricans with hypertension surveyed did not know that they were hypertensive (Munoz, Lecca, and Goldstein, 1988, cited in Council on Scientific Affairs, 1991). Caralis (1992) found that almost half of the study participants who knew that they were hypertensive did not take medication to regulate their blood pressure.

Various factors may contribute to cardiovascular disease among Hispanics, including obesity (Stern, Gaskill, and Hazuda, 1982; Stern *et al.*, 1981), lack of knowledge regarding hypertension and its prevention (Ailinger, 1982; Kumanyika *et al.*, 1989), physical inactivity (Friis, Najundappa, Prendergrast, and Welsh, 1981; Hazuda *et al.*, 1983), and smoking (Council on Scientific Affairs, 1991). Smoking is of particular concern. The HHANES data indicate that 43.6% of Mexican-American men smoked, compared to 41.8% of Cuban men and 41.3% of Puerto Rican men (Escobeda and Remington, 1989). Hispanic adolescents have been found to have higher prevalence rates of smoking compared to their white, African-American, and Asian counterparts (Moreno *et al.*, 1991). Studies have indicated that Hispanic women are less likely to smoke than are men (Perez-Stable, Marin, and Marin, 1994). Acculturation appears to affect smoking behaviors differentially by sex; less acculturated men are more likely to smoke, whereas more acculturated women are more likely to smoke (Marin *et al.*, 1989). Hispanics have been found more likely to be occasional smokers compared to other groups and are less likely to believe that smoking is addictive, despite knowledge of its harmful effects (Palinkas *et al.*, 1993).

Oral Health

Lack of knowledge about the importance of oral hygiene and lack of routine oral hygiene contribute to poor oral health (Watson and Brown, 1995). Children in low income families have been found to be twice as likely to have cavities (National Institute of Dental Research, 1989). Hispanics have been found twice as likely as whites to have untreated dental disease and to have a higher prevalence of calculus, gingivitis, attachment loss, and periodontal pockets than non-Hispanic whites (Watson and Brown, 1995).

Mental Health and Illness

Substance Use and Misuse

Hispanics have been found to have a slightly higher rate of heavy alcohol use compared with whites and African-Americans (Department of Health and Human Services, 1997). Alcoholism and cirrhosis are prevalent among Mexican Americans and Puerto Ricans in particular (Schinke *et al.*, 1988). Hispanic males often abstain from alcohol use for a period of time and then engage in binge drinking (Perez-Stable, Marin, and Marin, 1994). Hispanic youth have also been found to engage in extensive alcohol use. A recent study of 1500 high school students in San Francisco found that over one quarter of the Hispanic students used some type of alcohol at least once a week, while 13% drank to the point of intoxication on a daily basis (Morales, 1990).

Research indicates that Hispanics experience a disproportionate number of deaths due to narcotic use (Burge, Felts, Chenier, and Parrillo, 1995). Compared to other Hispanic groups, marijuana and cocaine use are more prevalent among Puerto Ricans (Vega, 1994). In general, however, the rates of substance misuse among Hispanics are similar to those of whites and African-Americans (Department of Health and Human Services, 1997). A recent study of maternal drug use in New York City found that drug use was less common among foreign-born Hispanic mothers. Puerto Ricans had the highest percentage of reported drug use among island-born and mainland-born mothers, while Mexican mothers had the lowest rate of drug use among mainland-born mothers (Lederman and Sierra, 1994). Previous research has demonstrated low rates of maternal drug use among Hispanic women compared to whites (Vega, Kolody, Hwang, and Noble, 1993). Young Hispanic males have rates of drug use similar to those of their white counterparts and somewhat higher in comparison with African-American youth. By contrast, Hispanic adolescent females use drugs at a rate lower than do their white counterparts, but somewhat higher than do African-American youth (Adams *et al.*, 1995).

Suicide

Although Hispanics in general appear to have low rates of suicide, Cuba-born and Puerto Rico-born men have higher rates of suicide compared to non-Hispanic men, while the rates among Mexican-American men are lower than among non-Hispanic men and higher than among African-American men (Shai and Rosenwaike, 1988). Suicide rates are highest among Puerto Rican and Cuban-American men between the ages of 25 and 35 (Shai and Rosenwaike, 1988). High rates of suicide attempts have been documented. "Suicide fits" constitute one of the most prevalent socioemotional and behavioral mental health issues for Puerto Ricans (Zavala-Martinez, 1994). Identified risk factors for suicidal ideation include stress, depression, low self-esteem, family dysfunction, substance abuse, and for youth, poor academic performance (Burge *et al.*, 1995). Immigrant status has also been linked to suicidal ideation (Zavala-Martinez, 1994: Vega *et al.*, 1993), with rates differing across various Hispanic ethnicities (Vega *et al.*, 1993).

Exercises

1. Many health researchers distinguish between whites, African-Americans, and Hispanics/ Latinos. What are the difficulties associated with this classification scheme? What alternatives can you propose? Should data be analyzed according to any racial/ethnic classification? Why or why not?
2. Data indicate that HIV transmission among non-Puerto Rican Hispanics is attributable primarily to unprotected male–male sex, while among Puerto Ricans, transmission is more likely to result from injection drug use.
   a. What factors might account for this difference in transmission pattern between various Hispanic subgroups?
   b. Design a study to assess whether the hypothesized factors indicated in (a) are, in fact, related to a different transmission pattern.

References

Adams, P., Schoenhorn, C., Moss, A., Warren, C., & Kann, L. (1995). Health-risk behaviors among our nation's youth: United States, 1992. *Vital and Health Statistics, Series 10, Data from the National Health Interview Survey, 192*, 1–51.

Ailinger, R.L. (1982). Hypertension knowledge in a Hispanic community. *Nursing Research, 31*, 207–210.

Anderson, R. (1987). The treatment of musculoskeletal disorders by a Mexican bonesetter (sobador). *Social Science and Medicine, 24*, 43–46.

Anonymous. (1996a). Tuberculosis morbidity—United States, 1995. *Morbidity and Mortality Weekly Report, 45*, 365–370.

Arfaa, F. (1981). Intestinal parasites among Indochinese refugees and Mexican immigrants resettled in Contra Costa County, California. *Journal of Family Practice, 12*, 223–226.

Baca, J.E. (1969). Some beliefs of the Spanish speaking. *American Journal of Nursing, 69*, 2172–2176.

Barrios, E., Iler, E., Mulloy, K., Goldstein, J., Chalfin, D., & Munoz, E. (1987). Hypertension in the Hispanic and black population in New York City. *Journal of the National Medical Association, 79*, 749–752.

Bass, J., Mehta, K., & Eppes, B. (1992). Parasitology screening of Latin American children in a primary care clinic. *Pediatrics, 89*, 279–283.

Bassford, T.L. (1995). Health status of Hispanic elders. *Clinics in Geriatric Medicine, 11*, 25–38.

Bonilla, F., & Campos, R. (1981). A wealth of poor: Puerto Ricans in the new economic order. *Daedalus, 110*, 133–176.

Brandon, G. (1991). The uses of plants in healing in an Afro-Cuban religion, santeria. *Journal of Black Studies, 22*, 55–76.

Browner, C.H. (1985). Criteria for selecting herbal remedies. *Ethnology, 24*, 13–32.

Burge, V., Felts, M., Chenier, T., & Parrillo, A. (1995). Drug use, sexual activity, and suicidal behavior in U.S. high school students. *Journal of School Health, 65*, 222–227.

Burgess, A., & Dean, R.F.A. (1962). *Malnutrition and Food Habits*. London: Tavistock.

Cantell, M., Snider, D., Cauthen, G., & Onorato, I. (1995). Epidemiology of tuberculosis in the United States, 1985 through 1992. *JAMA, 272*, 535–539.

Caralis, P.V. (1992). Coronary artery disease in Hispanic Americans. How does this ethnic background affect risk factors and mortality rates? *Postgraduate Medicine, 91*, 179–182, 185–188, 193.

Centers for Disease Control. (1987). *Tuberculosis in the United States*. Washington, DC: Department of Health and Human Services [DHHS Publ. No. (CDC) 89-8322].

Chenault, L. (1970). *The Puerto Rican Migrant in New York City*. New York: Columbia University Press.

Cheung, F., & Dobkin de Rios, M.F. (1982). Recent trends in the study of the mental health of Chinese immigrants to the United States. *Research in Race Relations, 3*, 145–163.

Clark, M., & Bartholomew, Inc. for the American Cancer Society. (1985). *A Study of Hispanics' Attitudes Concerning Cancer and Cancer Prevention*, 1–28.

Commonwealth Fund. (1995). *National Comparative Survey of Minority Health Care*. Commonwealth Fund. Unpublished manuscript. Cited in S. Guendelman (1998). Health and disease among Hispanics. In S. Loue (Ed.), *Handbook of Immigrant Health* (pp. 277–301). New York: Plenum.

Council on Scientific Affairs. (1991). Hispanic health in the United States. *JAMA, 265*, 248–252.

Cuellar, J.B. (1990). Hispanic-American aging: Geriatric education curriculum developed for selected health professionals. In M.S. Harper (Ed.), *Minority Aging: Essential Curricula Content for Selected Health and Allied Health Professionals* (pp. 365–413). Washington, DC: U.S. Government Printing Office [DHHS Publ. No. HRS P-DV-90-4].

Currier, R.L. (1966). The hot-cold syndrome and symbolic balance in Mexican and Spanish-American folk medicine. *Ethnology, 5*, 251–263.

DeLaCancela, V., Guarnaccia, P.J., & Carrillo, E. (1986). Psychosocial distress among Latinos: A critical analysis of *ataques de nervios*. *Humanity Soc., 10*, 431–447.

DeLaRosa, M. (1989). Health care needs of Hispanic Americans and the responsiveness of the health care system. *Health and Social Work, 14*, 104–113.

Department of Health and Human Services. (1997, January 8). Patterns: Patterns of drug use in 1994 [www.health.org/pubs/94hhs/patterns.htm].

Diaz, J. (1992, October). *Hispanic Children and AIDS: National Council of La Raza Center for Health Promotion Fact Sheet*. Washington, DC: National Council of La Raza.

Diaz, T., Buehler, J., Castro, K., & Ward, J. (1993). AIDS trends among Hispanics in the United States. *American Journal of Public Health, 83*, 504–509.

Diehl, A.K., & Stern, M.P. (1989). Special health problems of Mexican-Americans: Obesity, gallbladder disease, diabetes mellitus, and cardiovascular disease. *Advances in Internal Medicine, 34*, 73–96.

Edgerton, R.B., Karno, M., & Fernandez, I. (1970). Curanderismo in the metropolis: The diminished role of folk psychiatry among Los Angeles Mexican-Americans. *American Journal of Psychotherapy, 24*, 124–134.

Ehrlich, P.R., Bilderback, L., & Ehrlich, A.H. (1979). *The Golden Door: International Migration, Mexico, and the United States*. New York: Ballantine Books.

Escobedo, L.G., & Remington, P.L. (1989). Birth cohort analysis of prevalence of cigarette smoking among Hispanics in the United States. *JAMA, 261*, 66–69.

Foster, G.M. (1985). How to get well in Tzintzuntzan. *Social Science and Medicine, 21*, 807–818.

Foster, G.M. (1984). How to stay well in Tzintzuntzan. *Social Science and Medicine, 19*, 523–533.

Foster, G.M. (1988). The validating role of humoral theory in traditional Spanish-American therapeutics. *American Ethnologist, 15*, 120–135.

Friis, R., Nanjundappa, G., Prendergrast, T.J., Jr., & Welsh, M. (1981). Coronary heart disease mortality and risk among Hispanics and non-Hispanics in Orange County, California. *Public Health Reports, 96*, 418–422.

Fulton, J.P., Rakowski, B., & Jones, A.C. (1995). Determinants of breast cancer screening among inner-city Hispanic women in comparison with other inner-city women. *Public Health Reports, 110*, 476–482.

Furino, A. (Ed.). (1992). *Health and Policy and the Hispanic*. Boulder, CO: Westview Press.

Garcia-Palmieri, M.R., Solie, P., Tillotson, J., Costas, R., Jr., Codero, E., & Rodriguez, M. (1980). Relationship of dietary intake to subsequent coronary heart incidence: The Puerto Rican heart health program. *American Journal of Clinical Nutrition, 33*, 1818–1827.

Gillum, R.F. (1997). Sudden cardiac death in Hispanic Americans and African Americans. *American Journal of Public Health, 87*, 1461–1466.

Gonzalez, A.J. (1966, March). La economia y el status politico. *Revista de Ciencias Sociales, 10*, 5–50.

Guendelman, S. (1998). Health and disease among Hispanics. In S. Loue (Ed.), *Handbook of Immigrant Health* (pp. 277–301). New York: Plenum Press.

Guendelman, S., & English, P. (1995). The effect of United States residence on birth outcomes among Mexican immigrants: An exploratory study. *American Journal of Epidemiology, 142*, 530–538.

Handlin, O. (1959). *The Newcomers: Negroes and Puerto Ricans in a Changing Metropolis*. Cambridge, MA: Harvard University Press.

Hazuda, H.P., Stern, M.P., Gaskill, S.P., Haffner, S.M., & Gardner, L.I. (1983). Ethnic differences in health knowledge and behavior related to the prevention and treatment of coronary heart disease: The San Antonio Heart Study. *American Journal of Epidemiology*, *117*, 717–728.

Hispanic Health Alliance. (1990). *Crosscultural Medicine: Clinical and Cultural Dimensions in Health Care Delivery to Hispanic Parents*. Chicago, IL: Crosscultural Pathways and the Hispanic Health Alliance.

Hu, D.J., & Covell, R.M. (1986). Health care usage by Hispanic outpatients as a function of primary language. *Western Journal of Medicine*, *144*, 490–493.

Kay, M.A. (1977). Health and illness in a Mexican barrio. In E.A. Spencer (Ed.), *Ethnic Medicine in the Southwest* (pp. 96–166). Tucson, AZ: University of Arizona Press.

Kay, M., & Yoder, M. (1987). Hot and cold in women's ethnotherapeutics: The American-Mexican West. *Social Science and Medicine*, *25*, 347–355.

Kirkman-Liff, B., & Jacobs Kronenfeld, J. (1992). Access to cancer screening services for women. *American Journal of Public Health*, *82*, 733–735.

Kumanyika, S., Savige, D.D., Ramirez, A.J., Hutchinson, J., Trevino, M.M., Aams-Campbell, L.L., & Watkins, L.O. (1989). Beliefs about high blood pressure prevention in a survey of Blacks and Hispanics. *American Journal of Preventive Medicine*, *5*, 21–26.

Lederman, S.A., & Sierra, D. (1994). Characteristics of childbearing Hispanic women in New York City. In G. Lamberty & G. Coll (Eds.), *Puerto Rican Women and Children: Issues in Health, Growth, and Development* (pp. 85–102). New York: Plenum Press.

Liao, Y., Cooper, R.S., Cao, G., Durazo-Arrizu, R., Kaufman, J.S., Luke, A., & McGee, D.L. (1998). Mortality patterns among adult Hispanics: Findings from the NHIS, 1986 to 1990. *American Journal of Public Health*, *88*, 227–232.

Lipton, B., & Katz, M. (1989). Understanding the Hispanic market. *Medical Market Media*, *24*, 9–10, 12, 18.

Logan, M.H. (1977). Anthropological research on the hot-cold theory of disease: Some methodological reflections. *Medical Anthropology*, *1*, 87–108.

Los Angeles County Department of Health Services. (1993). *Los Angeles County Vital Statistics: Summary Report on Births, Deaths and Fetal Deaths 1988–1991*. Los Angeles, CA: Data Collection and Analysis Unit, Los Angeles County Department of Health Services.

Ludman, E.K., Newman, J.H., & Lynn, L.L. (1989). Blood-building foods in contemporary Chinese populations. *Journal of the American Dietetic Association*, *89*, 1122–1124.

Maldonado, M. (1998). The HIV/AIDS epidemic among Latinos in the United States. *Update, October*, 1–7.

Marcell, A. (1994). Understanding ethnicity, identity formation, and risk behavior among adolescents of Mexican descent. *Journal of School Health*, *64*, 323–327.

Marin, G., Perez-Stables, E.J., & Marin, B.V. (1989). Cigarette smoking among San Francisco Hispanics: The role of acculturation and gender. *American Journal of Public Health*, *79*, 196–199.

Marks, G., Garcia, M., & Solis, J.M. (1990). Health risk behaviors of Hispanics in the United States: Findings from HHANES, 1982–1984. *American Journal of Public Health*, *80*(Suppl.), 20–26.

Marks, G., Solis, J., Richardson, J.L., Collins, L.M., Birba, L., & Hisserich, J.C. (1987). Health behavior of elderly Hispanic women: Does cultural assimilation make a difference? *American Journal of Public Health*, *77*, 1315–1319.

Martin, H.W., Martinez, C., & Leon, R.L. (1985). Folk illnesses reported to physicians in the lower Rio Grande Valley: A binational comparison. *Ethnology*, *24*, 229–236.

Martinez, C., & Martin, H.W. (1966). Folk diseases among urban-Mexican Americans. *JAMA*, *196*, 147–150.

Mathews, H.F. (1983). Context-specific variation in humoral classification. *American Anthropologist*, *85*, 826–847.

Mayers, R.S. (1989). Use of folk medicine by elderly Mexican American women. *The Journal of Drug Issues*, *19*, 283–295.

Mendoza, F.S. (1994). The health of Latino children in the United States. *Critical Health Issues for Children and Youth*, *4*, 43–72.

Messer, E. (1981). Hot-cold classification: Theoretical and practical implications of a Mexican study. *Social Science and Medicine*, *15B*, 133–145.

Moore, J., & Devitt, M. (1989). The paradox of deviance in addicted Mexican American mothers. *Gender and Society*, *3*, 53–70.

Morales, E. (1990). *Cadre Evaluation Report: (Year Three). Demonstration Project*. Funded by the Office of Substance Abuse Prevention, U.S. Department of Health. San Francisco, CA: Community Substance Abuse Services, San Francisco Department of Health.

Morales, J. (1986). *Puerto Rican Poverty and Migration: We Just Had to Try Elsewhere*. New York: Praeger.

Moreno, C., Larriado-Laborin, R., Sallis, J., Elder, J., De Moon, C., Castro, F., & Devsaransingh, T. (1991). Parental influences to smoke in Latino youth. *Preventive Medicine*, *23*, 48–53.

Nall, F.C., II, & Spielberg, J. (1967). Social and cultural factors in the responses of Mexican Americans to medical treatment. *Journal of Health and Social Behavior*, *8*, 299–308.

National Cancer Institute. (1985). *Cancer Rates and Risks* (3rd ed.). Atlanta, GA: National Cancer Institute [Publ. No. 85-691].

National Cancer Institute. (1989, May). *Cancer Statistics Review 1973–1986, Including a Report on the Status of Cancer Control*. Bethesda, MD: National Cancer Institute. [NIH Publ. No. (NIH) 89-2789].

National Center for Health Statistics. (1989). Advance report of final mortality statistics, 1987. *Monthly Vital Statistics Report, 38*(Suppl.).

National Center for Health Statistics. (1995). *Health, United States, 1994*. Hyattsville, MD: National Center for Health Statistics.

National Institute of Dental Research. (1989). *Oral Health of United States Children: 1986–87*. Bethesda, MD: National Institutes of Health [NIH Publ. No. 89-2247].

Ortiz de Montellano, B. (1987). *Caida de mollera*: Aztec sources for a Mesoamerican disease of alleged Spanish origin. *Ethnohistory, 34*, 381–399.

Palinkas, L., Pierce, J., Rosbrook, B., Pickwell, S., & Bal, D. (1993). Cigarette smoking behavior and beliefs of Hispanics in California. *American Journal of Preventive Medicine, 9*, 331–337.

Perez-Stable, E., Marin, G., & Marin, B. (1994). Behavioral risk factors: A comparison of Latinos and non-Latino whites in San Francisco. *American Journal of Public Health, 84*, 971–976.

Perez-Stable, E.J., Otero-Sabogal, R., Sabogal, F., McPhee, S.J., & Hiatt, R.A. (1994). Self-reported use of cancer screening tests among Latinos and Anglos in a prepaid health plan. *Archives of Internal Medicine, 154*, 1073–1081.

Public Health Service. (1987). *Cancer and Minorities: Closing the Gap*. Washington, DC: Department of Health and Human Services.

Rodriguez, C.E. (1994). A summary of Puerto Rican migration to the United States. In G. Lamberty & C.G. Coll (Eds.), *Puerto Rican Women and Children: Issues in Health, Growth, and Development* (pp. 11–28). New York: Plenum Press.

Rubel, A.J. (1964). The epidemiology of a folk illness: Susto in Hispanic America. *Ethnology, 3*, 268–283.

Saint-Germain, M.A., & Longman, A. (1993). Resignation and resourcefulness: Older Hispanic women's responses to breast cancer. In S.E. Cayleff & B. Bair. (Eds.), *Minority Women and Health: Gender and the Experience of Illness*. Detroit, MI: Wayne State University Press.

Samet, J.M., Hunt, W.C., & Goodwin, J.S. (1990). Determinants of cancer stage. A population-based study of elderly New Mexicans. *Cancer, 66*, 1302–1307.

Samora, J. (1971). *Los Mojados: The Wetback Story*. Notre Dame, IN: University of Notre Dame Press.

Scheper-Hughes, N., & Stewart, D. (1983). Curanderismo in Taos County, New Mexico—A possible case of anthropological romanticism? *Western Journal of Medicine, 139*, 875–884.

Schinke, S.P., Moncher, M.S., Palleja, J., Zayas, L.H., & Schilling, R.F. (1988). Hispanic youth, substance abuse, and stress: Implications for prevention research. *International Journal of the Addictions, 23*, 809–826.

Schreiber, J.M., & Homiak, J.P. (1981). Mexican-Americans. In A. Harwood (Ed.), *Ethnicity and Medical Care* (pp. 264–336). Cambridge, MA: Harvard University Press.

Secretary's Task Force on Black and Minority Health. (1986a). *Cancer, III*. Washington, DC: U.S. Department of Health and Human Services.

Secretary's Task Force on Black and Minority Health. (1986b). *Cardiovascular and Cerebrovascular Disease, IV*. Washington, DC: U.S. Department of Health and Human Services.

Selik, R.M., Castro, K.G., Pappaioanou, M., & Buehler, J.W. (1989). Birthplace and the risk of AIDS among Hispanics in the United States. *American Journal of Public Health, 79*, 836–839.

Shai, D. (1986). Cancer mortality, ethnicity, and socioeconomic status: Two New York City groups. *Public Health Reports, 101*, 547–552.

Shai, D., & Rosenwaike, I. (1988). Violent deaths among Mexican-, Puerto Rican-, and Cuban-born migrants in the United States. *Social Science and Medicine, 26*, 269–276.

Signorini, I. (1982). Patterns of fright: Multiple concepts of susto in a Mahua-Ladino community of the Sierra de Pueblo (Mexico). *Ethnology, 21*, 313–323.

Stern, M.P., Gaskill, S.P., Allen, C.R., Garza, V., Gonzales, J.L., & Waldrop, R.H. (1981). Cardiovascular risk factors in Mexican Americans in Laredo, Texas. III. Prevalence and control of hypertension. *American Journal of Epidemiology, 113*, 556–562.

Stern, M.P., Gaskill, S.P., & Hazuda, H. (1982). Knowledge, attitudes and behavior related to obesity and dieting in Mexican Americans and Anglos: The San Antonio Heart Study. *American Journal of Epidemiology, 115*, 916–928.

Stevens-Arroyo, A., & Diaz-Stevens, M. (1982). Puerto Ricans in the United States: A struggle for identity. In A.G. Dworkin & R.J. Dworkin (Eds.), *The Minority Report: An Introduction to Racial, Ethnic, and Gender Relations* (2nd ed.). New York: CBS Publishing, Holt, Rinehart, & Winston.

Steward, J. (1965). *The People of Puerto Rico*. Chicago, IL: University of Illinois Press.

Trevino, F.M., Bruhn, J.G., & Bunce, H. (1979). Utilization of community mental health services in a Texas-Mexico border city. *Social Science and Medicine, 13A*, 331–334.

Trevino, F.M., & Moss, A.J. (1983). Insurance coverage and physician visits among Hispanic and non-Hispanic people. In *Health, United States, 1983*. Washington, DC: Public Health Service [Publ. No. PHS 84-1232].

Trevino, F.M., Moyer, M.E., Burciaga Valdez, R., & Stroup-Benham, C.A. (1991). Health insurance coverage and utilization of health services by Mexican Americans, mainland Puerto Ricans, and Cuban Americans. *JAMA, 265*, 233–237.

Trotter, R.T. (1985). Folk medicine in the Southwest: Myths and medical facts. *Folk Medicine, 78*, 167–179.

U.S. Bureau of the Census. (1988). *The Hispanic Population in the United States: March 1988*. Current Population Reports (Population Characteristics). Washington, DC: Government Printing Office [Series P-20, No. 438].

U.S. Bureau of the Census. (1989). *Statistical Abstract of the United States, 1989*. Washington, DC: U.S. Bureau of the Census.

U.S. Bureau of the Census. (1990). *The Hispanic Population in the United States: March 1989*. Current Population Reports (Population Characteristics). Washington, DC: Government Printing Office [Series P-20, No. 444].

U.S. Bureau of the Census. (1992). *Statistical Abstract of the United States, 1992*. Washington, DC: U.S. Bureau of the Census.

U.S. Bureau of the Census. (1993). *The Hispanic Population in the United States: March 1993*. Current Population Reports (Population Characteristics). Washington, DC: Government Printing Office.

U.S. Department of Health and Human Services. (1996). *Health United States, 1995*. Washington, DC: U.S. Department of Health and Human Services [DHHS Publ. No. PHS 96-1232].

Valdez, R.B., Morgenstern, H., Brown, E.R., Wyn, R., Wang, C., & Cumberland, W. (1993). Insuring Latinos against the costs of illness. *JAMA, 269*, 233–237.

Vega, W. (1994). Latino Outlook: Good health, uncertain prognosis. *Annual Review of Public Health, 15*, 39–67.

Vega, W.A., Gil, A., Warhelt, G., Apospori, E., & Zimmerman, R. (1993). The relationship of drug use to suicide ideation and attempts among African American, Hispanic, and white non-Hispanic male adolescents. *Suicide and Life Threatening Behavior, 23*, 110–119.

Vega, W.A., Kolody, B., Hwang, J., & Noble, A. (1993). Prevalence and magnitude of perinatal substance exposures in California. *New England Journal of Medicine, 329*, 850–854.

Villar, H., & Menck, H. (1994). The National Cancer Data Base Report on Cancer in Hispanics. *Cancer, 74*, 2386–2395.

Wagenheim, K., & Jimenez de Wagenheim, O. (1994). *The Puerto Ricans: A Documentary History*. Princeton: Marcus Winer Publishers.

Watson, M., & Brown, L. (1995). The oral health of U.S. Hispanics: Evaluating their needs and their use of dental services. *Journal of the American Dental Association, 126*, 789–795.

Weller, S.C. (1983). New data on intracultural variability: The hot-cold concept of medicine and illness. *Human Organization, 42*, 249–257.

Wells, K.B., Golding, J.M., Hough, R.L., Burnam, M.A., & Karno, M. (1989). Acculturation and the probability of use of health services by Mexican Americans. *Health Services Research, 24*, 237–257.

Zambrana, R.E., Scrimshaw, S.C.M., Collins, N., & Dunkel-Schetter, C. (1997). Prenatal health behaviors and psychosocial risk factors in pregnant women of Mexican origin: The role of acculturation. *American Journal of Public Health, 87*, 1022–1026.

Zavala-Martinez, I. (1994). Entremundos: The psychological dialectics of Puerto Rican migration and its implications for health. In G. Lamberty & C.G. Loll (Eds.), *Puerto Rican Women and Children: Issues in Health, Growth, and Development* (pp. 29–38). New York: Plenum.

9

The Health of Native Americans

Introduction

Origin and Culture Areas

The term "Native American" refers to the indigenous population of North America prior to the arrival of European settlers (Young, 1994). The term includes American Indians, Eskimos (also known as Inuit), and Aleuts (Young, 1994). Native Americans are believed to have originated in Asia, although the date, duration, and point of entry of this migration remain in dispute (Dillehay and Meltzer, 1991; Greenberg, Turner, and Zegura, 1986).

Prior to the arrival of European settlers, Native Americans' communities were distinguishable by "culture area," reflective of the varying climatic and geographical conditions and individuals' attempts to adapt to these varied conditions. These 13 culture areas included the Arctic, the Sub-Arctic, the Northwest Coast, the Plateau, the Plains, the Prairies, the East, California, the Great Basin, Baja California, the Southwest, Northeast Mexico, and Meso-America (Driver, 1969).

The Arctic, encompassing portions of Alaska, Canada, and Greenland, was generally characterized by its access to the sea. The Sub-Arctic included the interior portions of Canada and Alaska; moose and caribou were the primary food sources. The Northwest Coast, which extended from southeastern Alaska's panhandle to California's northwest corner, is now known for its plank houses and totem poles. In the Plateau region, which includes portions of British Columbia, fish were plentiful.

The Plains area, extending southward from central Alberta in Canada to Mexico, is bounded by the Rocky Mountains and the Missouri River. The Plains Indians included the Sioux, the Blackfoot, the Crow, and the Cheyenne. Unlike the predominantly nomadic Plains Indians, the Native Americans of the Prairies lived in villages near their farms, in areas that correspond to what is now the Midwest. Tribes of the Eastern culture area, which encompassed portions of New York, the Middle Atlantic states, and some portion of the southern states, included the Iroquois. The California culture area covered approximately two thirds of what is now the state of California. The Great Basin area, which includes areas of California, Oregon, Idaho, Wyoming, and Colorado and all of Nevada and Utah, was characterized by extreme dryness. Native American groups in this area included the Ute, the Paiutes, and the Shoshone. Like the Great Basin, Baja California has large areas of desert, but also has areas of heavy rainfall. Most settlements in this area were located less than 50 miles from the ocean. Many were missionized by the Spanish. Both the Southwest and the Northwest Mexico areas are characterized by desert. The Southwest, which encompasses what is now Arizona, New Mexico, the Mexican states of Sonora and Sinaloa, and portions of Chihuahua and Durango, was home to the Hopi, the Zuni, the Navaho, the Apache, the Mohave, the Yuma, and the Yaqui. The Meso-American culture area, best known for the Aztecs and the Mayas, extends from southern Mexico through Guatemala, Honduras, El Salvador, and portions of Nicaragua (Driver, 1969).

Current Demographics

The 1990 census reported that there were 1,959,234 Native Americans, Eskimos, and Aleuts in the United States (Paisano, 1995), constituting almost 1% of the total population. This represents a 38% increase in the Native American population between 1980 and 1990 (McKenney and Bennett, 1994). This increase has been attributed to improvements in counting individuals on reservations, reliance on self-identification, and improved outreach programs and promotion campaigns in connection with the census (Paisano, 1995).

The ten largest tribes included the Cherokee (19% of all Native Americans), Navaho (11.6%), Sioux (5.5%), Chippewa (5.5%), Choctaw (4.5%), Pueblo (2.9%), Apache (2.8%), Iroquois (2.7%), Lumbee (2.6%), and Creek (2.4%) (Bureau of the Census, 1994). A large proportion (27%) live on reservations, tribal trust lands, and in Alaskan Native villages (Bureau of the Census, 1993). Of those living on reservations, almost 20% of households disposed of sewage by means other than public sewer, septic tank, or cesspool; almost 20% lacked complete plumbing facilities in their homes (Bureau of the Census, 1995). Over time, an increasing proportion of Native Americans have moved to urban areas (Young, 1994). The largest proportion of Native Americans live in Oklahoma, California, Arizona, New Mexico, Alaska, Washington, North Carolina, Texas, New York, and Michigan (Paisano, 1995).

Compared to the entire U.S. population, Native Americans are more likely to be younger, poorer, and less educated. The median age of the Native American population at the time of the 1990 census was 26 years, compared to a median age of 36 years for the entire U.S. population (Paisano, 1995). Thirty-nine percent of the Native American population was under the age of 20, compared with 29% of the entire U.S. population. Thirty-one percent of Native Americans lived below the poverty level in 1989, compared with 13% of the entire U.S. population. The median family income of Native Americans, Eskimos, and Aleuts in 1990 was $21,750, compared to $35,225 for the entire U.S. population. Over half of Native Americans living on reservations and trust lands in 1989 were living below the poverty level (Bureau of the Census, 1993). Moreover, although the educational attainment of Native Americans has improved significantly, as of 1990 only 9% of Native Americans had completed a bachelor's degree or higher, compared with 20% of the total U.S. population (Paisano, 1995).

Cultural and Historical Context

Language

We know of a total of 221 mutually distinct Native American languages. The various culture areas correlate to a high degree with the areas in which specific languages are spoken. For example, the Eskimo-Aleut language coincides with the culture areas of the Arctic (Driver, 1969).

Traditional Lifestyles

The culture areas were distinguished not only by language, but also by various aspects of health, such as nutritional status and patterns of health behaviors. In the Arctic culture area, for example, Eskimos relied on sea mammals, such as the seal and the walrus, for their primary source of nutrition. Approximately half of their meat was eaten raw.

Sub-Arctic Native Americans relied primarily on caribou and small mammals, such as beaver, rabbit, and deer, for food. Their diet was supplemented with shellfish and fish. Eskimos and Native Americans in both the Arctic and Sub-Arctic areas boiled their food both by direct-fire boiling or placing heated stones in the liquid to be boiled (Driver, 1969).

Native Americans of the Northwest Coast relied predominantly on fish as a source of nutrition. Fish were preserved by burying them in pits and allowing them to decay or by smoking them. The addition of roots and berries supplemented their protein-rich diet with carbohydrates, sugar, iron, and copper.

The diet in the Plateau culture area included game, such as moose, elk, and deer, as well as wild plants and roots. Native Americans of the Plains relied heavily on the buffalo for sustenance, supplemented by elk, antelope, and bear, as well as by roots. In the Prairie culture area, Native Americans depended heavily on buffalo or deer, although maize, beans, squashes, and sunflowers were also cultivated. Food was often prepared by direct boiling (Driver, 1969).

Famines in the East culture area were rare due to the diversity of the food sources, which included fish, hunted animals, and crops, such as beans, squashes, and corn. Similarly, small game was secondary to other sources of food in the California culture area. There, the diet was based primarily on the acorn and smaller seeds, although fish, small game, and invertebrates, such as grasshoppers and earthworms, also provided nutrition (Driver, 1969).

In contrast, wild plants served as the dominant food source in the Great Basin area. Deer and the mountain sheep were the most common animals, and rabbits and other game were hunted. Salt was obtained from the surface of the land in and around the lake beds. Native Americans in Northeast Mexico and Baja California similarly emphasized plants in their diet, including mesquite pods and cactus fruits. Although fish and shellfish were available to inhabitants near the coast, this was not true for those further inland, who often faced the possibility of famine and who suffered from chronic malnutrition (Driver, 1969).

The extent of farming varied across the Native American groups in the Southwest culture area. As much as 80% of the Pueblos' diet may have consisted of maize in its various forms. Meat was seldom available due to the scarcity of game, often resulting in protein deficiency. Reliance on wild plants, however, provided high fiber, carbohydrates, and micronutrients (Teufel, 1996). Famine and drought occurred not infrequently. The Navaho acquired farming from the Pueblos and by the 19th century were also relying on maize as the cornerstone of their diet. Farm crops also constituted an important part of the diet of the Mohave and the Yuma.

Maize was also an important crop to the Native Americans of the Meso-America culture area. Seeds were often dried and cooked by parching. Residents of this area also relied on various animals as a source of nutrition, including turkey, goose, duck, and quail. Salt was obtained by evaporating salt water.

Explanatory Models of Health and Illness

Explanatory models of health and illness differed across the various culture areas. Depending on the culture area and the specific type of disease in question, disease was believed to be caused by soul loss, natural origins, a supernatural being, contact with the dead, and violations of taboos (Driver, 1969). Cures often required the intervention of a shaman (Driver, 1969) and/or the application or ingestion of specific remedies, such as plants and teas (Chamberlin, 1909; Driver, 1969; Grinnell, 1905; Hridlicka, 1932; Landes, 1963; Vogel, 1970).

Despite the apparent success of some of the Native-American curative remedies (Driver, 1969), the white settlers often displayed little regard for the abilities of the Native American medicine men and shamans. One writer characterized the medicine man as "an influence antagonistic to the rapid absorption of new ideas and the adoption of new customs" (Bourke, 1887:451). Only by "thoroughly [routing] the medicine men from their entrenchments and [making] them the object of ridicule" could whites "bend and train the minds of our Indian wards in the direction of civilization" (Bourke, 1887:594).

Historical Context

Leacock and Lurie (1971) have delineated four phases of Native American history following the arrival of the Europeans:

1. *Early contact*. This interchange, which was often on an equal footing, generally occurred through trade or missionaries.
2. *Conflict-disruption*. This phase was characterized by the large-scale settlement of the European settlers and resulting conflict, often due to the forcible displacement of Native American communities and the breach of treaty agreements.
3. *Government controls*. This phase is notable for the imposition of government controls and the establishment of reservations.
4. *Cultural revival*. This period reflects new forms of political organization in the context of industrial society.

Conflict and Disruption

These four periods are distinguishable in even the brief review of Native American history that follows. This synopsis begins with the 1600s, in what Leacock and Lurie would characterize as a period of conflict-disruption. Several continuing themes are apparent in this brief overview: settlers' betrayal of negotiated agreements with various tribes; the decimation of tribes by disease and war; and the settlers' disdain for Native Americans, reflected in broken agreements, enslavement, corporal punishment for refusal to convert to Christianity, prohibitions against intermarriage, and in some cases, a policy of extermination.

In 1600, members of the Apache, Navaho, and Ute tribes were captured by Spaniards, with the assistance of the Pueblos, to be used as slave labor and household servants. These kidnapping raids by the Spanish continued into the 1900s (Nies, 1996). In 1609, British settlers in Jamestown, Virginia, burned Powhatan villages and captured the Powhatan as slaves. In 1614, English sea captain Thomas Hunt captured 24 New England coastal Indians and sold them as slaves in Spain (Nies, 1996).

New England Indians, from Massachusetts to Maine, suffered a smallpox epidemic from 1616 to 1619. The infection was believed to be transmitted from European fishermen on the coast. More than 190,000 Huron died between 1633 and 1635 due to a smallpox epidemic. Indian oral history tells us that during this epidemic, French Jesuit missionaries advised the Huron that those who were baptized as Catholics would be spared. The missionaries gave the unbaptized blankets from smallpox victims, resulting in transmission of the infection. Various tribes were decimated by other epidemics in later years.

By 1660, approximately 1,000 British settlers per year were arriving in Massachusetts Bay. The Indians interpreted the gifts that they received from the British as a rental fee for land use; the British believed that these exchanges represented the purchase price to a tract of land which was private property. This misunderstanding constituted the source of much conflict to follow.

In 1622, after years of conflict over land and other issues, the Powhatan attacked the Jamestown Colony. The royal British Virginia Company ordered that the Powhatan be exterminated and prohibited all peace negotiations. In 1623, the English invited the Powhatan leaders to a peace conference, where the Powhatan were served poisoned wine. Those who survived were shot. The Powhatan–British conflicts continued for at least a decade (Nies, 1996).

Numerous other attempts by Native Americans to negotiate peace with the European settlers also met with failure. In 1641, the Five Nations of the Iroquois attempted to reach a settlement with the French. Their efforts were rebuffed because the French believed that such an agreement would not further their economic interests. In 1649, Virginia settlers disregarded the terms of an agreement with the Powhatan and encroached further onto lands guaranteed to the Powhatan.

By the mid- to late 1600s, numerous Native American rebellions occurred against the British, French, and Spanish settlers. These rebellions were often provoked by settlers' kidnapping raids, infringements on Native American lands, breaches of agreements, and physical punishment of Native American leaders for "idolatry" (Nies, 1996). In 1691, Virginia banished all English who married Native Americans, blacks, or anyone with mixed ancestry (Nies, 1996).

The 1700s were characterized by continuing conflict between Native American tribes and various European groups and between Native American tribes with differing loyalties to the European settlers. French, British and Spanish colonists continued to appropriate land as their own. The British, in particular, were known for their kidnapping raids to capture Native Americans for sale as slaves (Francis, 1996). The sale of alcohol to Native Americans had become an issue; the Powhatan leader Anne complained of this practice to the Virginia legislature in 1715, to no avail. Sir Jeffrey Amherst, a British commander, became known for his genocidal policy toward the natives: "Could it not be contrived to send the smallpox among the disaffected tribes of Indians? We must on this occasion [smallpox outbreak] use every stratagem in our power to reduce them" (Nies, 1996:191). Amherst had blankets taken from smallpox victims and given to healthy Indians, ensuring the transmission of the epidemic.

Life under the new United States appeared to be no better for Native Americans than it had been under the colonists and European powers. Large numbers of Great Lakes Indians died during a smallpox epidemic from 1780 to 1782 (Nies, 1996). Numerous tribes and confederacies, such as the Iroquois Six Nations, were forced to cede their lands. The new government respected negotiated agreements no more than the previous authorities had (Francis, 1996; Nies, 1996).

Contact with the Native Americans continued to be regulated. The third Trade and Intercourse Act, passed in 1799, provided for the appointment of federal agents to tribes and restricted those without a license from trading with Indians.

Government Controls

The 1800s witnessed the imposition of further government controls on Native Americans. The new government continued to breach agreements, in their desire for greater amounts of land. Conflicts between the settlers and the Indians continued as a result. Federal policy toward Native Americans was clearly one of assimilation and removal. The government prohibited traditional religious observances and required that Native American children attend boarding schools, cut their hair, learn English, and convert to Christianity. The Indian Allotment Act of

1887 dissolved the previously established reservation system and tribal landholding, converting much reservation land into large parcels in an attempt to make the natives individual landowners and to promote their assimilation (Nies, 1996).

Cultural Revival

The 1900s have been called an Indian renaissance. The release of the Meriam Report of 1928 harshly criticized the allotment policy and recommended reforms in land management and support for communally held tribal lands. The allotment policy had resulted in the reduction of Indian-held lands from 155 million acres in 1881 to approximately 69 million acres in 1934, when the government officially abandoned the policy. At this time, there was almost a complete lack of health, education, and employment facilities for Native Americans.

Following the federal termination of 13 tribes between 1948 and 1960, resulting in their loss of federal recognition, annuities, and services, numerous Native American groups organized programs and actions to renegotiate land deals and address problems on the reservations (Nies, 1996). Native American publications were established in various communities (Francis, 1996).

Native American Health Status

Overview

Numerous theories have been advanced in an attempt to explain the decline in the Native American population over time. One of the better known theories posits the decline of the Native American population as the result of disease transmission resulting from contact with infected and infectious European settlers (Ashburn, 1947). Others have argued, however, that low population levels among some groups resulted from periods of starvation and the practice of female infanticide (Helm, 1980). Johansson (1982) has delineated four phases in the mortality of Native Americans. The first phase, which predated contact with European settlers, was characterized by a birth rate slightly greater than the death rate. During the initial contact period, the birth rate declined and the mortality rate increased. The birth rate eventually exceeded the death rate toward the end of the 19th century. Finally, during the 20th century, the mortality rate and the birth rate have declined.

Compared to all groups in the United States, Native Americans have a higher rate of potential years of life lost due to injuries, and a lower rate of mortality due to chronic diseases such as cancer or circulatory problems (U.S. Department of Health and Human Services [USDHHS], 1990). Native Americans experience a higher rate of restricted activity days compared to all U.S. groups (USDHHS, 1990). During the period from October 1994 through January 1995, almost one third of all Indians and Alaska Natives age 15 and older reported having a disability; of those over the age of 65, 50% reported having a disability (Bureau of the Census, 1997).

Infectious Disease

Sexually Transmitted Disease

National rates of sexually transmitted disease, such as syphilis and gonorrhea, tend to be lower among Native American populations compared to other U.S. groups (Young, 1994), although the rates may be higher in certain geographic areas (Toomey, Oberschelp, and Greenspan, 1989; Rice, Roberts, Handsfield, and Holmes, 1991). Although few cases of AIDS have been reported among Native Americans, the majority of reported cases have been attributable to unprotected sexual intercourse (Metler, Conway, and Stehr-Green, 1991). At least one writer has identified a number of potential vulnerabilities to HIV transmission among the Navaho, including refusal to officially acknowledge homosexuality among the Navaho, the use of alcohol and marijuana which serve as disinhibitors and lead to greater risk-taking, and the high rate of suicide (Sullivan, 1991).

Hepatitis

In comparison to non-Native Americans, Native Americans experience a high prevalence of both hepatitis A and hepatitis B (Williams, 1986; Schreeder *et al.*, 1983). Hepatitis A infection results from both the consumption of contaminated water and foods and from person-to-person transmission via the oral–fecal route (Benenson, 1995). In contrast, infection with hepatitis B results from person-to-person transmission through sexual transmission or contact with contaminated blood or blood products, such as blood transfusions, contact with blood through shared use of injection equipment, or hemodialysis (Benenson, 1995).

Tuberculosis

Although tuberculosis has been documented among Native Americans prior to the arrival of the European settlers (Paulsen, 1987), it is believed that both the incidence and the virulence of tuberculosis among Native Americans increased in the postcontact period (Clark, Kelley, Grange, and Hill, 1987). Various recent studies have documented high rates of tuberculosis among specific Native American populations. Breault and Hoffman (1997) found in their study of the Oglala Sioux on the Pine Ridge reservation in South Dakota that the relative risk of tuberculosis for a Pine Ridge Native American was 18.9 compared to the South Dakota population. The age-specific relative risk for the Pine Ridge population age 65 and older was 65.7. Tuberculin tests were positive in 70% of the diabetic patients on the reservation.

Parasitic Infections

Numerous gastrointestinal diseases have affected the Native American populations, often resulting from *Shigella, Salmonella, E. coli, Yersinia, Campylobacter*, and *Clostridium botulinum* (Young, 1994). A study of 535 patients at the Fort Apache Indian reservation in Whiteriver, Arizona, for example, found that Rotavirus, enterotoxigenic *Escherichia coli*, and Shigella were the most common agents of infection (Sack *et al.*, 1995). Such infections may be due to bacterial contamination of water (Woodward *et al.*, 1974), or may be associated with the proximity of animals (Engelberg *et al.*, 1982) or the consumption of specific fermented food products (Shaffer, Wainwright, Middaugh, and Tauxe, 1990). Infection by various helminths and protozoa, such as Echinococcus, has been linked to close contact with infected animals (Pappaioanou, Schwabe, and Sard, 1977; Schantz *et al.*, 1977).

Chronic Disease

In contrast to the decline in infectious disease, Native Americans have been experiencing an increase in various chronic diseases.

Cancer

Researchers have reported a lower risk of cancer among Native Americans compared to other groups (Creagan and Fraumeni, 1973; Smith, 1957). A more recent meta-analysis, which included Native American populations in two Canadian provinces as well as four states in the United States, found a lower overall incidence of cancer among Native Americans (Mahoney and Michalek, 1991). The apparently low cancer incidence among some Native American groups as compared to whites may be suspect, however, due to misclassification of race/ethnicity (Frost, Taylor, and Fries, 1992). Native American women have been found to have an increased risk of cancer of the gallbladder, cervix, and kidneys; Native American men have a higher risk of cancer of the kidneys. Eskimos are at higher risk of nasopharyngeal cancer, cancer of the salivary gland, and esophageal cancer (Hildes and Schaefer, 1984). Native Americans seem to have poorer survival compared to whites (Young, Ries, and Pollock, 1984), although this may be related to presentation at a later stage of disease (Samet, Key, Hunt, and Goodwin, 1987).

Native Americans experience the same risk factors for cancer as do other groups. A recent study of 982 Native Americans of the Lumbee tribe in North Carolina found that 20.6% of the women used smokeless tobacco, while 23.7% were smokers (Spangler, Bell, Dignan, and Michielutte, 1997). Users of smokeless tobacco were more likely to be older, to have had less education, to report poor or fair health, to be widowed, and to report having a large number of friends. Cigarette smokers, in contrast, were more likely to be of a younger age, to have higher levels of education, to report excellent or good health, to use alcohol, and to be separated or divorced. Byers (1996) found that the current diet of Native Americans and Alaska Natives tends to be high in fat and low in fruits and vegetables, and speculated that nutrition-related cancers may increase as a result. A recent study of attendance at mammography appointments found that Native American women were less likely to appear for mammography compared to women in other groups, although the reasons for this were unclear (Margolis, Lurie, McGovern, and Slater, 1993).

Cardiovascular Disease

In general, rates of cardiovascular disease have been lower among Native Americans compared to the U.S. population in general. For example, Sievers, Nelson, and Bennett (1990) found in their study of the Pima that the age-standardized mortality ratio for heart disease among the Pima compared to the U.S. population was 0.6. For stroke, however, the ratio was 1.3. Becker, Wiggins, Key, and Samet (1988) found in their study of Native Americans in New Mexico that the age-standardized mortality ratio for ischemic heart disease (comparing Native Americans and U.S. whites) was 0.2 during all periods from 1958 through 1982. However, the rates may be increasing. Klain, Covlehan, Arena, and Jannett (1988) observed an increase in rates of acute myocardial infarction among the Navaho. Gillum (1995), using data from the U.S Vital Statistics System and two National Health and Nutrition Examination Surveys, found that stroke was the cause of 6% of deaths among Native Americans over the age of 45 in 1990, compared to 7% of the deaths among whites.

The prevalence of risk factors for cardiovascular disease appears to be high among some groups. A recent study of 230 randomly selected adults ages 25 to 65 of the Pascua Yaqui tribe found that 69% of the women and 40% of the men were obese, 39% of the women and 35% of the men had diabetes, and 24% of the women and 43% of the men were smokers (Campos-Outcalt et al., 1995). Over one half of the participants reported more than one risk factor.

Diabetes

Diabetes among Native Americans is most often of the non-insulin dependent type (Young, 1994). It appears to have been extremely rare prior to World War II (West, 1974). Since that time, the prevalence of diabetes has increased among a number of groups, including the Pima (Knowler, Pettit, Saad, and Bennett, 1990) and the Navaho (Sugarman, Hickey, Hall, and Gohdes, 1990). Wide geographical variations in the prevalence of diabetes have been noted (Schraer et al., 1988). Identified risk factors for diabetes include having a diabetic parent (Knowler, Pettit, Savage, and Bennett, 1981), older age (Knowler et al., 1990), and obesity (Knowler et al., 1981). Native Americans appear to be at higher risk than whites for various complications of diabetes, including end stage renal disease (Newman, Marfin, Eggers, and Helgerson, 1990) and lower extremity amputations (Nelson et al., 1988). Carter and colleagues (1993) found that the age-adjusted mortality rates for Native Americans in New Mexico over a 30-year period far exceeded the rates for non-Hispanic whites during the same period.

Mental Health and Illness

Adolescent Health

Little research has been conducted to examine the prevalence or nature of eating disorders among Native American groups (Davis and Yager, 1992). One of the few studies to do so found that compared to Hispanics and non-Hispanic whites, Native American high school students displayed a higher prevalence of abnormal eating behaviors and attitudes (Smith and Krejci, 1991).

Among adolescents in the United States, rates of suicide are highest among Native Americans. The 1988 Indian Health Service Adolescent Health Survey, administered to 7,254 students in grades 6 through 12, found that nearly 15% of the respondents had tried to commit suicide at least once (Grossman, Milligan, and Deyo, 1991). Several factors were found to be associated with a suicide attempt: a history of mental problems, a feeling of alienation from family and community, having a friend who attempted suicide, weekly consumption of hard liquor, a family history of suicide or a suicide attempt, poor self-perception of health, a history of physical abuse, being female, and sexual abuse.

Alcohol Use

Alcohol misuse has taken its toll on Native American communities. Alcohol has been associated with as much as 90% of all homicides involving Native Americans and has been implicated as a factor in many suicides, accidental-injury deaths (Bachman, 1991; Gallaher, Fleming, Berger, and Sewell, 1992; Goodman et al., 1991), and vehicular accidents (Chang, Lapham, and Barton, 1996). Children of parents who misuse alcohol are at higher risk of abuse and neglect (Berger and Kitzes, 1989; Lujan, DeBruyn, May, and Bird, 1989).

It appears that initially, at least, the colonists provided alcohol to Native Americans in much the same way that they offered it to each other, as a welcome or as a gift (Mancall, 1995). Later, however, the sale of alcohol to Native Americans was prohibited due to the perceived adverse effects of alcohol on Native Americans, such as accidents, and the colonial perception that drinking by Native Americans was a threat to society. Both the Dutch and the English imposed monetary penalties and/or corporal punishment on those found selling alcohol to Native Americans. Despite these prohibitions, Native Americans were able to obtain alcohol during this temperance period (Mancall, 1995). Native American use of alcohol continued, both because they wanted the alcohol and because the colonists were ambivalent about the alcohol trade. However, the sale of alcohol served a need much deeper than mere commercial benefit. As Mancall (1995:170) notes,

> [Alcohol] became, especially in the last decades of the colonial period, crucial to the way colonists and Indians understood each other. Indians' responses to liquor reinforced colonists' notions about their cultural and racial inferiority; colonists' desire to maintain the trade despite its all too apparent costs reinforced Indians' notions about the deeply rooted problems of colonial culture.... The liquor trade joined with the growing colonial population and recurring epidemics to destabilize Indian villages, and perhaps contributed to the decision of countless Indians to sell their land to colonists and move westward, beyond colonial settlements.... The alcohol trade plagued relations between Indians and colonists precisely because each group interpreted its existence as a sign of the other's failings.

Numerous theories have been advanced in an attempt to explain the prevalence of alcohol misuse among Native Americans. One theory posits that the availability of alcohol is determinative, noting the increased use of alcohol among Native Americans living near urban areas and the increased usage among those who are more assimilated into non-Native American society (Levy and Kunitz, 1974). Others have argued that alcohol is an escape from problems, including the forcible relocation of many Native American communities, the loss of a traditional way of life, and the attempted imposition of new spiritual beliefs by the missionaries (Dozier, 1966). Others have suggested that drinking serves to release repressed aggression and to solidify group bonds (Littmen, 1970).

Whether there exists a genetic basis for alcohol misuse remains undetermined and controversial. Study results have yielded conflicting findings, some indicating that Native Americans actually metabolize ethanol more quickly than Caucasians (Segal and Duffy, 1992; May, 1994), while at least one study observed a slower rate of disappearance of blood alcohol (Fenna, Mix, Schaefer, and Gilbert, 1971). These studies are also difficult to interpret due to reliance on varying definitions and measurement techniques (Schaefer, 1981).

Exercises

1. Research seems to indicate that Native American groups identified themselves as independent nations and became "tribes" as the result of federal court decisions. Various federal statutes and regulations recognize individuals' identity as Native American based on a "blood quantum," mandating that individuals have a certain proportion of "Indian blood" to be recognized as Native American for the purpose of eligibility under various programs (Jaimes, 1994).
    a. What are the implications of these policies for our ability to conduct health research with Native American groups? Consider, at a minimum, the following aspects of research in your response: recruitment, bias, and generalizability.
    b. What are the implications in the health context of collapsing the various diverse Native American nations into one classification? How does this compare with our compression of various groups under the headings of "Latino/Hispanic," and "Asian and Pacific Islander"?
2. Research has implicated alcohol as a factor in a high proportion of homicides, suicides, accidental-injury deaths, and vehicular accidents among Native Americans.
    a. What explanations might exist? Consider the following in your response: study design, biological factors, and cultural factors.
    b. Design a study to determine whether the rate of alcohol-related injury differs among Native Americans compared to non-Native Americans. What are the methodological difficulties, including classification issues, in designing such a study?

c. Assume for the purpose of this question only that your research has detected a difference in the rate of alcohol-related injury among Native Americans and non-Native Americans (and that you have addressed appropriately or have overcome the methodological issues that you identified in (b) above). Design a study to identify the variables contributing to this difference. What are the methodological difficulties in designing this study?

References

Ashburn, P.M. (1947). *The Ranks of Death: A Medical History of the Conquest of the Americas.* New York: Coward-McCann.

Bachman, R. (1991). The social causes of American Indian homicide as revealed by the life experiences of thirty offenders. *American Indian Quarterly, 15,* 471–487.

Becker, T.M., Wiggins, C.R., Key, R., & Samet, J.M. (1988). Ischemic heart disease mortality in Hispanics, American Indians, and non-Hispanic whites in New Mexico. *Circulation, 78,* 302–309.

Benenson, A.S. (Ed.) (1995). *Control of Communicable Disease Manual* (16th ed.). Washington, DC: American Public Health Association.

Berger, L.R., & Kitzes, J. (1989). Injuries to children in a Native American community. *Pediatrics, 84,* 152–156.

Bourke, J. (1888). The medicine men of the Apache. *Ninth Annual Report, Bureau of American Ethnology, 1887–1888.* Cited in V.J. Vogel. (1970). *American Indian Medicine.* Oklahoma City, OK: University of Oklahoma Press.

Breault, J.L., & Hoffman, M.G. (1997). A strategy for reducing tuberculosis among Oglala Sioux Native Americans. *American Journal of Preventive Medicine, 13,* 182–188.

Bureau of the Census. (1994). *1990 Census of Population.* Washington, DC: Government Printing Office.

Bureau of the Census, U.S. Department of Commerce, Economics and Statistics Administration. (1993). *We the ... First Americans.*

Bureau of the Census, U.S. Department of Commerce, Economics and Statistics Administration. (1995). *Bureau of the Census Statistical Brief: Housing of American Indians on Reservations—Plumbing* [SB/95-9].

Bureau of the Census, U.S. Department of Commerce, Economics and Statistics Administration. (1997, October 31). *Census Bureau Fact Sheet for Native American Month* [http://www.census.gov/Press-Release/fs97-ll.html].

Byers, T. (1996). Nutrition and cancer among American Indians and Alaska Natives. *Cancer, 78,* 1612–1616.

Campos-Outcalt, D., Ellis, J., Aickin, M., Valencia, J., Wunsch, M., & Steele, L. (1995). Prevalence of cardiovascular disease risk factors in a southwestern Native American tribe. *Public Health Reports, 110,* 742–748.

Carter, J.S., Wiggins, C.L., Becker, T.M., Key, C.R., & Samet, J.M. (1993). Diabetes mortality among New Mexico's American Indian, Hispanic, and non-Hispanic white populations, 1958–1987. *Diabetes Care, 16,* 306–309.

Chamberlin, R.V. (1909). Some plant names of the Ute Indians. *American Anthropologist, 11,* 27–40.

Chang, I., Lapham, S.C., & Barton, K.J. (1996). Drinking environment and sociodemographic factors among DWI offenders. *Journal of Studies of Alcohol, 57,* 659–669.

Clark, G.A., Kelley, M.A., Grange, J.M., & Hill, M.C. (1987). The evolution of mycobacterial disease in human populations. *Current Anthropology, 28,* 45–62.

Creagan, E.T., & Fraumeni, J.F. (1973). Cancer mortality among American Indians, 1950–67. *Journal of the National Cancer Institute, 49,* 959–967.

Davis, C., & Yager, J. (1992). Transcultural aspects of eating disorders: A critical literature review. *Culture, Medicine, & Psychiatry, 16,* 377–394.

Dillehay, T.D., & Meltzer, D.J. (1991). *The First Americans: Search and Research.* Boca Raton, FL: CRC Press.

Dozier, E.P. (1966). Problem drinking among American Indians: The role of sociocultural deprivation. *Quarterly Journal of Studies on Alcohol, 27,* 72–87.

Driver, H.E. (1969). *Indians of North America* (2nd ed., rev.). Chicago, IL: University of Chicago Press.

Engelberg, N.C., Holburt, E.N., Barrett, T.J., Gary, G.W., Trujillo, M.H., Feldman, R.A., & Hughes, J.M. (1982). Epidemiology of diarrhea due to rotavirus on an Indian reservation: Risk factors in the home environment. *Journal of Infectious Disease, 145,* 894–898.

Fenna, D., Mix, L., Schaefer, O., & Gilbert, J.A. (1971). Ethanol metabolism in various racial groups. *Canadian Medical Association Journal, 105,* 472–475.

Francis, L. (1996). *Native Time: A Historical Time Line of Native America.* New York: St. Martin's Griffin.

Frost, F., Taylor, V., & Fries, E. (1992). Racial misclassification of Native Americans in a surveillance, epidemiology, and end results cancer registry. *Journal of the National Cancer Institute, 84,* 957–962.

Gallaher, M.M., Fleming, D.W., Berger, L.R., & Sewell, M. (1992). Pedestrian and hypothermia deaths among Native Americans in New Mexico. *JAMA, 267,* 1345–1348.

Gillum R.F. (1995). The epidemiology of stroke in Native Americans. *Stroke, 26,* 514–521.

Goodman, R., Hernson, J.L., Jordan, F.B., Herndon, J.L., & Kelaghan, J. (1991). Alcohol and fetal injuries in Oklahoma. *Journal of Studies on Alcohol, 52,* 156–161.

Greenberg, J.H., Turner, C.G., & Zegura, S.L. (1986). The settlement of the Americas: A comparison of the linguistic, dental, and genetic evidence. *Current Anthropology, 27,* 447–497.

Grinnell, G.B. (1905). Some Cheyenne plant medicines. *American Anthropologist, 7,* 38–43.

Grossman, D.C., Milligan, B.C., & Deyo, R.A. (1991). Risk factors for suicide attempts among Navajo adolescents. *American Journal of Public Health, 81,* 870–874.

Helm, J. (1980). Female infanticide, European diseases, and population levels among the MacKenzie Dene. *American Ethnologist, 7,* 259–285.

Hildes, J.A., & Schaefer, O. (1984). The changing picture of neoplastic disease in the Western and Central Canadian Arctic. *Canadian Medical Association Journal, 130,* 25–32.

Hridlicka, A. (1932). Disease, medicine, and surgery among the American aborigines. *JAMA, 99,* 1661–1666.

Jaimes, M.A. (1994). American racism: The impact on American-Indian identity and survival. In S. Gregory & R. Sanjek (Eds.), *Race* (pp. 41–61). New Brunswick, NJ: Rutgers University Press.

Johansson, S.R. (1982). The demographic history of the native peoples of North America: A selective bibliography. *Yearbook of Physical Anthropology, 25,* 133–152.

Klain, M., Coulehan, J.L., Arena, V.C., & Jannett, R. (1988). More frequent diagnosis of acute myocardial infarction among Navajo Indians. *American Journal of Public Health, 78,* 1351–1352.

Knowler, W.C., Pettit, D.J., Saad, M.F., & Bennett, P.H. (1990). Diabetes mellitus in the Pima Indians: Incidence, risk factors, and pathogenesis. *Diabetes Metabolic Review, 6,* 1–27.

Knowler, W.C., Pettit, D.J., Savage, P.J., & Bennett, P.H. (1981). Diabetes incidence in Pima Indians: Contributions of obesity and parental diabetes. *American Journal of Epidemiology, 113,* 144–156.

Landes, R. (1963). Potawatomi medicine. *Transactions, Kansas Academy of Science, 66,* 553–599.

Leacock, E.B., & Lurie, N.O. (Eds.) (1971). *North American Indians in Historical Perspective.* New York: Random House.

Levy, J.E., & Kunitz, S.J. (1974). *Indian Drinking: Navajo Practices and Anglo-American Theories.* New York: Wiley.

Littman, G. (1970). Alcoholism, illness, and social pathology among American Indians in transition. *American Journal of Public Health, 60,* 1769–1778.

Lujan, C., DeBruyn, L.M., May, P.A., & Bird, M.E. (1989). Profile of abused and neglected American Indian children in the Southwest. *Child Abuse and Neglect, 13,* 449–461.

Mahoney, M.C., & Michalek, A.M. (1991). A meta-analysis of cancer incidence in United States and Canadian native populations. *International Journal of Epidemiology, 20,* 323–327.

Mancall, P.C. (1995). *Deadly Medicine: Indians and Alcohol in Early America.* Ithaca, NY: Cornell University Press.

Margolis, K.L., Lurie, N., McGovern, P.G., & Slater, J.S. (1993). Predictors of failure to attend scheduled mammography appointments at a public teaching hospital. *Journal of General Internal Medicine, 8,* 602–605.

May, P.A. (1994). The epidemiology of alcohol abuse among American Indians: The mythical and real properties. *American Indian Culture and Research Journal, 18,* 121–143.

McKenney, N.R., & Bennett, C.E. (1994). Issues regarding data on race and ethnicity: The Census Bureau experience. *Public Health Reports, 109,* 16–25.

Metler, R., Conway, G.A., & Stehr-Green, J. (1991). AIDS surveillance among American Indians and Alaska Natives. *American Journal of Public Health, 81,* 1469–1471.

Nelson, R.G., Gohdes, D.M., Everhart, J.E., Hartner, J.A., Zwemer, F.L., Pettitt, D.J., & Knowler, M.C. (1988). Lower-extremity amputation in NIDDM: 12 year follow-up study in Pima Indians. *Diabetes Care, 11,* 8–16.

Newman, J.M., Marfin, A.A., Eggers, P.W., & Helgerson, S.D. (1990). End state renal disease among Native Americans, 1983–1986. *American Journal of Public Health, 80,* 318–319.

Nies, J. (1996). *Native American History: A Chronology of a Culture's Vast Achievements and Their Links to World Events.* New York: Ballantine Books.

Paisano, E.L. (1995). The American Indian, Eskimo, and Aleut population. In Bureau of the Census, *Population Profile of the United States, 1995.* Washington, DC: U.S. Government Printing Office. [Current Population Reports, Series 23-189].

Pappaioanou, M., Schwabe, C.W., & Sard, D.M. (1977). An evolving pattern of human hyatid disease transmission in the United States. *American Journal of Tropical Medicine and Hygiene, 26,* 732–742.

Paulsen, H.J. (1987). Tuberculosis in the Native American: Indigenous or introduced? *Review of Infectious Disease, 9,* 1180–1186.

Rice, R.J., Roberts, P.L., Handsfield, H.H., & Holmes, K.K. (1991). Sociodemographic distribution of gonorrhea incidence: Implications for prevention and behavioral research. *American Journal of Public Health, 81,* 1252–1258.

Sack, R.B., Santosham, M., Reid, R., Black, R., Croll, J., Yolken, R., Aurelian, L., Wolff, M., Chan, E., & Garrett, S. (1995). Diarrhoeal diseases in the White Mountain Apaches: Clinical studies. *Journal of Diarrhoeal Disease Research, 13,* 12–17.

Samet, J.M., Kay, C.R., Hunt, W.C., & Goodwin, J.S. (1987). Survival of American Indian and Hispanic cancer patients in New Mexico and Arizona. *Journal of National Cancer Institute, 79,* 457–463.

Schaefer, J.M. (1981). Firewater myths revisited: Review of findings and some new directions. *Journal of Studies of Alcohol, 42*(Suppl. 9), 99–117.

Schantz, P.M., Von Reye, C.F., Welty, T., Andersen, F.L., Schultz, M.G., & Kagan, I.G. (1977). Epidemiologic investigation of echinococcosis in American Indians living in Arizona and New Mexico. *American Journal of Tropical Medicine and Hygiene, 26,* 121–126.

Schraer, C.D., Lanier, A.P., Boyko, E.J., Gohdes, D., & Murphy, N.J. (1988). Prevalence of diabetes mellitus in Alaskan Eskimos, Indians, and Aleuts. *Diabetes Care, 11,* 693–700.

Schreeder, M.T., Bender, T.R., McMahon, R.J., Moser, M.R., Murphy, B.L., Sheller, M.J., Heyward, W.L., Hall, D.B., & Maynard, J.E. (1983). Prevalence of hepatitis B in selected Alaskan Eskimo villages. *American Journal of Epidemiology, 118,* 543–549.

Segal, B., & Duffy, L.K. (1992). Ethanol elimination among different racial groups. *Alcohol, 9,* 213–217.

Shaffer, N., Wainwright, R.B., Middaugh, J.P., & Tauxe, R.V. (1990). Botulism among Alaska natives: The role of changing food preparation and consumption practices. *Western Journal of Medicine, 153,* 390–393.

Sievers, M.L., Nelson, R.G., & Bennett, P.H. (1990). Adverse mortality experience of a southwestern American Indian community: Overall death rates and underlying causes of death in Pima Indians. *Journal of Clinical Epidemiology, 43,* 1231–1242.

Smith, J.E., & Krejci, J. (1991). Minorities join the majority: Eating disturbances among Hispanic and Native American youth. *International Journal of Eating Disorders, 10,* 179–186.

Smith, R.L. (1957). Recorded and expected mortality among the Indians of the United States with special reference to cancer. *Journal of the National Cancer Institute, 18,* 385–396.

Spangler, J.G., Bell, R.A., Dignan, M.B., & Michielutte, R. (1997). Prevalence and predictors of tobacco use among Lumbee Indian women in Robeson County, North Carolina. *Journal of Community Health, 22,* 115–125.

Sugarman, U.R., Hickey, M., Hall, T., & Gohdes, D. (1990). The changing epidemiology of diabetes mellitus among Navajo Indians. *Western Journal of Medicine, 153,* 140–145.

Sullivan, C. (1991). Pathways to infection: AIDS vulnerability among the Navajo. *AIDS Education and Prevention, 3,* 241–257.

Toomey, K.E., Oberschelp, A.G., & Greenspan, J.R. (1989). Sexually transmitted diseases and Native Americans: Trends in reported gonorrhea and syphilis morbidity, 1984–88. *Public Health Reports, 104,* 566–572.

Teufel, N.I. (1996). Nutrient characteristics of Southwest Native American pre-contact diets. *Journal of Nutritional and Environmental Medicine, 3,* 273–284.

United States Department of Health and Human Services. (1990). *Trends in Indian Health 1990.* Rockville, MD: U.S. DHHS/PHS/Indian Health Service.

Vogel, V.J. (1970). *American Indian Medicine.* Norman, OK: University of Oklahoma Press.

West, K.M. (1974). Diabetes in American Indians and other native populations of the New World. *Diabetes, 23,* 841–855.

Williams, R. (1986). Prevalence of hepatitis A virus antibody among Navajo school children. *American Journal of Public Health, 76,* 282–283.

Woodward, W.E., Hirschhorn, N., Sack, R.B., Cash, R.A., Brownlee, I., Chickadonz, G.H., Evans, L.K., Shepard, R.H., & Woodward, R.C. (1974). Acute diarrhea on an Apache Indian reservation. *American Journal of Epidemiology, 99,* 281–290.

Young, J.L., Jr., Ries, L.G., & Pollack, E.S. (1984). Cancer patient survival among ethnic groups in the United States. *Journal of the National Cancer Institute, 73,* 341–352.

Young, T.K. (1994). *The Health of Native Americans: Towards a Biocultural Epidemiology.* New York: Oxford University Press, Inc.

10

Women and Health

Background

Some might assert that a separate chapter devoted to women's health is superfluous. Yet, this focus is critical for a variety of reasons. First, biological sex and societally constructed and imposed gender roles have often been inextricably intertwined throughout history, resulting in the construction of specified spheres of acceptable activity for women. An understanding of women and health research requires an examination of this relationship (Clarke, 1990).

Second, various health concerns exist that are either unique to women, such as ovarian and cervical cancer, hysterectomy, and cesarean section, or that affect women to a far greater degree than men, such as eating disorders and certain autoimmune disorders. Third, various issues relating to access to care and the quality of that care are critical to women, including the greater reliance on psychoactive medications for the treatment of women's complaints as compared to those of men (Ogur, 1986). Finally, women and men differ biologically and with respect to health indicators. Women tend to have higher rates of illness and disability than men but tend to live longer than men (Centers for Disease Control and Prevention [CDC], 1995). Sex differences have been attributed to one or more of the following factors, all of which are relevant in the research context: (1) biological factors, such as hormones; (2) acquired risks through work and leisure activities; (3) psychosocial aspects of symptoms and care; (4) health-reporting behavior; and (5) the effect of previous health care on future health (Verbrugge, 1990).

Health indicators vary substantially, however, across subgroups of women. For example, all-cause age-adjusted mortality among Asian and Pacific Islander women during the period 1993 through 1995 was 229.3 per 100,000. Mortality during the same period was 1.2 times as high for Hispanic women, 1.6 times as high among whites and Native Americans, and 2.5 times as high among blacks (CDC, 1995).

This chapter begins with an overview of the role of biological sex in the determination of gender role and the impact of that relationship on women's health care and health research. Various health issues of concern to women are discussed, including reproductive health, chronic diseases, and intentional injury.

Cultural and Historical Context: Sex and Gender

Prior to the late 18th century, women in the United States were viewed as fundamentally similar to men, but inferior, due to the underdevelopment of their reproductive organs. Beginning with the late 18th century, women were seen as biologically different from men, but still inferior, as evidence by their smaller skulls and resulting smaller brain capacity (Fee, 1979). A division of labor by biological sex, it was argued, was justified and necessary because women's lives were tyrannized and controlled by their reproductive systems, from menstruation, through childbearing and childrearing, through menopause. Consequently, women were not only debilitated but disabled and unsuited for larger societal roles (Smith-Rosenberg, 1973).

Unlike men, who, as believed in the 19th century, had the power to indulge in or repress their sexual impulses (Skene, 1889, cited in Smith-Rosenberg, 1973), women were subject to cyclical periods of pain, weakness, irritability, and insanity (Wiltbank, 1854, cited in Smith-Rosenberg, 1973). Puberty represented a precipitous crossing into womanhood, fraught with danger of disease should there be either an "excess or a deficiency of the proper influence of these organs [ovaries] over the other parts of the system" (Kellogg, 1895:371, cited in Smith-Rosenberg, 1973). The preservation of health, then, demanded full attention to the development of healthy reproductive organs, which could be accomplished by adherence to a regimen of rest, a simple diet, and an unchallenging routine of domestic tasks (Smith-Rosenberg, 1973). Menopause was similarly ominous, resulting in numerous diseases including diarrhea, vaginal inflammation, paralysis, tuberculosis, diabetes, depression, hysteria, and insanity, due to the cessation of menstruation and the "violation of the physiological and social laws dictated by [a woman's] ovarian system" (Smith-Rosenberg, 1973:192). Such violations included education, attempts at birth control or abortion, a failure to adequately attend to the needs of one's husband or children, an overly indulgent lifestyle, and engaging in sexual intercourse during or after menopause (Smith-Rosenberg, 1973).

Hysteria, in particular, was believed to be an affliction specific to women. Hysteria was brought on by feelings of depression, nervousness, or crying and could manifest in the form of a hysterical "fit" similar to an epileptic seizure. Gradually, the seizure was eliminated as a diagnostic criterion of the illness, so that hysteria could be diagnosed on the basis of any number of symptoms, including loss of sensation, nausea, headache, pain, or contracture or paralysis of an extremity (Smith-Rosenberg, 1973). The onset of hysteria was attributed to "the indolent, vapid and unconstructive life of the fashionable middle- and upper-class woman, or by the ignorant, exhausting, and sensual life of the lower- or working-class woman" (Smith-Rosenberg, 1985:205).

It has been postulated that the diagnosis of hysteria, defined by the medical profession as a disease, enabled women to assume a sick role and, concomitantly, to renegotiate their roles within their families. The restructuring of domestic activities to accommodate the illness essentially permitted a woman to opt out of her traditional role, without provoking the disapproval and confrontation that a more overt rejection of role would have entailed (Smith-Rosenberg, 1973).

The emergence, then, in the late 1800s and through the mid-1900s of the "New Woman" clearly violated existing taboos. "New Women" abandoned the domestic setting, seeking an education not equal, but identical, to that received by men (Smith-Rosenberg, 1973). It was predicted that such women would disrupt a delicate psychological balance through the emphasis on the mind rather than the ovaries. Within men, however, the brain and heart were dominant, permitting them to pursue such intellectual activities. One physician predicted:

> The nervous force, so necessary at puberty for the establishment of the menstrual function, is wasted on what may be compared as trifles to perfect health, for what use are they without health? The poor sufferer only adds another to the great army of neurasthenics and sexual incompetents, which furnish neurologists and gynecologists with so much of their material.... Bright eyes have been dulled by the brain-fag and sweet temper transformed into irritability, crossness and hysteria, while the womanhood of the land is deteriorating physically.
>
> She may be highly cultured and accomplished and shine in society, but her future husband will discover too late that he has married a large outfit of headaches, backaches and spine aches, instead of a woman fitted to take up the duties of life. (Darnall, 1901:490)

Men who stimulated their sexual organs through masturbation rather than their brains through intellectual pursuits would meet a similar fate (Smith-Rosenberg, 1978).

The late 19th century medical view of women and their role, then, rested on four assumptions: (1) a closed energy system, whereby the use of the brain resulted, essentially, in the theft of energy from the ovaries; (2) a hierarchy of bodily functions which, as indicated, placed the ovary in a position superior to that of the brain; (3) the physiological fragility of the female; and (4) the dichotomization or polarization of male (brain/mind) and female (body/ovaries) function (Smith-Rosenberg, 1973). Women who rejected these premises were characterized by physicians as an "intermediate sex," fusing the female and male to become the "mannish lesbian" (Smith-Rosenberg, 1985:265).

Medical discourse which had previously focused on homosexuality in men to the almost complete exclusion of women now began to address female homosexuality. Von Krafft-Ebing (1908) delineated four categories of homosexual women. Those in the first category were not recognizable as lesbians based on their physical characteristics, but would respond to the overtures of more masculine women. The second category encompassed those lesbians who preferred to wear male garments. Those in the third category were "inverted," having assumed a masculine role. Women in the fourth category, "gynandry," had reached the epitome of degenerative homosexuality:

> The woman of this type possesses of the feminine qualities only the genital organs; thought, sentiment, action, even external appearance are those of a man. Often enough one does come across in life such characters whose frame, pelvis, gait, appearance, coarse masculine features, rough, deep voice, etc. betrayed rather the man than the woman. (Von Krafft-Ebing, 1908:333–336)

Such women, Von Krafft-Ebing reported, avoided the women's fashion and pursued, instead, male sports. In addition, the desire for privileges and power traditionally associated with men exceeded a sexual desire for other women (Von Krafft-Ebing, 1908). Women who rejected traditional female gender norms were, in essence, abnormal.

Unlike Von Krafft-Ebing, the sexologist Ellis attributed "inversion" to biological and hereditary factors, concluding that it was irreversible. He distinguished between those women who were congenitally inverted and those with a genetic disposition, for whom homosexuality was an acquired, preventable, and curable trait (Ellis, 1895). Definitions of masculinity and femininity arose directly from the biological basis for sex. Like Krafft-Ebing, Ellis concluded that departures from socially determined roles were abnormal. Those who were congenitally inverted were not only sexually active, unlike normal women, but also competed aggressively with men for their sexual partners (Ellis, 1895–1896). By the 1920s, charges of lesbianism became a common strategy to discredit female professionals and reformers (Smith-Rosenberg, 1985).

The women's health movement was to have a lasting impact on women's health and health care and, not surprisingly, their social roles as well. Eagan (1994) has traced the beginning of the movement to 1970, when women protested their exclusion from congressional hearings on the use of birth control pills. Numerous events converged to alert women to the dangers of relying on physicians as their only source of information in making health care decisions. The first printing of *Our Bodies, Ourselves* was released in 1971, providing women with a basic source of information. Abortion was legalized in 1973 with the decision in Roe v. Wade. In 1971, it was revealed that diethylstilbestrol (DES), used by millions of women to prevent miscarriage, was linked to a rare form of vaginal cancer in the daughters of women who had ingested the drug (Herbst, Ulfelder, and Poskanzer, 1971). The publication of *Why Me?* challenged medicine's reliance on the Halsted radical mastectomy to treat breast cancer (Kushner, 1975). That procedure had required the removal of the entire breast, the axillary lymph nodes, and the underlying chest wall muscle.

Health Status

Human Immunodeficiency Virus

In 1988, seven years after the HIV epidemic was first recognized, the proportion of AIDS cases attributable to women was 10%. By 1994, that figure had risen to 18%, representing a 151% increase compared to a 105% increase among men for the same time period (Anonymous, 1994). Although African-American and Hispanic women comprise 21% of the U.S. population, 74% of cumulative AIDS cases in women occur among these groups (Chu, Buehler, and Berkelman, 1990). In 1992, AIDS became the fourth leading cause of death among women ages 25 to 44 years, but had been the leading cause of death among African-American women since 1987 (Guinan & Leviton, 1995). The majority of AIDS cases among women have resulted from heterosexual intercourse and drug injection (Guinan and Leviton, 1995).

Chronic Disease

Cancer

From 1982 through 1993, malignant neoplasms were the leading cause of death among women ages 25 to 44 years (Guinan and Leviton, 1995). Cancer death rates among women from 1930 through 1991 have been highest for lung, breast, colon/rectal, uterine, and stomach cancers (Husten, Chrisman, and Reddy, 1996). Lung cancer deaths among women have been increasing since the 1960s, and lung cancer is now the leading cause of cancer deaths among white and African-American women (CDC, 1993). Not surprisingly, cancer has been found to be the most feared disease among women due to its perceived incurability and associated suffering (Gordon *et al.*, 1991; Murray and McMillan, 1993).

A recent study by Hahn and colleagues (1998) found that cancer-related risk behaviors vary greatly across subgroups of women. Among women who were 50 years of age or older, approximately 30% of Asian and Pacific Islander women had never had a mammography or had not had a mammography within the previous 2 years, compared to almost 38% of Hispanic women. Among women 20 years of age and older, 12.2% of African-American women who had not had a hysterectomy had not had a Pap smear during the previous 3 years, compared with 29.1% of Asian and Pacific Islander women.

Cardiovascular Disease

The incidence of coronary heart disease has increased among women since 1950, although it has decreased among men (Eleveback, Connolly, and Milton, 1986). Access to care may be an issue for women suffering from coronary heart disease. Tobin and colleagues (1987) found that among patients with presumed coronary heart disease, women with positive radionuclide exercise tests were referred for coronary angiography less frequently than men. Khan and associates (1990) found that women are referred for coronary artery bypass surgery at a more advanced stage of disease than men, resulting in higher perioperative mortality. Ayanian and Epstein (1991) concluded from their examination of 49,623 discharges in Massachusetts and 33,159 discharges in Maryland that women who were hospitalized for coronary heart disease underwent fewer diagnostic and therapeutic procedures than men. The authors were unable to ascertain whether these differences represented underuse by women or overuse by men.

Autoimmune Disease

Women are disproportionately affected by certain autoimmune diseases, including systemic lupus erythematosus, thrombocytopenic purpura, multiple sclerosis, primary biliary cirrhosis, thyroiditis, and Grave's disease (Beeson, 1994; Lockshin, 1988). Several unconfirmed hypotheses have been advanced to explain the increased frequency of these diseases in women: (1) that gonadal hormones lower the threshold for clinical illness; (2) that gonadal hormones increase autoantibodies and lower the threshold for clinical illness; (3) that nonhormonal factors lower the threshold for clinical illness; and (4) that women are exposed more frequently to factors resulting in illness (Lockshin, 1988). Systemic lupus erythematosus (SLE) is considered in more detail here.

SLE is a chronic, multi-system disease that affects women nine times more frequently than men (Petri, 1995). The etiology of SLE is unknown. Studies have suggested that genetic and environmental risk factors exist (Miller, 1995). Both the incidence and the prevalence of the disease are higher among African-Americans compared to whites (McCarty et al., 1995). This increased incidence among African-Americans has been attributed to genetic factors (Hochberg, Petri, Machan, and Bias, 1991) and to environmental factors (Kardestuncer and Frumkin, 1997; Strom et al., 1994).

Differences have also been noted in the manifestation of SLE across subgroups of women. White women are more frequently affected by photosensitivity, malar rash, and Sjögren's syndrome (Petri, 1998), whereas African-American women experience a greater frequency of nephritis (Gioud-Paquet et al., 1988; Hochberg et al., 1985; Reveille, 1989; Reveille, Bartolucci, and Alarcon, 1990; Ward and Studenski, 1990), cardiac involvement, discoid lupus, and musculoskeletal and organ damage (Petri, 1998). These various differences have been attributed to genetics (Salmon et al., 1996), environmental factors such as smoking (Brown, Petri, and Goldman, 1996), and other factors including older age at diagnosis, longer duration of SLE, poor nutrition, and increased disease activity at time of diagnosis (Karlson et al., 1997).

Reproductive Health

Reproductive health has often focused on issues relating to birth control and contraception. Although numerous methods had been used throughout time to prevent pregnancy, it was not until the mid-19th century that birth control gained public attention in the United States. As a response to growing concern with falling birth rates among middle- and upper-class whites,

Congress in 1863 passed the Comstock Law. This law defined contraception as obscene and prohibited distribution of birth control information through the mail (Poirier, 1990).

Margaret Sanger championed the efforts of women to control their bodies through the control of contraception. She was arrested twice, once in 1912 for the distribution of information through the mail and again in 1916, following the opening of a clinic that fitted women with diaphragms (Sanger, 1938). Ultimately, Sanger advocated laws that permitted only physicians to prescribe and fit diaphragms; the reasons for her position remain subject to debate (Kennedy, 1970; Reed, 1978).

The Comstock Law was not overturned until 1938. In the interim, however, many states had implemented legislation prohibiting birth control. It was not until the 1965 Supreme Court decision in Griswold v. Connecticut that women were permitted access to birth control information, subsumed under a right to privacy (Dienes, 1972). The contraceptive pill was released in the U.S. market in the 1960s.

The testing and use of birth control has raised numerous ethical issues. The first anovulatory drugs were tested on poor women in Puerto Rico. At least one author has raised concerns regarding the nature of the informed consent, given the economic and political context at the time (Gordon, 1976). U.S. government-sponsored family programs emerged during the Depression and often targeted its sterilization efforts at poor women. Numerous reports have documented the involuntary sterilizations of poor women and women of color (Davis, 1981; Dreifus, 1977; Larson, 1995; Rodrigues-Trias, 1978). The use among poor women of Depo-Provera®, a long-term contraceptive injection, has raised similar ethical concerns (Cassidy, 1980; Levine, 1980).

It was not until the mid-1880s that most states made most abortions illegal, including abortions performed by physicians. Prior to that time, many states permitted abortion until "quickening" (Smith-Rosenberg, 1985). It was in response to the lobbying of the American Medical Association (AMA) that harsh anti-abortion laws were enacted. As chairman of an AMA committee formed to ascertain the number of abortions performed in the United States, Horatio Stover opined against the availability of abortions to married middle- and upper-class women, who "prefer to devastate with poison and with steel their wombs rather than ... forego the gaieties of a winter's balls, parties, and plays, or the pleasure of a summer's trips and amusements" (Stover and Heard, 1865:72). The efforts of Stover and the AMA, together with the Protestant clergy and Roman Catholic church, effectively ended the availability of legal abortion until the 1970s. The anti-abortion rhetoric and efforts were supported through the Comstock Law which, as noted above, prohibited the distribution of birth control information through the mail. In 1964 alone, 10,000 women were admitted to New York City hospitals for treatment of severe complications resulting from criminal abortions.

At least one author has asserted that the intensity of this anti-abortion movement was a direct outgrowth of obstetricians' and gynecologists' concern over their low professional status, public reputation, and relative lack of knowledge and their perceived lack of financial power at the hands of the bourgeois matrons who sought their services (Smith-Rosenberg, 1985). The husbands and fathers of the unborn child were exonerated from all responsibility in the decision to abort. Speaking of the women seeking an abortion, an AMA committee observed:

> She becomes unmindful of the course marked out for her by Providence, she overlooks the duties imposed on her by the marriage contract. She yields to the pleasures—but shrinks from the pains and responsibilities of maternity; and, destitute of all delicacy and refinement, resigns herself, body and soul, into the hands of unscrupulous and wicked men. Let not the

husband of such a wife flatter himself that he possesses her affection. (Atlee and O'Donnell, 1871:241)

During the 1960s, various groups lobbied for relaxed abortion laws. The 1973 Supreme Court decision in Roe v. Wade relegated first-trimester abortion decisions to a woman and her physician; only after the first trimester could the state regulate or prohibit abortion. Later court decisions restricted the case's impact. For example, Maher v. Roe resulted in a prohibition against the use of federal funds to perform abortions (Poirier, 1990).

Intentional Injury

Domestic Violence

Because definitions vary across studies, it becomes difficult to compare incidence and prevalence rates. The proportion of women reporting severe domestic violence in a one-year period (being kicked, bitten, hit, choked, threatened by a gun, or wounded by a gun or knife) ranges from 0.27% in a probability sample of 60,000 women (Klaus and Rand, 1984) to 5% in a nonprobability sample of 304 women (Meredith, Abbott, and Adams, 1986). Total domestic violence, including severe domestic violence, has ranged in a one-year period from 8.4% in a stratified random sample of 1,324 women (Plitcha and Weisman, 1995) to 22% in the non-probability sample noted previously (Meredith *et al.*, 1986). Lifetime prevalence of severe domestic violence has been reported to range from 9% in a stratified random sample of 602 women (Petersen, 1980) to 12.6% in a stratified random sample of 2,143 women (Straus, Gelles, and Steinmetz, 1980). Lifetime prevalence of total domestic violence has ranged from 7.3% (McFarlane *et al.*, 1991) to 30% (Straus and Gelles, 1990; Teske and Parker, 1983). Domestic violence has been found to be more prevalent among younger persons (Straus *et al.*, 1980; Straus and Gelles, 1990; Teske and Parker, 1983) and among those with lower incomes (Stark and Flitcraft, 1988). Domestic violence has also been associated with alcohol use (Eberle, 1982; Teske and Parker, 1983).

Injuries resulting from domestic violence include bruises, cuts, concussions, broken bones, miscarriages, loss of hearing or vision, and scars from burns, bites, or knife wounds (Council on Scientific Affairs, 1992). Reactions to domestic violence include shock, denial, withdrawal, confusion, psychological numbing, and fear. Long-term effects include fear, anxiety, fatigue, sleeping and eating disturbances, depression, and suicidal thoughts or attempts (Stark and Flitcraft, 1988).

Rape

Epidemiological data indicate that the prevalence of rape is high; at least 20% of adult women, 15% of college women, and 12% of adolescent girls have experienced sexual abuse and assault during their lifetimes (Koss, 1988). Reports indicate that rape victims may initially experience shock, numbness, withdrawal, and denial. Longer-term effects include chronic anxiety, nightmares, sexual dysfunction, physical distress (Koss and Harvey, 1991), phobias, depression, hostility (Resick, Calhoun, Atkeson, and Ellis, 1981), and suicidal thoughts (Kilpatrick, Veronen, and Best, 1985).

Work-Related Homicide

Homicide accounts for 40% of work-related deaths among women (Bell, 1991; Bell *et al.*, 1990). The highest work-related homicide rates are among African-Americans (Bell, 1991) and women over the age of 65 (Bell, 1991; Davis, Honchar, and Suarez, 1987). Settings with a higher risk for homicide include gasoline service stations, food stores, and eating and drinking places—sites all characterized by an exchange of money (Bell, 1991; Davis *et al.*, 1987; Kraus, 1987).

Exercises

1. You are conducting a study to identify the risk factors for breast cancer among women.
   a. Explain your study design. Include the following elements in your response:
      i. *type of study design to be utilized*
      ii. *inclusion and exclusion criteria, including your definition of "women" and how that definition will be operationalized*
      iii. *choice of control or comparison group*
      iv. *diagnostic criteria to be applied*
   b. What are the scientific and ethical arguments for and against restricting this study to only women?
2. Various diseases and injuries have been found to affect disproportionately certain subgroups of women. For example, African-American women are more likely to experience certain effects of SLE, and are at greater risk of HIV infection and death by homicide compared to white women.
   a. What does it mean to say that African-American women are at increased risk? Is this a function of skin color, genetics, or environmental factors?
   b. What benefit is derived by relating risk factors to racial or ethnic classifications? Include in your response a discussion of the implications for the development of effective prevention and intervention programs emphasizing racial or ethnic classification as a risk factor.

References

Anonymous. (1994). Update: Impact of the expanded AIDS surveillance case definition for adolescents and adults on case reporting—United States, 1993. *Morbidity and Mortality Weekly Report, 43*, 160–170.

Atlee, W.L., & O'Donnell, D.A. (1871). Report of the Committee on Criminal Abortion. *Transactions of the American Medical Association, 22*.

Ayanian, J.Z., & Epstein, A.M. (1991). Differences in the use of procedures between women and men hospitalized for coronary heart disease. *New England Journal of Medicine, 325*, 221–225.

Beeson, P.B. (1994). Age and sex associations of 40 autoimmune diseases. *American Journal of Medicine, 96*, 457–462.

Bell, C.A. (1991). Female homicides in United States workplaces, 1980–1985. *American Journal of Public Health, 81*, 729–732.

Bell, C.A., Stout, N.A., Bender, T.R., Conroy, C.S., Crouse, W.E., & Myers, J.R. (1990). Fatal occupational injuries in the United States, 1980 though 1985. *JAMA, 263*, 3047–3050.

Brown, K., Petri, M., & Goldman, D. (1996). Cutaneous manifestations of SLE: Associations with other manifestations of SLE and with smoking [abstract]. *Arthritis and Rheumatism, 39*, S291.

Cassidy, M.M. (1980). Depo-Provera and sterilization overview. In H.B. Holmes, B.B. Hoskins, & M. Gross. (Eds.), *Birth Control and Controlling Birth*. Clifton, NJ: Humana Press.

Centers for Disease Control. (1993). Mortality trends for selected smoking-related cancers and breast cancer—United States, 1950–1990. *Morbidity and Mortality Weekly Report, 42*, 857, 863–866.

Centers for Disease Control and Prevention. (1995). *Health United States 1996–97*. Hyattsville, MD: Department of Health and Human Services [DHHS Publ. (PHS) 95-1232].

Chu, S.Y., Buehler, J.W., & Berkelman, R.L. (1990). Impact of the human immunodeficiency virus epidemic on mortality in women of reproductive age in the United States. *JAMA, 117,* 523–544.

Clarke, A.F. (1990). Women's health: Life cycle issues. In R.D. Apple (Ed.), *Women, Health, and Medicine in America: A Historical Handbook* (pp. 3–39). New York: Garland Publishing, Inc.

Council on Scientific Affairs. (1992). Violence against women: Relevance for medical practitioners. *JAMA, 267,* 3184–3189.

Darnall, W.E. (1901).. The pubescent schoolgirl. *American Gynecological and Obstetrical Journal, 18,* 488–493.

Davis, A.Y. (1981). Racism, birth control, and reproductive rights. In A.Y. Davis (Ed.), *Women, Race, and Class* (pp. 202–221). New York: Random House.

Davis, H., Honchar, P.A., & Suarez, L. (1987). Fatal occupational injuries of women, Texas 1975–1984. *American Journal of Public Health, 77,* 1524–1527.

Dienes, C.T. (1972). *Law, Politics, and Birth Control.* Urbana, IL: University of Illinois Press.

Dreifus, C. (1977). Sterilizing the poor. In C. Dreifus (Ed.), *Seizing Our Bodies: The Politics of Women's Health* (pp. 105–20). New York: Random House.

Eagan, A.B. (1994). The women's health movement and its lasting impact. In E. Friedman (Ed.), *An Unfinished Revolution: Women and Health Care in America* (pp. 15–27). New York: United Hospital Fund of New York.

Eberle, P.A. (1982). Alcohol abusers and non-abusers: A discriminant analysis of differences between 2 subgroups of batterers. *Journal of Health and Social Behavior, 23,* 260–271.

Eleveback, L.R., Connolly, D.C., & Milton, L.J., III. (1986). Coronary heart disease in residents of Rochester, Minnesota. VII. Incidence, 1950 through 1982. *Mayo Clinic Proceedings, 61,* 896–900.

Ellis, H. (1895). Sexual inversion in women. *Alienist and Neurologist, 16,* 141–158.

Ellis, H. (1895–1896). Sexual inversion with an analysis of thirty-three new cases. *Medico-Legal Journal, 13,* 255–267.

Fee, E. (1979). Nineteenth century craniology: The study of the female skull. *Bulletin of the History of Medicine, 53,* 415–433.

Gioud-Paquet, M., Chamot, A.M., Bourgeois, P., Meyer, O., & Kahn, M.F. (1988). Ethnic differences in the symptoms and prognosis of systemic lupus erythematosus. A controlled study in 3 populations. *Presse Medicale, 17,* 103–106.

Gordon, D.R., Venturini, A., Del Tucco, M.R., Palli, D., & Paci, E. (1991). What healthy women think, feel, and do about cancer, prevention and breast cancer screening in Italy. *European Journal of Cancer, 27,* 913–917.

Gordon, L. (1976). *Woman's Body, Woman's Right: A Social History of Birth Control in America.* New York: Grossman.

Guinan, M.E., & Leviton, L. (1995). Prevention of HIV infection in women: Overcoming barriers. *Journal of the American Medical Women's Association, 50,* 74–77.

Hahn, R.A., Teutsch, S.M., Franks, A.L., Chang, M.H., & Lloyd, E.E. (1998). The prevalence of risk factors among women in the United States by race and age, 1992–1994: Opportunities for primary and secondary prevention. *Journal of the American Medical Women's Association, 53,* 96–104, 107.

Herbst, A.L., Ulfelder, H., & Poskanzer, D.C. (1971). Adenocarcinoma of the vagina. Association of maternal stilbestrol therapy with tumor appearance in young women. *New England Journal of Medicine, 284,* 878–881.

Hochberg, M.C., Boyd, R.E., Ahearn, J.M., Arnett, F.C., Bias, W.B., Provost, T.T., & Stevens, M.B. (1985). Systemic lupus erythematosus: A review of clinico-laboratory features and immunogenetic markers in 150 patients with emphasis on demographic subsets. *Medicine, 64,* 285–295.

Hochberg, M.C., Petri, M., Machan, C., & Bias, W.B. (1991). HLA class II alleles DrB1*1501/15.3 and DqB1*0602 are associated with systemic lupus erythematosus (SLE) in African-Americans [abstract]. *Arthritis and Rheumatism, 34,* S140.

Husten, C.G., Chrisman, J.H., & Reddy, M.N. (1996). Trends and effects of cigarette smoking among girls and women in the United States, 1965–1993. *Journal of the American Medical Women's Association, 51,* 11–18.

Kardestuncer, T., & Frumkin, H. (1997). Systemic lupus erythematosus in relation to environmental pollution: An investigation in an African-American community in North Georgia. *Archives of Environmental Health, 52,* 85–90.

Karlson, E.W., Daltroy, L.H., Lew, R.A., Wright, E.A., Partridge, A.J., Fossel, A.H., Roberts, W.N., Stern, S.H., Straaton, K.V., Wacholtz, M.C., Kavanaugh, A.F., Grosflam, J.M., & Liang, M.H. (1997). The relationship of socioeconomic status, race, and modifiable risk factors to outcomes in patients with systemic lupus erythematosus. *Arthritis and Rheumatism, 40,* 47–56.

Kellogg, J.H. (1895). *Ladies' Guide in Health and Disease.* Battle Creek, MI: Modern Medicine Publishing Co. Cited in C. Smith-Rosenberg. (1985). *Disorderly Conduct: Visions of Gender in Victorian America.* New York: Alfred A. Knopf, Inc.

Kennedy, D.M. (1970). *Birth Control in America: The Career of Margaret Sanger*. New Haven, CT: Yale University Press.

Khan, S.S., Nessim, S., Gray, R., Czer, L.S., Chaux, A., & Matloff, J. (1990). Increased mortality of women in coronary artery bypass surgery: Evidence for referral bias. *Annals of Internal Medicine, 112*, 561–567.

Kilpatrick, D.G., Veronen, L.J., & Best, V.L. (1985). Factors predicting psychological distress among rape victims. In C.R. Figley (Ed.), *Trauma and Its Wake*. New York: Brunner/Mazel.

Klaus, P.A., & Rand, M.R. (1984). *Family Violence. Special Report by the Bureau of Justice Statistics*. Washington, DC: U.S. Department of Justice.

Koss, M.P. (1988). Hidden rape: Sexual aggression and victimization in a national sample of students in higher education. In A.W. Burgess (Ed.), *Rape and Sexual Assault* (Vol. 2, pp. 3–25). New York: Garland Publishing.

Koss, M.P., & Harvey, M. (1991). *The Rape Victim: Clinical and Community Approaches to Treatment*. Beverly Hills, CA: Sage Publications.

Kraus, J.F. (1987). Homicide while at work: Persons, industries, and occupations at high risk. *American Journal of Public Health, 77*, 1285–1289.

Kushner, R. (1975). *Why Me?* New York: Saunders.

Larson, E.J. (1995). *Sex, Race, and Science: Eugenics in the Deep South*. Baltimore, MD: Johns Hopkins University Press.

Levine, C. (1980). Depo-Provera: Some ethical questions about a controversial contraceptive. In H.B. Holmes, B.B. Hoskins, & M. Gross (Eds.), *Birth Control and Controlling Birth* (pp. 101–106). Clifton, NJ: Humana Press.

Lockshin, M.D. (1998). Why women? *Journal of the American Medical Women's Association, 53*, 4–12.

McCarty, D.J., Manzi, S., Medsger, T.A. Jr., Ramsey-Goldman, R., LaPorte, R.E., & Kwoh, C.K. (1995). Incidence of systemic lupus erythematosus. Race and gender differences. *Arthritis and Rheumatism, 38*, 1260–1270.

McFarlane, J., Christoffel, K., Bateman, L., Miller, V., & Bullock, L. (1991). Assessing for abuse: Self-report versus nurse interview. *Public Health Nursing, 8*, 245–250.

Meredith, A.W., Abbott, D., & Adams, S. (1986). Family violence: Its relation to marital and parental satisfaction and family strengths. *Journal of Family Violence, 1*, 299–305.

Miller, F.W. (1995). Genetics of autoimmune diseases. *Experimental and Clinical Immunogenetics, 12*, 182–190.

Murray, M., & McMillan, C.L. (1993). Gender differences in perceptions of cancer. *Journal of Cancer Education, 8*, 53–62.

Ogur, B. (1986). Long day's journey into night: Women and prescription drug abuse. *Women and Health, 11*, 99–115.

Petersen, R. (1980). Social class, social learning, and wife abuse. *Social Service Review, 54*, 390–406.

Petri, M. (1995). Gender-based differences in autoimmunity and autoimmune disease. *Journal of Women's Health, 44*, 433–436.

Petri, M. (1998). The effect of race on incidence and clinical course in systemic lupus erythematosus: The Hopkins lupus cohort. *Journal of the American Medical Women's Association, 53*, 9–12.

Plitcha, S.B., & Weisman, C.S. (1995). Spouse or partner abuse, use of health services, and unmet need for medical care in U.S. women. *Journal of Women's Health, 4*, 45–54.

Poirier, S. (1990). Women's reproductive health. In R.D. Apple (Ed.), *Women, Health, and Medicine in America: A Historical Handbook* (pp. 217–245). New York: Garland Publishing, Inc.

Reed, J. (1978). *From Private Vice to Public Virtue: The Birth Control Movement and American Society Since 1830*. New York: Basic Books.

Resick, P., Calhoun, K., Atkeson, B., & Ellis, E. (1981). Adjustment in victims of sexual assault. *Journal of Consulting and Clinical Psychology, 49*, 705–712.

Reveille, J.D. (1989). The impact of race in SLE. *Lupus News, 9*, 4–5.

Reveille, J.S., Bartolucci, A., & Alarcon, G.S. (1990). Prognosis in systemic lupus erythematosus: Negative impact of increasing age at onset, black race, and thrombocytopenia, as well as causes of death. *Arthritis and Rheumatism, 33*, 37–48.

Rodrigues-Trias, H. (1978). Sterilization of abuse. *Women's Health, 3*, 10–15.

Roe v. Wade, 410 U.S. 113 (1973).

Salmon, J.E., Millard, S., Schachter, L.A., Arnett, F.S., Ginzler, E.M., Gourley, M.F., Ramsey-Goldman, R., Peterson, M.G.E., & Kimberly, R.P. (1996). Fc gamma RIIA alleles are heritable risk factors for lupus nephritis in African Americans. *Journal of Clinical Investigations, 97*, 1348–1354.

Sanger, M. (1938). *Margaret Sanger: An Autobiography*. Elmsford, NY: Maxwell Reprint Company.

Skene, A.J.C. (1889). *Education and Culture as Related to the Health and Diseases of Women*. Detroit, MI: George S. Davis. Cited in C. Smith-Rosenberg. (1973). The cycle of femininity: Puberty to menopause in nineteenth century America. *Feminist Studies, 1*, 58–72. Reprinted in C. Smith-Rosenberg. (1985). *Disorderly Conduct: Visions of Gender in Victorian America*. New York: Alfred A. Knopf, Inc.

Smith-Rosenberg, C. (1973). The cycle of femininity: Puberty to menopause in nineteenth century America. *Feminist Studies, 1,* 58–72. Reprinted in C. Smith-Rosenberg. (1985). *Disorderly Conduct: Visions of Gender in Victorian America.* New York: Alfred A. Knopf, Inc.

Smith-Rosenberg, C. (1978). Sex as symbol in Victorian purity: An ethnohistorical analysis of Jacksonian America. *American Journal of Sociology, 134,* Suppl. 212–247.

Smith-Rosenberg, C. (1985). *Disorderly Conduct: Visions of Gender in Victorian America.* New York: Oxford University Press.

Stark, E., & Flitcraft, A. (1988). Violence among intimates: An epidemiological review. In V.B. Van Heselt, R.L. Morrison, A.S. Bellack, & M. Hersen (Eds.), *Handbook of Family Violence* (pp. 293–317). New York: Plenum Press.

Stover, H.R., & Heard, F.F. (1865). *Criminal Abortion: Its Nature, Evidence, and Its Law.* Boston, MA: Little, Brown, and Company.

Straus, M.A., & Gelles, R.J. (1990). *Physical Violence in American Families.* New Brunswick, NJ: Transaction Publishers.

Straus, M.A., Gelles, R.J., & Steinmetz, S.K. (1980). *Behind Closed Doors: Violence in the American Family.* New York: Anchor Books.

Strom, B.L., Reidenberg, M.M., West, S., Snyder, E.S., Freundlich, B., & Stolley, P.D. (1994). Shingles, allergies, family medical history, oral contraceptives, and other potential risk factors for systemic lupus erythematosus. *American Journal of Epidemiology, 140,* 632–642.

Teske, R.H.C., & Parker, M.L. (1983). *Spouse Abuse in Texas: A Study of Women's Attitudes and Experiences.* Huntsville, TX: Criminal Justice Center, Sam Houston State University.

Tobin, J.N., Wassertheil-Smoller, S., Wexler, J.P., Steingart, R.M., Budner, N., Lense, L., & Wachpress, J. (1987). Sex bias in considering coronary bypass surgery. *Annals of Internal Medicine, 107,* 19–25.

Verbrugge, L.M. (1990). Pathways of health and death. In R.D. Apple (Ed.), *Women, Health, and Medicine in America: A Historical Handbook* (pp. 41–79). New York: Garland Publishing, Inc.

Von Krafft-Ebing, R. (1908). *Psychopathia Sexualis with Especial Reference to the Antipathic Sexual Instinct* (F.J. Rebman, Trans.). Brooklyn, NY: Physicians and Surgeons Book Club.

Ward, M.M., & Studenski, S. (1990). Clinical manifestations of systemic lupus erythematosus: Identification of racial and socioeconomic influences. *Archives of Internal Medicine, 150,* 849–853.

11

Sexual Orientation and Health

Introduction

It is believed that between 2 and 10% of the U.S. population is gay or lesbian (Gadpaille, 1995). However, relatively little is known about the demographic characteristics of those who identify themselves as gay, lesbian, or bisexual. Some data are available from the National Lesbian Health Care Survey, which involved 1,917 volunteers recruited primarily through lesbian and gay health organizations and practitioners and numerous professional organizations (Ryan and Bradford, 1988). Survey findings indicated that respondents were 17 years of age and older; that over one quarter had completed college and more than one third held an advanced degree; and that over one half were employed in a professional capacity on a full-time basis. The majority of respondents self-identified as non-Hispanic white with no religious affiliation.

Relatively little research has been devoted to an examination of the health issues confronting non-heterosexuals and transsexuals. Numerous methodological problems have been identified in the research conducted to date. For example, there exists no consensus among clinicians and behavioral scientists regarding the definition of homosexuality (Friedman, 1988) and multiple definitions of the labels "bisexual," "gay," and "lesbian" exist (Francoeur, Perper, and Scherzer, 1991). Only a minority of researchers define the population being investigated, and the methods of identifying eligible respondents vary considerably across studies (Sell and Petrulio, 1996). Researchers often fail to recognize the distinction between sexual identity (I am a gay/lesbian), sexual behavior (I have sex with men/women), and community participation (I am a member of a gay/lesbian community) (Golden, 1987; Rothblum, 1994). Second, probability sampling is rarely used to assemble study participants, often resulting in selection bias (Platzer and James, 1997; Sell and Petrulio, 1996). Instead, participants are often recruited from gay or lesbian organizations or based on their self-identity as gay/lesbian or their involvement in same-sex sexual activity. These three dimensions, while somewhat overlapping, are not synonymous, and emphasis on the inappropriate dimension in recruitment efforts will affect the ability to address the research question at issue (Rothblum, 1994). Third, individuals' self-identity may change over time and context (Rothblum, 1994). It is important to reflect on these issues in evaluating the summary that follows.

Cultural and Historical Context

The U.S. society's displeasure with homosexuality and lesbianism is evident from its earliest beginnings. Thomas Jefferson, for example, proposed in 1779 that "whoever shall be guilty of sodomy shall be punished if a man by castration, if a woman by cutting through the cartilage of her nose a hole one-half inch in diameter" (Quoted in Abramson, 1980:187).

By the end of the 19th century, homosexuality and lesbianism had become a medical concern rather than only a moral or theological one. Von Krafft-Ebing attributed homosexuality to degeneracy, as did Westphal and Charcot (Bullough, 1976; Miller, 1995; Schmidt, 1984). Others, however, were more sympathetic. Ulrichs, a German lawyer, conceived of homosexuals as a third sex, whose gender characteristics and choice of sexual object were inverted due to developments in the uterus (Miller, 1995). Ellis, a British sexologist, also believed that homosexuality was inherited and rejected its characterization as a sign of moral degeneracy. He further rejected the stereotyping of homosexuals (Miller, 1995).

Freud's psychoanalytic model of homosexuality, however, came to dominate American medical thought. Freud initially postulated that all individuals are essentially bisexual and that homosexuality was neither an illness nor a form of degeneracy. He characterized homosexuality as an arrested stage of development (Miller, 1995). American psychoanalysts, rejecting Freud's observation that homosexuals generally functioned well and ignoring his skepticism regarding its curability, often depicted homosexuality as a disease and a form of moral corruption (Berg and Allen, 1958; Bergler, 1957; Chideckel, 1935; Rado, 1933; Stekel, 1946). Lesbians, for example, were characterized as hostile (Bene, 1965), fearful of disappointment, guilt-ridden (Deutsch, 1932), fearful of pregnancy and childbirth (Rado, 1933), aggressive and domineering (Bene, 1965; Caprio, 1954; Fenichel, 1945), sadistic (Socarides, 1968), and homicidal (Caprio, 1954). Their specific "condition" was said to result from rape, incest, tomboyish behavior, seduction by an older woman, masturbation, and fear of dominance (Rosen, 1974). Numerous strategies were adopted in an effort to cure individuals of their homosexuality, including castration, hormone therapy, and hypnosis (Miller, 1995).

During the 1910s and 1920s, despite these views, Greenwich Village in New York provided a relatively tolerant environment, which permitted same-sex relationships and homosexuality (Miller, 1995). By the 1920s, gay balls had become an accepted event in the Village. Police crackdowns, however, were quite common during the 1920s. These raids abated somewhat during the 1930s, when the New York police permitted gays to socialize in public so long as they didn't draw attention to themselves. That tolerance, however, was somewhat short-lived (Miller, 1995).

The notion of homosexuals as sick became entrenched through the work of Rado, Bieber, Wilbur, and Socarides. Rado (1933) attributed homosexuality to fears of the opposite sex, while Bieber (1965) characterized homosexuality as resulting from life with a detached and hostile father and a seductive mother. Socarides (1968) insisted that the majority of homosexuals were either neurotic or psychotic. The apparent consensus viewing homosexuality as a pathology resulted in the inclusion of homosexuality as a sociopathic personality disturbance in the 1952 edition of the American Psychiatric Association's *Diagnostic and Statistical Manual of Mental Disorders* (DSM-I).

Military recruits in the United States were asked about their sexual orientation during World War II recruitment efforts. Homosexual men and women were labeled "sexual psychopaths" (Berube, 1990). Gradually, the military toughened its policies against homosexuals. Concurrently, various agencies and individuals within the federal government, including the

Federal Bureau of Investigation and the attorney Roy Cohn, embarked on a campaign to eliminate homosexuals from government service (Miller, 1995). "Sexual perversion" became a sufficient basis for the exclusion of an individual from federal employment.

The pathological nature of homosexuality was put into question as a result of studies by Kinsey and colleagues (Kinsey, Wardell, and Martin, 1948; Kinsey, Wardell, Martin, and Gebhard, 1953), which indicated that homosexual behavior was more widespread than had been thought. The 1968 edition of the *Diagnostic and Statistical Manual* reclassified homosexuality as an "other non-psychotic mental disorder," together with fetishism, pedophilia, voyeurism, exhibitionism, sadism, and masochism (Miller, 1995). The June 27, 1969 raid of the Stonewall Inn in Greenwich Village in New York City marked the commencement of what was to become the gay and lesbian liberation movement (Miller, 1995). Instead of leaving, the bar patrons resisted the police raid, creating "the Boston Tea Party of the Gay Movement" (Altman, 1973). This movement constituted a transformation of approach within the gay communities, from one of reconciliation and adjustment (gay people can fit into American society) to one of self-acknowledgement and assertiveness (American society needs to change). The impact of this movement is reflected in the 1973 de-classification of homosexuality as a mental disorder following the vote of the American Psychiatric Association membership to remove homosexuality *per se* from the nosology (Miller, 1995).

Despite these milestones, state laws continued to prohibit homosexual behavior. Although there were many monogamous gay couples, urban male culture of the 1970s was characterized by anonymous sexual encounters with multiple partners. The emergence of what was to become known as AIDS provoked marked changes in individual behaviors, including the adoption of safe sex practices, and in community values, such as the initiation of benefit coverage for domestic partners and the implementation by the Food and Drug Administration of procedures to expedite the approval of drug treatments (Miller, 1995).

Access to Health Care

Access to health care that is both necessary and sensitive has been identified as a major issue confronting gay, lesbian, bisexual, and transsexual patients. The majority of lesbians often do not reveal their sexual orientation to health care providers (Cochran and Mays, 1988; Reagan, 1981) due to the perceived or actual risk of hostility, neglect, denial of care, condescension, or other negative response from the health care provider (Bradford and Ryan, 1987; Denenberg, 1992; Perrin and Kulkin, 1996; Raymond, 1988; Stevens and Hall, 1988; Stevens, 1995; Trippet and Bain, 1992).

These fears are far from misplaced. A recent study of 278 nursing students' attitudes toward lesbian patients found that a large proportion (38%) believed that lesbians seek to seduce heterosexual women; that lesbians can be identified on the basis of their relatively masculine appearance (31%); and that lesbians provide a negative role model for children (11%) (Eliason, Donelan, and Randall, 1992). Randall (1989) found in her survey of 100 nursing educators that 24% believed that lesbian behavior is wrong, 23% believed that lesbianism is immoral, and 15% indicated that lesbians are perverted. Almost one fifth of the respondents (19%) indicated that state laws punishing lesbians for their sexual behavior should be preserved. Heterosexist and homophobic attitudes have also been noted among social workers (Berkman and Zinberg, 1997) and physicians (Douglas, Kalman, and Kalman, 1985; Matthews, Booth, Turner, and Kessler, 1986; Oriel, Maldon-Kay, Govaker, and Mersy, 1996). Such attitudes have been found to affect both the quality of the care provided (Schatz and O'Hanlan, 1994; Wise and Bowman, 1997) and the perception by heterosexual physicians of the competency of their homosexual colleagues (Oriel *et al.*, 1996). They may extend so far as to interfere with the ability of gay or lesbian parents to obtain pediatric care for their children (Perrin and Kulkin, 1996). Such attitudes and practices are not, unfortunately, surprising in view of the scant training provided to medical school students (Robinson and Cohen, 1996; Townsend, Wallick, Pleak, and Cambre, 1997; Wallick, Cambre, and Townsend, 1992) and nursing students (Leifer and Young, 1997) on the topics of homosexuality and bisexuality.

In response to such attitudes, lesbian patients may adopt any number of protective strategies, including rallying support, screening providers, seeking mirrors of their experience, maintaining vigilance, controlling information, bringing a witness, challenging mistreatment, and escaping perceived danger (Hitchcock and Wilson, 1992; Stevens, 1993; Stevens, 1994).

Various additional barriers to health care for gay men and lesbian women have been identified, including lack of insurance (Stevens, 1993), ceilings on coverage, exclusions due to preexisting conditions, "gatekeepers" at health maintenance organizations (Stevens, 1993), lack of financial resources (Bradford and Ryan, 1988; Stevens, 1993), and providers' lack of attention to preventive care and education (Trippet and Bain, 1992).

Cancer

Various studies have suggested that lesbians may be at lower risk of cervical cancer, due to lower rates of dysplasia and abnormal Pap smears compared to bisexual and heterosexual women (Johnson, Smith, and Guenther, 1987; Robertson and Schachter, 1981; Sadeghi *et al.*, 1989). Perhaps because of this relatively low risk and incorrect assumptions relating to screening (Rankow, 1997), many lesbian women fail to receive regular Pap tests (Bradford and Ryan, 1988; Johnson, Guenther, Lauber, and Keettel, 1981; Johnson *et al.*, 1987; Rankow, 1995, Zeidenstein, 1990), although cancer screening has been identified as a high priority among lesbian women (Lucas, 1992). Providers may also mistakenly believe that women in same-sex relationships never had heterosexual intercourse and do not need Pap smear testing (Ferris *et al.*, 1996).

Various researchers and writers have speculated that lesbians as a group may be at increased risk of breast, endometrial, and ovarian cancers (National Gay and Lesbian Task Force, 1993; Rankow, 1997; Roberts and Sorenson, 1995; White and Levinson, 1995). Epidemiologic studies have noted an increased risk of breast cancer among nulliparous women who have never breastfed and women of older age at the time of their first child's birth (Byers, Graham, Rzepka, and Marshall, 1985; Kelsey, 1979; Haynes, 1993, cited in Roberts and Sorenson, 1995), categories applicable to many lesbian women (Rankow, 1997; White and Levinson, 1995). In addition, rates of breast self-examination have been found to be low among lesbian women (Michigan Organization for Human Rights, 1991; Roberts and Sorenson, 1994, cited in Roberts and Sorenson, 1995). The risk of ovarian cancer may be increased due to nonuse of oral contraceptives and nulliparity (Cancer and Steroid Hormone Study of the Centers for Disease Control and the National Institute of Child Health and Development, 1987; Cramer *et al.*, 1983). Nulliparity may also increase lesbians' risk of endometrial cancer (White and Levinson, 1995).

Gay men may be at increased risk of anal cancer due to human papillomavirus infection (Rankow, 1997). Routine digital examinations have been recommended, as well as periodic cytologic screening and annual anoscopy in high-risk patients (O'Neill and Shalit, 1992).

Sexually Transmitted Diseases

Sexually transmitted diseases (STDs) appear to be less common among lesbian women than among heterosexual men or women or homosexual men (White and Levinson, 1995). The reasons for this are unclear. Accordingly, women who are sexually active with women experience lower incidence rates of gonorrhea and syphilis than all other groups except those who have never been sexually active (Degan and Waitkevicz, 1982). Certain other infections are also uncommon among women who are sexually active only with other women. These include chlamydia, herpes virus, and human papillomavirus (Johnson *et al.*, 1981; Johnson *et al.*, 1987). Female-to-female transmission of human immunodeficiency virus also appears relatively uncommon (Chu, Buehler, Fleming, and Berkelman, 1990; Harris, Thiede, McGough, and Gordon, 1993; Marmor *et al.*, 1986; Monzon and Capellon, 1987; Sabatini, Patel, and Hirschman, 1984). However, bacterial vaginosis, candidiasis, and *Trichomonas vaginalis* appear to be common (Degan and Waitkevicz, 1982; Johnson and Palermo, 1984; Johnson *et al.*, 1987; Sivakumar, DeSilva, and Roy, 1989; Trippet and Bain, 1993). Despite the apparently low risk of transmission of many of these infections, it is clear that they are transmissible between women (Berger *et al.*, 1995; Edwards and Thin, 1990; Simkin, 1993; Sivakumar *et al.*, 1989; Walters and Rector, 1986). Further, many lesbians may have had some heterosexual sexual contact and may continue to be sexually active with men on a regular or intermittent basis, while identifying themselves as lesbian (Einhorn and Polgar, 1994; Rankow, 1997).

Various strategies have been suggested to reduce the risk of STD transmission, including HIV, between female sexual partners. These include the use of female condoms, gloves, and dental dams (Kahn, 1987; White and Levinson, 1995); the avoidance of cervical and vaginal secretions, menstrual blood, and blood from vaginal and rectal trauma in partners (White and Levinson, 1995); the avoidance of fresh semen when undergoing artificial insemination (Chiasson, Stoneburner, and Joseph, 1990; Eskenazi *et al.*, 1989); and refraining from sharing sex toys (Rankow, 1997).

Gay men are at increased risk of specific gastrointestinal infections due to transmission through receptive anal intercourse and oral–anal sexual contact. These infections include *Giardia lamblia*, *Entamoeba histolytica*, Shigella species, *Campylobacter*, and hepatitis A (Rompalo, 1990). They are also at increased risk for transmission of hepatitis B virus, STDs, and HIV due to unprotected anogenital intercourse (de Wit, van Griensven, Kok, and Sandfort, 1993; Harrison and Silenzio, 1996).

Mental Health and Psychosocial Issues

"Coming Out"

Gay men and women must often address issues related to "coming out," the process of discovering one's homosexuality and revealing it to others. This process, which may begin at any age, is often associated with considerable emotional distress (Schneider, 1989). The process involves a shift in core identity and occurs in four phases: (1) awareness of homosexual feelings, (2) testing and exploration, (3) identity acceptance, and (4) identity integration and disclosure to others (Faderman, 1985; Walpin, 1997). The process of coming out appears to differ between males and females in that it is more abrupt and more likely to be associated with depression or suicide attempts in males (Gonsiorek, 1988). Prevailing social attitudes can affect the experience of coming out (Faderman, 1985; Schneider, 1989). Ethnic minority gays and lesbians may be minorities within minorities and may consequently face additional levels of discrimination (Greene, 1994).

Adolescents may be particularly vulnerable during this process. Confusion about sexual orientation may result in depression, poor school performance, substance misuse, acting out, and suicidal ideation (Feinleib, 1989). Coming out may provoke negative responses from others, including family conflict and rejection (Kreiss and Patterson, 1997), loss of friendships (Nelson, 1997), and verbal abuse from teachers (Uribe and Horbeck, 1992), exacerbating the youth's confusion and isolation (Kreiss and Patterson, 1997; Nelson, 1997).

Substance Use

Significant research has been conducted on the use of alcohol among gays and lesbians. Fifeld (1975) found in a study of individuals frequenting bars that the lesbian and gay respondents drank an average of six drinks per bar visit and frequented bars, on average, 19 times per month. McKirnan and Peterson (1989a, 1989b) found from their survey of 748 lesbians and 2,652 gay men that a higher proportion of gays and lesbians used alcohol, marijuana, and cocaine compared to the general population. Bradford, Ryan, and Rothblum (1994) found in their study of the health of 1,925 lesbians that almost one third used tobacco on a daily basis, 30% drank alcohol more than once a week, and 6% used alcohol on a daily basis. Nearly half of the women reported that they used marijuana at least occasionally, while almost one fifth reported having used cocaine. Other researchers have reported increased use of alcohol and drug use in lesbians compared with heterosexual women and women in the general population (Bradford et al., 1994; Lewis, Saghir, and Robins, 1982; Milman and Su, 1973; Roberts and Sorenson, 1994, cited in Roberts and Sorenson, 1995). Various explanations have been advanced in an attempt to understand the extensive use of alcohol and other substances: (1) dysfunctional families of origin (Gardner-Loulan, 1983; Glaus, 1988; Hepburn and Gutierrez, 1988; Swallow, 1983); (2) societal oppression (Cantu, 1983; Glaus, 1988; Martin and Lyon, 1972; Weathers, 1976; Willowroot, 1983); and (3) past trauma including incest (Bradford et al., 1994; Covington and Kohen, 1984; Evans and Schaefer, 1987; Perry, 1995). Earlier medical writings postulated that the high use of alcohol among lesbians was related to masculinity (Knight, 1937), guilt (Weijl, 1944), and the need to contain sexual drives (Clark, 1919; Stekel, 1946). Numerous approaches have been used to address excessive alcohol use among gays and lesbians, including psychotherapy, 12-step programs, and Alcoholics Anonymous (Hall, 1993).

Suicide

Numerous studies have documented high rates of suicidal behavior among gays and lesbians in comparison with heterosexuals. A 1979 study by Jay and Young of more than 5,100 lesbians and gay men found that 40% of the gay men and 39% of the lesbians had attempted or seriously considered suicide. Bell and Weinberg (1978) reported from their study of 979 gays and lesbians that significantly higher percent ages of gays than heterosexuals had attempted or seriously contemplated suicide. Saunders and Valente (1987) concluded that lesbians had 2.5 times more suicidal behavior than heterosexuals. Bradford and coworkers (1994) found in their study involving 1,925 lesbians that 19% had thought about suicide sometimes and 2% had thought about it often. Eighteen percent of the respondents had attempted suicide, often through the use of drugs, razor blades, alcohol, weapons, gas, or a car.

Gay, lesbian, and bisexual youth may be at especially high risk for suicide (Gibson, 1989; Proctor and Groze, 1994; Remafedi, 1990). Proctor and Groze (1994) found in their study of 221 gay, lesbian, and bisexual youth that over 40% had attempted suicide. Gibson (1989) has found in his study that 20 to 35% of gay youths interviewed had attempted suicide and 50% had experienced suicidal ideation. Saghir and Robins (1973) found that five out of six homosexual men who attempted suicide did so before they reached the age of 20. Numerous factors associated with suicide and suicide attempts have been identified, including depression (Remafedi, Farrow, and Deisher, 1991), social isolation, anger, feelings of inadequacy (Sears, 1991), paternal alcoholism, familial physical abuse, familial suicide attempts (Schneider, Farberow, and Kruks, 1989), violence directed against gays (Hunter, 1990), lack of support (Gonsiorek, 1988), and sexual experience before the age of 14 (Jay and Young, 1979).

Physical and Sexual Abuse

Relatively few studies have been conducted on the use of physical or sexual violence within same-sex relationships. These studies have consistently noted such violence among a high proportion of study respondents.

One of the earlier studies, conducted by Brand and Kidd (1986), found that 30% of the 55 lesbian respondents reported ever having been "physically abused." Later studies found even higher proportions. Bologna, Waterman, and Dawson (1987) used the Conflict Tactics Scale (Straus, Gelles, and Steinmetz, 1980) in their survey of 70 lesbian women and gay men. Fifty-six percent of the lesbian women and 25% of the gay male respondents reported abuse by their current or most recent partner. Over one half of the 1,099 lesbians participating in Lie and Gentlewarrior's (1991) survey reported physical abuse by their current partner. Lie and colleagues (1991), using the Conflict Tactics Scale (Straus et al., 1980) found that 25% of the 174 lesbian respondents were experiencing abuse by their then-current partner and 75% had ever experienced abuse. A more recent study by Lockhart, White, Causby, and Isaac (1994), which also used the Conflict Tactics Scale, found that almost one third of the 284 lesbian respondents had been physically abused during the previous year. Similar findings have been noted by Schilit, Lie, and Montagne (1990). A high prevalence of abuse was also noted by Waldner-Haugrud, Gratch, and Magruder (1997) among their 283 gay and lesbian participants. Results indicated that 47.5% of the lesbians and 29.7% of the gay men had been victimized by a same-sex partner at some time. Lesbians reported an overall prevalence rate for violence of 38%, compared to a rate of 21.8% for gay men. Both lesbians and gay men most frequently reported pushing, receiving threats, and slapping as the primary forms of abuse. Thirty-eight percent of the lesbians and 21.8% of the gay men reported using violence against their partners. The National Lesbian Health Care Survey results indicated that 15% of the 1,925 respondents suffered physical and/or sexual abuse as an adult (Bradford et al., 1994). More than half of the women reporting abuse as adults identified their lover (53%, gender unspecified) or their husbands (27%) as the perpetrator (Bradford et al., 1994).

Despite the apparently high prevalence of physical abuse, lesbian victims have been found less likely to seek help in shelters or from counselors (Morrow and Hawxhurst, 1989). Dissatisfaction has been reported with several sources of assistance, including the clergy, police, and private physicians (Bradford et al., 1994).

Exercises

1. You are conducting a study to examine the likelihood of female-to-female transmission of HIV, hepatitis B, and various sexually transmitted diseases.

    a. How will you define your study population with this purpose in mind?

    b. Explain how you will recruit the population specified above (strategies, source, etc.) and identify any biases that may attend your approach.

    c. Design a study to answer the research question above. Explain your rationale for your choice of design.

2. You are conducting a study to identify risk factors for prostate cancer. Previous studies indicate that certain sexual behavior, such as early age at first heterosexual intercourse, are associated with this form of cancer. You are interested in examining the relationship between type of intercourse (vaginal vs. receptive anal vs. insertive anal) and the risk of prostate cancer.

    a. How will you define your study population for the purpose of this study?

    b. How will you recruit the population identified to participate?

    c. Design a questionnaire or interview form to assess and measure sexual behaviors of your study participants. Consider the following in designing the study instrument:

        i. *possible confounders and effect modifiers*

       ii. *induction and latency periods*

      iii. *reliability and validity*

References

Abramson, H.A. (1980). The historical and cultural spectra of homosexuality and their relationship to the fear of being lesbian. *Journal of Asthma Research, 17,* 177–188.

Altman, D. (1973). *Homosexual Oppression and Liberation.* New York: Avon Books.

Bell, A.P., & Weinberg, M.S. (1978). *Homosexualities.* New York: Simon & Schuster.

Bene, E. (1965). On the genesis of female sexuality. *British Journal of Psychiatry, 111,* 815–821.

Berg, C., & Allen, C. (1958). *The Problem of Homosexuality.* New York: Citadel.

Berger, B.J., Kolton, S., Zenilman, J.M., Cummings, M.C., Feldman, J., & McCormack, W.M. (1995). Bacterial vaginosis in lesbians: A sexually transmitted disease. *Clinics of Infectious Disease, 21,* 1402–1405.

Bergler, E. (1957). *Homosexuality: Disease or Way of Life.* New York: Hill & Wang.

Berkman, C.S., & Zinberg, G. (1997). Homophobia and heterosexism in social workers. *Social Work, 42,* 319–332.

Berube, A. (1990). *Coming Out Under Fire.* New York: Free Press.

Bieber, I. (1965). Clinical aspects of male homosexuality. In J. Marmor (Ed.), *Sexual Inversion.* New York: Basic Books.

Bologna, M.J., Waterman, C.K., & Dawson, L.J. (1987, July). Violence in gay male and lesbian relationships: Implications for practitioners and policy makers. Paper presented at the Third National Conference for Family Violence Researchers, Durham, New Hampshire.

Bradford, J., & Ryan, C. (1988). *The National Lesbian Health Care Survey.* Washington, DC: National Lesbian and Gay Health Foundation.

Bradford, J., & Ryan, C. (1989). *The National Lesbian Health Care Survey: Final Report.* Washington, DC: National Lesbian and Gay Health Foundation.

Bradford, J., Ryan, C., & Rothblum, E.D. (1994). National Lesbian Health Care Survey: Implications for mental health care. *Journal of Consulting and Clinical Psychology, 62,* 228–242.

Brand, P.A., & Kidd, A.H. (1986). Frequency of physical aggression in heterosexual and female homosexual dyads. *Psychological Reports, 59,* 1307–1313.

Bullough, V.L. (1976). Homosexuality and its confusion with the "secret sin" in pre-Freudian America. In V.L. Bullough (Ed.), *Sex, Society, and History* (pp. 112–124). New York: Science History.

Byers, T., Graham, S., Rzepka, T., & Marshall, J. (1985). Lactation and breast cancer—Evidence for a negative association in premenopausal women. *American Journal of Epidemiology, 121,* 664–674.

Cancer and Steroid Hormone Study of the Centers for Disease Control and the National Institute of Child Health and Human Development. (1987). The reduction in risk of ovarian cancer associated with oral contraceptive use. *New England Journal of Medicine, 316,* 650–655.

Cantu, C. (1983). In sobriety you get life. In J. Swallow. (Ed.), *Out from Under: Sober Dykes and Our Friends.* San Francisco, CA: Spinsters/Aunt Lute.

Caprio, F.S. (1954). *Female Homosexuality: A Psychodynamic Study of Lesbianism.* New York: Citadel.

Chiasson, M.A., Stoneburner, R.L., & Joseph, S.C. (1990). Human immunodeficiency virus transmission through artificial insemination. *Journal of Acquired Immune Deficiency Syndromes, 3,* 69–72.

Chideckel, M. (1935). *Female Sex Perversion: The Sexually Aberrated Woman As She Is.* New York: Eugenics.

Chu, S.Y., Buehler, J.W., Fleming, P.L. & Berkelman, R.L. (1990). Epidemiology of reported cases of AIDS in lesbians, United States 1980–89. *American Journal of Public Health, 80,* 1380–1381.

Clark, L.P. (1919). Some psychological aspects of alcoholism. *New York Medical Journal, 109,* 930–933.

Cochran, S.D., & Mays, V.M. (1988). Disclosure of sexual preference to physicians by black lesbian and bisexual women. *Western Journal of Medicine, 149,* 616–619.

Covington, S.S., & Kohen, J. (1984). Women, alcohol, and sexuality. *Advances in Alcohol and Substance Abuse, 4,* 41–56.

Cramer, D.W., Hutchinson, G.B., Welsh, W.R., Scully, R.E., & Ryan, K.J. (1983). Determinants of ovarian cancer risk. I. Reproductive experiences and family history. *Journal of the National Cancer Institute, 71,* 711–716.

Degen, K., & Waitkevicz, H.J. (1982). Lesbian health issues. *British Journal of Sexual Medicine, May,* 40–47.

Denenberg, R. (1992). Invisible women. Lesbians and health care. *Health PAC Bulletin, 22,* 14–21.

Deutsch, H. (1932). On female homosexuality. *Psychoanalytic Quarterly, 1,* 484–510.

de Wit, J.B.F., van Griensven, G.J.P., Kok, G., & Sandfort, T.G.M. (1993). Why do homosexual men relapse into unsafe sex? Predictors of resumption of unprotected anogenital intercourse with casual partners. *AIDS, 7,* 1113–1118.

Douglas, C.J., Kalman, C.M., & Kalman, T.P. (1985). Homophobia among physicians and nurses: An empirical study. *Hospital and Community Psychiatry, 36,* 1309–1311.

Edwards, A., & Thin, R.N. (1990). Sexually transmitted diseases in lesbians. *International Journal of STD and AIDS, 1,* 178–181.

Einhorn, L., & Polgar, M. (1994). HIV-risk behavior among lesbians and bisexual women. *AIDS Education and Prevention, 6,* 514–523.

Eliason, M., Donelan, C., & Randall, C. (1992). Lesbian stereotypes. *Health Care for Women International, 13,* 131–144.

Eskenazi, B., Pies, C., Newstetter, A., Shepard, C., & Pearson, K. (1989). HIV serology in artificially inseminated lesbians. *Journal of Acquired Immune Deficiency Syndromes, 2,* 187–193.

Evans, S., & Schaefer, S. (1987). Incest and chemically dependent women: Treatment implications. *Journal of Chemical Dependency Treatment, 1,* 141–172.

Faderman, L. (1985). The "new gay" lesbians. *Journal of Homosexuality, 10,* 85–95.

Feinleib, M.R. (1989). *Report of the Secretary's Task Force on Youth Suicide.* Rockville, MD: U.S. Department of Health and Human Services.

Fenichel, O. (1945). *On the Psychoanalytic Theory of Neurosis.* New York: W.W. Norton.

Ferris, D.G., Batish, S., Wright, T.C., Cushing, C., & Scott, E.H.J. (1996). A neglected lesbian health concern: Cervical neoplasia. *Journal of Family Practice, 43,* 581–584.

Fifeld, L. (1975). On My Way to Nowhere: Alienated, Isolated, Drunk. Los Angeles: Gay Community Services Center. (Unpublished manuscript.). Cited in Bradford, J., Ryan, C., & Rothblum, E.D. (1994). National Lesbian Health Care Survey: Implications for mental health care. *Journal of Consulting and Clinical Psychology, 62,* 228–242.

Francoeur, R.T., Perper, T., & Scherzer, N.A. (1991). *A Descriptive Dictionary and Atlas of Sexology.* New York: Greenwood Press.

Friedman, B.C. (1988). *Male Homosexuality: A Contemporary Psychoanalytic Perspective.* New Haven, CT: Yale University Press.

Gadpaille, W. (1995). Homosexuality and homosexual activity. In H.I. Kaplan, & B.J. Sadock (Eds.), *Comprehensive Textbook of Psychiatry* (6th ed., Vol. 1, pp. 1321–1333). Baltimore, MD: Williams and Wilkins.

Gardner-Loulan, J. (1983). It's a wonder we have sex at all. In J. Swallow (Ed.), *Out from Under: Sober Dykes and Our Friends.* San Francisco, CA: Spinsters/Aunt Lute.

Gibson, P. (1989). Gay male and lesbian youth suicide. In *Report of the Secretary's Task Force on Youth Suicide* (Vol. 3, pp. 110–142). Washington, DC: Department of Health and Human Services. [DHHS Publ. No. [ADM] 89-1623].

Glaus, K.O. (1988). Alcoholism, chemical dependency and the lesbian client. *Women and Therapy, 8,* 131–144.

Golden, C. (1987). Diversity and variability in women's sexual identities. In the Boston Lesbian Psychologies Collective (Eds.), *Lesbian Psychologies: Explorations and Challenges* (pp. 18–34). Urbana, IL: University of Illinois Press.

Gonsiorek, J.C. (1988). Mental health issues of gay and lesbian adolescents. *Journal of Adolescent Health Care, 9,* 114–122.

Greene, B. (1994). Ethnic-minority lesbians and gay men: Mental health and treatment issues. *Journal of Consulting and Clinical Psychology, 62,* 243–251.

Hall, J.M. (1993). Lesbians and alcohol: Patterns and paradoxes in medical notions and lesbians' beliefs. *Journal of Psychoactive Drugs, 25,* 109–119.

Harris, N.V., Thiede, H., McGough, J.P., & Gordon, D. (1993). Risk factors for HIV infection among injection drug users: Results of blinded surveys in drug treatment centers, King County, Washington 1988–1991. *Journal of Acquired Immune Deficiency Syndromes, 6*, 1275–1282.

Harrison, A.E., & Silenzio, V.M.B. (1996). Comprehensive care of lesbian and gay patients and families. *Models of Ambulatory Care, 23*, 31–46.

Haynes, S. (1993). Lesbian and breast cancer. Paper presented at Fenway Community Health Center. Cited in Roberts, S.J., & Sorenson, L. (1995). Lesbian health care: A review and recommendations for health promotion in primary care settings. *Nurse Practitioner, 20*, 42–47.

Hepburn, C., & Gutierrez, B. (1988). *Alive and Well: A Lesbian Health Guide.* Freedom, CA: Crossing Press.

Hitchcock, J.M., & Wilson, H.S. (1992). Personal risking: Lesbian self-disclosure of sexual orientation to professional health care providers. *Nursing Research, 41*, 178–183.

Hunter, J. (1990). Violence against lesbian and gay male youths. *Journal of Interpersonal Violence, 5*, 295–300.

Jay, K., & Young, A. (1979). *The Gay Report: Lesbians and Gay Men Speak Out About Sexual Experiences and Lifestyles* (2nd ed.). New York: Summit Books.

Johnson, S.R., Guenther, S.M., Laube, D.W., & Keettel, W.C. (1981). Factors influencing lesbian gynecological care: A preliminary study. *American Journal of Obstetrics and Gynecology, 140*, 20–28.

Johnson, S.R., & Palermo, J.L. (1984). Gynecologic care for the lesbian. *Clinical Obstetrics and Gynecology, 27*, 724–730.

Johnson, S.R., Smith, E.M., & Guenther, S.M. (1987). Comparison of gynecologic health care problems between lesbians and bisexual women. *Journal of Reproductive Medicine, 32*, 805–811.

Kahn, E. (1987, Fall). Lesbians and AIDS: Let's go safe. *On Our Backs*, 12–14, 42–45.

Kelsey, J.L. (1979). A review of the epidemiology of human breast cancer. *Epidemiology Review, 1*, 74–109.

Kinsey, A.C., Wardell, B., & Martin, C. (1948). *Sexual Behavior in the Human Male.* Philadelphia, PA: Saunders.

Kinsey, A.C., Wardell, B., Martin, C., & Gebhard, P. (1953). *Sexual Behavior in the Human Female.* Philadelphia, PA: Saunders.

Knight, R.P. (1937). The dynamics and treatment of chronic alcohol addiction. *Bulletin of the Menninger Clinic, 1*, 233–250. Cited in J.M. Hall, (1993). Lesbians and alcohol: Patterns and paradoxes in medical notions and lesbians' beliefs. *Journal of Psychoactive Drugs, 25*, 109–119.

Kreiss, J.L., & Patterson, D.L. (1997). Psychosocial issues in primary care of lesbian, gay, bisexual, and transgender youth. *Journal of Pediatric Health Care, 11*, 166–274.

Leifer, C., & Young, E.W. (1997). Homeless lesbians: Psychology of the hidden, the disenfranchised, and the forgotten. *Journal of Psychosocial Nursing, 35*, 28–33.

Lewis, C.E., Saghir, M.T., & Robins, E. (1982). Drinking patterns in homosexual and heterosexual women. *Journal of Clinical Psychology, 43*, 277–279.

Lie, G., & Gentlewarrior, S. (1991). Intimate violence in lesbian relationships: Discussion of survey findings and practice implications. *Journal of Social Service Research, 15*, 41–59.

Lie, G., Schilit, R., Bush, J., Montagne, M., & Reyes, L. (1991). Lesbians in currently aggressive relationships: How frequently do they report aggressive past relationships? *Violence and Victims, 6*, 121–135.

Lockhart, L.L., White, B.A., Causby, V., & Isaac, A. (1994). Letting out the secret: Violence in lesbian relationships. *Journal of Interpersonal Violence, 9*, 469–492.

Lucas, V.A. (1992). An investigation of the health care preferences of the lesbian population. *Health Care for Women International, 13*, 221–228.

Marmor, M., Weiss, L.R., Lyden, M., Weiss, S.H., Saxinger, W.C., Spira, T.J., & Feorino, P.M. (1986). Possible female-to-female transmission of human immunodeficiency virus. *Annals of Internal Medicine, 105*, 969.

Martin, D., & Lyon, P. (1972). *Lesbian/Woman.* New York: Bantam Books.

Matthews, W.C., Booth, M.W., Turner, J.D., & Kessler, L. (1986). Physicians' attitudes towards homosexuality—A survey of a California medical society. *Western Journal of Medicine, 144*, 106–110.

McKirnan, D.J., & Peterson, P.L. (1989a). Alcohol and drug use among homosexual men and women: Epidemiology and population characteristics. *Addictive Behaviors, 14*, 545–553.

McKirnan, D.J., & Peterson, P.L. (1989b). Psychosocial and cultural factors in alcohol and drug abuse: An analysis of a homosexual community. *Addictive Behaviors, 14*, 555–563.

Michigan Organization for Human Rights. (1991, August). *The Michigan Lesbian Health Survey.* Lansing, MI: Michigan Organization for Human Rights.

Miller, N. (1995). *Out of the Past: Gay and Lesbian History from 1869 to the Present.* New York: Vintage.

Milman, D.H., & Su, E.H. (1973). Patterns of drug usage among university students. *Journal of the American College Health Association, 21*, 181–87.

Monzon, O.T., & Capellon, J.M.B. (1987). Female-to-female transmission of human immunodeficiency virus. *Lancet, 2*, 40–41.

Morrow, S.K., & Hawxhurst, D.M. (1989). Lesbian partner abuse: Implications for therapists. *Journal of Counseling and Development, 68,* 58–62.

National Gay and Lesbian Task Force. (1993, April). *Lesbian Health Issues and Recommendations.* Washington, DC: National Gay and Lesbian Task Force.

Nelson, J.A. (1997). Gay, lesbian, and bisexual adolescents: Providing esteem-enhancing care to a battered population. *Nurse Practitioner, 22,* 94–109.

O'Neill, J.F., & Shalit, P. (1992). Health care of the gay male patient. *Primary Care, 19,* 191–201.

Oriel, K.A., Maldon-Kay, D.J., Govaker, D., & Mersy, D.J. (1996). Gay and lesbian physicians in training: Family practice program directors' attitudes and students' perceptions of bias. *Family Medicine, 28,* 720–725.

Perrin, E.C., & Kulkin, H. (1996). Pediatric care for children whose parents are gay or lesbian. *Pediatrics, 97,* 629–635.

Perry, S.M. (1995). Lesbian alcohol and marijuana use: Correlates of HIV risk behaviors and abusive relationships. *Journal of Psychoactive Drugs, 27,* 413–419.

Platzer, H., & James, T. (1997). Methodological issues conducting sensitive research on lesbian and gay men's experience of nursing care. *Journal of Advanced Nursing, 25,* 626–633.

Proctor, C.D., & Groze, V.K. (1994). Risk factors for suicide among gay, lesbian, and bisexual youth. *Social Work, 39,* 504–513.

Rado, S. (1933). Fear of castration in women. *Psychoanalytic Quarterly, 2,* 425–475.

Randall, C.E. (1989). Lesbian phobia among BSN educators: A survey. *Journal of Nursing Education, 28,* 302–306.

Rankow, E.J. (1995). Lesbian health issues for the primary health care provider. *Journal of Family Practice, 40,* 486–493.

Rankow, E.J. (1997). Primary medical care of the gay or lesbian patient. *North Carolina Medical Journal, 58,* 92–96.

Raymond, C.A. (1988). Lesbians call for greater physician awareness, sensitivity to improve patient care. *JAMA, 259,* 18.

Reagan, P. (1981). The interaction of health professionals and their lesbian clients. *Patient Counseling and Health Education, 3,* 21–25.

Remafedi, G. (1990). Fundamental issues in the care of homosexual youth. *Medical Clinics of North America, 74,* 1169–1179.

Remafedi, G., Farrow, J.A., & Deisher, R.W. (1991). Risk factors for attempted suicide in gay and bisexual youth. *Pediatrics, 87,* 869–875.

Roberts, S.J., & Sorenson, L. (1994). Health promotion and early disease detection among lesbians: Results from the Boston Lesbian Health Project. Unpublished manuscript. Cited in S.J. Roberts & L. Sorenson (1995). Lesbian health care: A review and recommendations for health promotion in primary care settings. *Nurse Practitioner, 20,* 42–47.

Roberts, S.J., & Sorenson, L. (1995). Lesbian health care: A review and recommendations for health promotion in primary care settings. *Nurse Practitioner, 20,* 42–47.

Robertson, P., & Schachter, J. (1981). Failure to identify venereal disease in a lesbian population. *Sexually Transmitted Disease, 8,* 75–76.

Robinson, G., & Cohen, M. (1996). Gay, lesbian, and bisexual health care issues and medical curricula. *Canadian Medical Association Journal, 155,* 709–711.

Rompalo, A. (1990). Sexually transmitted causes of gastrointestinal symptoms in homosexual men. *Medical Clinics of North America, 74,* 1633–1646.

Rosen, D.H. (1974). *Lesbianism: A Study of Female Homosexuality.* Springfield, IL: Charles C. Thomas.

Rothblum, E.D. (1994). "I only read about myself on bathroom walls": The need for research on the mental health of lesbians and gay men. *Journal of Consulting and Clinical Psychology, 62,* 213–220.

Ryan, C., & Bradford, J. (1988). The National Lesbian Health Care Survey: An overview. In M. Shernoff & W.A. Scott (Eds.), *The Sourcebook on Lesbian/Gay Health Care* (2nd ed., pp. 30–40). Washington, DC: National Lesbian/Gay Health Foundation.

Sabatini, M.T., Patel, K., & Hirschman, R. (1984). Kaposi's sarcoma and T-cell lymphoma in an immunodeficient woman. *AIDS Research, 1,* 135–137.

Sadeghi, S.B., Sadeghi, A., Cosby, M., Olincy, A., & Robboy, S.J. (1989). Human papillovirus infection: Frequency and association with cervical neoplasia in a young population. *Acta Cytologica, 33,* 319–323.

Saghir, M.T., & Robins, E. (1973). *Male and Female Homosexuality: A Comprehensive Investigation.* Baltimore, MD: Wilkins & Wilkins.

Saunders, J.M., & Valente, S.M. (1987). Suicide risk among gay men and lesbians: A review. *Death Studies, 11,* 1–23.

Schatz, B., & O'Hanlan, K.A. (1994). *Anti-Gay Discrimination in Medicine: Results of a National Survey of Lesbian, Gay, and Bisexual Physicians.* San Francisco: American Association of Physicians for Human Rights.

Schilit, R., Lie, G., & Montagne, M. (1990). Substance use as a correlate of violence in intimate lesbian relationships. *Journal of Homosexuality, 19,* 51–65.

Schmidt, G. (1984). Allies and persecutors: Science and medicine in the homosexuality issue. *Journal of Homosexuality, 10*, 127–140.

Schneider, M. (1989). Sappho was a right-on adolescent: Growing up lesbian. *Journal of Homosexuality, 17*, 111–130.

Schneider, S.G., Farberow, N.L., & Kruks, G.N. (1988). Suicidal behavior in adolescent and young gay men. *Suicide and Life-Threatening Behavior, 19*, 381–394.

Sears, J.T. (1991). *Growing Up Gay in the South: Race, Gender, and Journeys of the Spirit.* New York: Harrington Park Press.

Sell, R.L., & Petrulio, C. (1996). Sampling homosexuals, bisexuals, gays, and lesbians for public health research: A review of the literature from 1990 to 1992. *Journal of Homosexuality, 30*, 31–47.

Simkin, R.J. (1993). Unique health concerns of lesbians. *Canadian Journal of Obstetrics, Gynecology, & Women's Health Care, 5*, 516–522.

Sivakumar, K., DeSilva, A.H., & Roy, R.B. (1989). *Trichomonas vaginalis* infection in a lesbian [letter]. *Genitourinary Medicine, 65*, 399–400.

Socarides, C.W. (1968). *The Overt Homosexual.* New York: Grune & Stratton.

Stekel, W. (1946). *The Homosexual Neurosis.* New York: Emerson Books.

Stevens, P.E. (1993). Marginalized women's access to health care: A feminist narrative analysis. *Advances in Nursing Science, 16*, 39–56.

Stevens, P.E. (1994). Protective strategies of lesbian clients in health care environments. *Research in Nursing and Health, 17*, 217–229.

Stevens, P.E. (1995). Structural and interpersonal impact of heterosexual assumptions on lesbian health care clients. *Nursing Research, 44*, 25–30.

Stevens, P.E., & Hall, J.M. (1988). Stigma, health beliefs and experiences with health care in lesbian women. *Image: Journal of Nursing Scholarship, 20*, 69–73.

Straus, M., Gelles, R., & Steinmetz, S. (1980). *Behind Closed Doors: Violence in the American Family.* New York: Doubleday.

Swallow, J. (1983). Recovery: The story of an ACA. In J. Swallow (Ed.), *Out from Under: Sober Dykes and Our Friends.* San Francisco, CA: Spinsters/Aunt Lute.

Townsend, M.H., Wallick, N.N., Pleak, R.R., & Cambre, K.M. (1997). Gay and lesbian issues in child and adolescent psychiatry training as reported by training directors. *Journal of the Academy of Child and Adolescent Psychiatry, 36*, 764–768.

Trippet, S.E., & Bain, J. (1992). Reasons American lesbians fail to seek traditional health care. *Health Care for Women International, 13*, 145–153.

Trippet, S.E., & Bain, J. (1993). Physical health problems and concerns of lesbians. *Women & Health, 20*, 59–70.

Uribe, V., & Horbeck, K.M. (1991). Addressing the needs of lesbian, gay, and bisexual youth: The origins of PROJECT 10 and school-based intervention. In K.M. Harbeck (Ed.), *Coming Out of the Classroom Closet: Gay and Lesbian Students, Teachers, and Curricula.* New York: Harrington Park Press.

Waldner-Haugrud, L.K., Gratch, L.V., & Magruder, B. (1997). Victimization and perpetration rates of violence in gay and lesbian relationships: Gender issues explored. *Violence and Victims, 12*, 173–184.

Wallick, N.M., Cambre, K.M., & Townsend, M.H. (1992). How the topic of homosexuality is taught at U.S. medical schools. *Academic Medicine, 67*, 601–fl03.

Walpin, L. (1997). Combating heterosexism: Implications for nursing. *Clinical Nurse Specialist, 11*, 126–132.

Walter, M.H., & Rector, W.G. (1986). Sexual transmission of hepatitis A in lesbians [letter]. *JAMA, 256*, 594.

Weathers, B. (1976). *Alcoholism and the Lesbian Community: Needs Report.* Los Angeles, CA: Alcoholism Center for Women. Cited in J.M. Hall (1993). Lesbians and alcohol: Patterns and paradoxes in medical notions and lesbians' beliefs. *Journal of Psychoactive Drugs, 25*, 109–119.

Weijl, S. (1944). Theoretical and practical aspects of psychoanalytic therapy of problem drinkers. *Quarterly Journal of Studies on Alcohol, 5*, 200–211.

White, J.C., & Levinson, W. (1995). Lesbian health care: What a primary care physician needs to know. *Western Journal of Medicine, 162*, 463–466.

Willowroot, A. (1983). Creativity, politics, and sobriety. In J. Swallow (Ed.). *Out from Under: Sober Dykes and Our Friends.* San Francisco, CA: Spinsters/Aunt Lute.

Wise, A.J., & Bowman, S.L. (1997). Comparison of beginning counselors' responses to lesbian vs. heterosexual partner abuse. *Violence and Victims, 12*, 127–135.

Zeidenstein, L. (1990). Gynecological and childbearing needs of lesbians. *Journal of Nurse Midwifery, 35*, 10–18.

III

Case Studies of Disease

12

Case Study One

Human Immunodeficiency Virus (HIV) and the Acquired Immunodeficiency Syndrome (AIDS)

Background

Rosenberg (1987:5n) has defined a disease as "[not an] absolute physical entity but a complex intellectual construct, an amalgam of biological state and social definition." This social definition or construction of disease involves four components: (1) identification of the disease's origin, (2) the assignation of responsibility for the disease and its transmission, (3) the identification or construction of the patient, and (4) the assignation of responsibility for a cure (Herek, 1990).

Various conflicts may develop in the process of socially constructing a disease. Herek (1990) has identified two such conflicts occurring during the social construction of the human immunodeficiency virus (HIV) and the acquired immunodeficiency syndrome (AIDS). The first pertains to the identification of the disease's origin and the assignation of responsibility for its transmission. This debate is occurring between the moralists, who view the disease as a divine punishment or test, and the pragmatists, who define the disease on the basis of its biological processes and manifestations. The second conflict relates to the identification or construction of the patient and the assignation of responsibility for a cure. Patients may be viewed, for example, as "innocent victims" or as individuals who refused to modify their voluntary behavior despite known health risks (Brandt, 1987; Herek, 1990).

This chapter first examines the physical entity known as HIV/AIDS, including its transmission and progression. The chapter then examines the use of sex, race, ethnicity, and sexual orientation in the social construction of HIV and AIDS, and the prevention and treatment of the disease.

A Biomedical Perspective of HIV/AIDS

Virus Transmission

HIV was identified in 1983–1984 as the causative agent of the acquired immune deficiency syndrome (AIDS) (Barre-Sinoussi *et al.*, 1983; Popovic, Sarngadharan, Read, and Gallo, 1984). HIV is transmitted by sexual intercourse, including vaginal (Laga, Taelman, Van der Stuyft, and Bonneux 1989; Peterman *et al.*, 1988), anal (Darrow *et al.*, 1987; Detels *et al.*, 1989; Moss *et al.*, 1987; Winkelstein *et al.*, 1987), and oral intercourse (Lifson *et al.*, 1990); injection drug use with shared needles and syringes (Hoffman, Larkin, and Samuel, 1989; Sasse, Salmaso, Conti, and First Drug User Multicenter Study Group, 1989; Schoenbaum *et al.*, 1989); transfusion with virus-contaminated blood or blood products; and from mother to child prior to birth or during breastfeeding. Vehicles of transmission include semen (Chiasson, Stoneburner, and Joseph, 1990; Ho *et al.*, 1984; Levy, 1989), vaginal and cervical secretions (Vogt *et al.*, 1986; Wofsy *et al.*, 1986), blood and blood products (Donegan *et al.*, 1990), tissue and organs from HIV-infected donors (Centers for Disease Control, 1987, 1988; Kumar *et al.*, 1987), and breast milk (Colebunders *et al.*, 1988; Thiry *et al.*, 1985; Ziegler, Cooper, Johnson, and Gold, 1985). Although HIV has been isolated from other body fluids, such as tears (Fujikawa *et al.*, 1985) and saliva (Ho *et al.*, 1985), HIV has not been found to be transmissible through casual and household contact (Friedland *et al.*, 1990; Rogers *et al.*, 1990).

Clinical Progression of Disease

Diagnosis of HIV-1 infection can be made by virus culture, antibody detection, antigen detection, viral genome amplification, and immune function tests (Saag, 1997b). Readers who would like additional information pertaining to testing and the body's immune response are urged to consult Berrios *et al.* (1995), Davey, Vasudevachari, and Lane (1992), Saag (1997b), Levy (1993), and Feinberg and Greene (1992).

Generally, a period of 2 to 4 weeks elapses from the time of HIV-1 infection until the onset of clinical illness, although the period can range from 6 days to 6 weeks (Vanhems *et al.*, 1997). The acute clinical illness generally lasts from 1 to 2 weeks. Symptoms during this time may include fever, lymphadenopathy, arthralgia, myalgia, lethargy or malaise, anorexia and weight loss, peripheral neuropathy, dermatologic manifestations such as alopecia and diffuse urticaria, and gastrointestinal symptoms such as nausea, diarrhea, and vomiting (Carr and Cooper, 1997).

Following this acute phase, individuals may be asymptomatic for a period of time ranging from months to years (Carr and Cooper, 1997). During this early stage, individuals generally have a CD4$^+$ T cell count greater than 500/mm^3 (Hollander, 1997). Numerous adverse prognostic factors have been identified, including neurologic involvement, acquisition of HIV from an individual with late-stage disease, higher HIV RNA viremia after seroconversion, a persistent low CD4$^+$ T cell count, and immunodeficiency at the time of infection. Skin diseases during this early phase of infection may include genital warts, oral hairy leukoplakia, and herpes zoster (Berger, 1997).

Middle-stage disease is characterized by a CD4$^+$ T cell count between 200 and 500/mm^3 (Hollander, 1997). Dermatologic manifestations during this phase include candidiasis, herpes zoster, oral hairy leukoplakia, psoriasis, and atopic dermatitis (Berger, 1997). Other clinical manifestations of HIV infection include neuropathy (Price, 1997) and tuberculosis (Hopewell, 1997).

Late-stage disease is defined by a CD4$^+$ T cell count of less than 200/mm^3 (Hollander,

1997). Complications become much more common and may include dermatologic complications such as cryptococcosis and histoplasmosis (Berger, 1997), neurologic manifestations such as encephalopathy and AIDS dementia complex (Price, 1997), respiratory difficulties such as *Pneumocystis carinii* pneumonia (Stansell and Huang, 1997), and various other bacterial (Jacobson, 1997) and fungal infections (Saag, 1997a).

Current Trends in the Epidemiology of HIV/AIDS in the United States

Initially defined on the basis of immune deficiency and the presence of certain specified severe illnesses, the case definition for AIDS was revised in 1985, 1987, and 1993 to incorporate additional severe illnesses that were found to be associated with HIV infection. The 1993 definition also included for the first time individuals with CD4$^+$ T-lymphocyte counts of less than 200/mm^3 or a percentage of total lymphocytes less than 14 (Centers for Disease Control, 1992).

As of December 30, 1997, the Centers for Disease Control and Prevention had received reports of 641,086 AIDS patients in the United States (Maldonado, 1998). The rate of AIDS differs across ethnic groups. Individuals classified as black and Hispanic who are living in the Northeast and Florida have been found to have the highest rates of AIDS (Centers for Disease Control, 1994). The incidence of AIDS and the specific risk behaviors for HIV transmission also vary by country of origin (Diaz, Buehler, Castro, and Ward, 1993; Metler, Hu, Fleming, and Ward, 1994). At least one research group has recognized that "race and ethnicity are not risk factors for HIV infection. Rather, race and ethnicity are surrogates for behavioral, socioeconomic, and other factors that influence HIV transmission" (Ward, Petersen, and Jaffe, 1997). It is also important to note that significant rates of disagreement have been found between surveillance data sources, such as AIDS case reports and death certificates, with respect to race/ethnicity classification (Kelly *et al.*, 1996).

Chu and colleagues (1992) reported that in 1989, the AIDS rate due to sex with a bisexual man was three times greater among Hispanic women compared to white women, and five times greater among black women compared to white women. Among women, AIDS is increasing most quickly among those with heterosexual contacts, so that the number of women in this category now exceeds the number related to injection drug use (Ward *et al.*, 1997). In 1993, HIV/AIDS was the fourth leading cause of death among women ages 25 to 44 years old. One report noted that the

> disproportionate impact of HIV/AIDS among women in racial/ethnic minority groups reflects social and economic factors that have not been completely defined. Despite the methodologic limitations associated with use of race/ethnicity, these data have assisted in the development and implementation of community-based prevention efforts. (Anonymous, 1995)

A total of 100,777 deaths among persons with AIDS had been reported through 1990. Although most of these deaths had occurred among individuals classified as white, death rates were the highest among blacks and Hispanics (Centers for Disease Control, 1991).

Examination of recent national trends reveals a smaller increase in the incidence of AIDS among individuals classified as homosexual/bisexual compared to males classified as injection drug users (Ward *et al.*, 1997). Individuals classified as black and Hispanic experienced a much greater increase in AIDS incidence than whites for the years 1990 through 1994 (73%, 49%, and 17%, respectively) (Ward *et al.*, 1997).

The Cultural Construction of HIV/AIDS

In 1981, *Pneumocystis carinii* pneumonia (PCP) was reported in five homosexual men (Centers for Disease Control, 1981a) and Kaposi's sarcoma was identified in 26 others (Centers for Disease Control, 1981b). Ultimately, both conditions were linked to an underlying immune deficiency (Gottlieb *et al.*, 1981; Masur *et al.*, 1981). The illness, initially known as gay-related immune deficiency (GRID) (Gottlieb *et al.*, 1982), was attributed to lifestyle choices: "the fact that these patients were all homosexuals suggests an association between some aspect of homosexual lifestyle or disease acquired through sexual contact and *Pneumocystis* pneumonia in this population" (Centers for Disease Control, 1986:2). The ailment was later noted among Haitians, hemophiliacs, and injection drug users (Shilts, 1987), prompting the identification of groups at risk for contracting HIV/AIDS: homosexuals, heroin users, Haitians, and hemo-philiacs (New York City Commission on Human Rights, 1986, 1987). On March 4, 1983, the Centers for Disease Control specifically referred to high-risk groups, defining them as groups whose members were both at higher risk of contracting HIV infection and of infecting others (Oppenheimer, 1992).

Those individuals identified as gay, bisexual, or intravenous drug users would henceforth be identified as members of a group with an increased risk of HIV infection, regardless of whether the individuals actually engaged in behavior linked to an increased risk of HIV transmission. AIDS risk groups were depicted as somehow culturally different as well as deviant. Diversity within groups was ignored and stereotyping became common (Schiller, Crystal, and Lewellen, 1994). Such stereotyping carries serious implications for HIV preven-tion, diagnosis, and care.

For example, homosexuals were perceived as harbingers of disease (New York City Commission on Human Rights, 1986, 1987; Wyatt, 1991). The culture of gay men was depicted as involving multiple sexual partners, frequent sexual activity in bath houses, use of sex-enhancing drugs, oral–genital contact, and anal intercourse, without regard to the variations in frequency and manner of sexual activity among gays (Schiller *et al.*, 1994). Such generaliza-tions carried serious implications for these individuals. First, negatively stereotyped patients might receive less than adequate care (Najman, Klein, and Munro, 1982) or may be viewed by their providers as more responsible for and deserving of their illness and less deserving of sympathy than other patients (Kelly *et al.*, 1987). Second, an emphasis on homosexuality, rather than on unprotected sexual intercourse between men, results in the exclusion and self-exclusion of men who have sex with men but who do not self identify as either homosexual and bisexual due to political, cultural, or other connotations (Jonsen and Stryker, 1993).

Similar difficulties have resulted with respect to HIV prevention, diagnosis, and care among other groups as a result of such stereotyping. For example, individuals infected via injection drug use, who may be viewed by providers as self-destructive, manipulative, or de-pendent (Groves, 1978), or whose use of drugs is perceived to be a lifestyle choice (Castro, 1993) have been found less likely to receive antiretroviral therapy than patients who contracted HIV via unprotected male–male sexual intercourse (Stein *et al.*, 1991). The perception of AIDS as a "gay white disease" (Goodman, 1986; Martin, 1985) impeded HIV prevention efforts in black communities (Mays and Cochran, 1987).

The initial construction of AIDS based on symptoms and manifestations noted in men has adversely affected women's care in a number of ways. Prior to the 1993 revision of the AIDS case definition (Centers for Disease Control, 1992), defining criteria for an AIDS diagnosis included PCP, toxoplasmosis, Kaposi's sarcoma and other cancers, oral candidiasis, and wasting (Institute of Medicine, 1988). These criteria did not include numerous other conditions that were noted among HIV-infected women, including cervical cancer, pelvic inflammatory disease, human papillomavirus, recurrent or persistent herpes simplex virus, and recurrent or persistent genital candidiasis (American Public Health Association, 1991; Anastos and Marte, 1989). Cervical dysplasia, which is more than eight times as likely to occur in HIV-infected women than in noninfected women (American Public Health Association, 1991), was similarly omitted as a diagnostic criterion until 1993 (Centers for Disease Control, 1992). This omission of conditions affecting HIV-infected women from the AIDS case definition resulted in under-diagnosis of AIDS among women and the inability of many women to qualify for publicly funded benefits such as Medicare and disability (American Public Health Association, 1991; Roper and Winkenwerder, 1988), and may have contributed to differential survival times among women due to lack of access to appropriate care (American Public Health Association, 1991).

Perhaps as a result of the development of risk group classifications and their associated stereotypes, Asians and Pacific Islanders were believed to be immune from the disease (Mandel and Kitano, 1989). In 1988, that belief was supported, in part, by a relatively low AIDS cumulative incidence rate of 13.9 per 100,000 compared to 26.3 for whites and 83.8 for blacks (Centers for Disease Control, 1990). Anecdotal reports suggesting sexual conservatism across Asian and Pacific Islander groups (Hirayama and Hirayama, 1986) lent further credence to the assumption that Asians and Pacific Islanders were not as vulnerable to HIV infection as others, whether due to some unidentified immunological mechanism or to behavioral differences. Reliance on a broad classification of many ethnicities under the general term "Asian and Pacific Islander," however, has obscured significant cultural differences between the subsumed groups that may be relevant to the transmission and prevention of HIV infection (Kitano, 1988; Loue, Lane, Lloyd, and Loh, in press;). Although recent data indicate that sexually active Asian and Pacific Islander homosexual and heterosexual adults display risk-taking behavior similar to adults of other ethnic groups (Carrier, Nguyen, and Su, 1992; Choi et al., 1995; Cochran, Mays, and Leung, 1991; Flaskerud and Nyamathi, 1988; Gellert et al., 1994; Murase, Sung, and Vuong, 1991), the rate of high-risk sexual activity appears to differ across Asian and Pacific Islander groups (Horan and DiClemente, 1993).

Differences relevant to the prevention and transmission of HIV among Hispanic subgroups have similarly been obscured (Singer et al., 1990). Diaz and colleagues (1993) reported differences in the predominant mode of HIV transmission between Hispanic subgroups, as defined by place of birth. They found that for non-Puerto Rican Hispanic men, the predominant mode of transmission was male-to-male sex, versus injection drug use among Puerto Rican males. HIV infection was attributed to injection drug use in 56% of the Hispanic women born in the United States and 46% of the Hispanic women born in Puerto Rico. Other researchers have reported similar findings (Diaz and Klevens, 1997). Magana (1991) found that the practice of "becoming milk brothers," in which several men have sexual intercourse with a single woman in rapid succession, is a not an uncommon practice among migrant undocumented workers from Mexico living in southern California. This practice has not been reported among other Hispanic groups. Loue and Oppenheim (1994) reported the use of shared equipment for injections of vitamins and medications among immigrants from Mexico and other Latin American countries. Although this practice had been reported previously (Lafferty, 1991), the reasons for and extent of this practice, as well as the risk that attends this practice, remain uninvestigated. Hispanic subgroups have been found to be associated with the likelihood of having multiple sexual partners (Sabogal, Faigeles, and Catania, 1993).

Porter and Bonilla (1991) have found that Mexican-Americans are significantly more likely to have incorrect knowledge about HIV transmission than Puerto Ricans, and that

Cubans are more likely to have been tested for HIV than Puerto Ricans. The underlying reasons for these differences are unclear. Hardy, Thornberry, and Dawson (1990) have also found lower levels of awareness about HIV among Mexican-Americans compared to Cubans and Puerto Ricans. Marin, Tschann, Gomes, and Kegeles (1993) have specifically noted that findings related to knowledge and risk behaviors among Mexicans and Central Americans in the United States may not be generalizable to other Hispanic subgroups. Murphy, Muller, and Whitman's (1995) study of the epidemiology of AIDS among Hispanics in Chicago revealed differences in the predominant transmission patterns between Puerto Rican (injection drug use) and Mexican men (men having sex with men). Based on these findings, the researchers recommended that "culturally sensitive interventions tailored to *Puerto Rican* IDUs [injection drug users] and their sex partners are needed ..." (emphasis added). The results are similar to those of Ford, Stoyanoff, Weber, and Kerndt (1993) who found that HIV seroprevalence and risk behaviors among Hispanic men in Los Angeles County differed by country of birth. Ford's group concluded that "[c]onceptualizing all Hispanics living in the U.S. obscures our understanding of how HIV is transmitted among individual subgroups and impedes prevention efforts."

Differences have also been detected between Hispanic subgroups with respect to HIV testing. In contrast to the findings of Porter and Bonilla (1991), Phillips (1993) found that Puerto Ricans are more likely to report having been tested or to plan to be tested than are either Mexicans or Cubans. Cubans, however, were found to be more likely to have undergone HIV testing or to plan to be tested than were Mexicans.

While some might argue that the more recent research findings noted above have challenged the previously existing generalizations and stereotypes of HIV and various ethnic groups and permitted the dissipation of such views, it is also likely that such research was regarded as unnecessary and superfluous precisely because of underlying assumptions and generalizations regarding susceptibility to infection across significantly diverse groups. Whether race and ethnicity should be used at all in the presentation of AIDS data is controversial. At least one researcher has asserted that race and ethnicity in reporting such things as prevalence rates serve as surrogate markers for socioeconomic status, which is one of the "root cause[s] of the high prevalence rates seen in minorities" (Rosenberg, 1996). Others have argued that the presentation of AIDS incidence data according to ethnic groups implies that ethnicity is causally related somehow to AIDS (McMillan, 1996). Also, emphasis on race/ ethnicity as a surrogate measure avoids examination of both the specific variable requiring examination and context factors that may be significant in the level of HIV risk (Singer *et al.*, 1992).

Exercises

1. The state of Woeisme is experiencing an alarming increase in the number of AIDS cases. The state department of health's most recent statistics, derived from a blinded serosurvey of delivering mothers in hospitals in the state's three largest cities, reveal that an alarmingly high proportion of these women are HIV-seropositive. The underlying reasons for this apparent increase are unclear.
   a. Keeping in mind that this was a blinded serosurvey, and the identities of the women tested for HIV are not available, indicate how you will determine the underlying explanations for this apparent increase. Note that you do not have to rely on the same sample of women to respond to this part of the question.
   b. Assume that the blinded serosurvey has revealed an increased prevalence of HIV among members of a specific ethnic group.

i. *What are the scientific, ethical, and political implications of these findings?*
ii. *How will you use these findings?*

2. Assume that the study you conduct in Exercise 1 above reveals that a growing proportion of the women infected not only engaged in high-risk sexual behaviors, but also shared "works" for their drug injections. Assume further that (1) needles and syringes are not available over the counter in the state of Woeisme and (2) a high proportion of these injecting women are not injecting heroin, for which methadone treatment is currently available at drug rehab programs with treatment slots open, but are instead injecting cocaine or methamphetamine, for which no outpatient, publicly funded treatment programs are available. Assume that you are charged with the responsibility of developing a program to reduce HIV transmission among similarly situated women.

   a. How will you estimate the population of "similarly situated women" in the state of Woeisme? Discuss the methodological techniques that you will use and the difficulties inherent in your approach.

   b. In view of your delineated responsibility, indicate your program priorities in order of the importance that you will place on each. In your response, include a discussion of the following: the (in)advisability of drug treatment; the (un)availability of drug treatment; your proposed method(s) for accessing this population; and your proposed methods for the delivery of services, if any, to this group.

   c. Assume that needles and syringes are to become available over the counter, either in conjunction with a legalized needle distribution program or through a change in state law. How will such a change affect your program priorities, if at all?

   d. HIV transmission and drug use are often seen as individual problems, involving individual choice and responsibility and necessitating an individual cure. Discuss the differences in approach to treatment and transmission prevention between an individual-based approach and a "community prevention" approach. How would your program priorities differ under each approach?

References

American Public Health Association. (1991). *Women and HIV Disease: A Report of the Special Initiative on AIDS of the American Public Health Association*. Washington, DC: American Public Health Association.

Anastos, K., & Marte, C. (1989). The missing persons in the AIDS epidemic. *Health PAC Bulletin*. Cited in S.C. Quinn. (1993). AIDS and the African American woman: The triple burden of race, class, and gender. *Health Education Quarterly, 20,* 305–320.

Anonymous. (1995). Update: AIDS among women—United States, 1994 (editorial comment). *Morbidity and Mortality Weekly Report, 44,* 81–84.

Barre-Sinoussi, F., Cherman, J.C., Rey, F., Chamaret, S., Gruest, J., Dauguet, C., & Axler-Blin, C. (1983). Isolation of a T-lymphotropic retrovirus from a patient at risk for acquired immune deficiency syndrome (AIDS). *Science, 220,* 868–870.

Berger, T.G. (1997). Dermatologic care in the AIDS patient. In M.A. Sande & P.A. Volberding (Eds.), *The Medical Management of AIDS* (5th ed., pp. 159–168). Philadelphia, PA: W.B. Saunders Company.

Berrios, D.C., Awins, A.L., Haynes-Sanstad, K., Eversley, R., & Woods, W.J. (1995). Screening for human immunodeficiency virus antibody in urine. *Archives of Pathology & Laboratory Medicine, 119,* 139–141.

Brandt, A.M. (1987). *No Magic Bullet: A Social History of Venereal Disease in the United States Since 1880* (expanded ed.). New York: Oxford University Press.

Carrier, J., Nguyen, B., & Su, S. (1992). Vietnamese American sexual behaviors & HIV infection. *Journal of Sex Research, 29,* 547–560.

Castro, K.G. (1993). Distribution of acquired immunodeficiency syndrome and other sexually transmitted diseases in racial and ethnic populations, United States: Influences of life-style and socioeconomic status. *Annals of Epidemiology, 3,* 181–184.

Centers for Disease Control. (1981a). Pneumocystis pneumonia—Los Angeles. *Morbidity and Mortality Weekly Report, 30*, 250–252.

Centers for Disease Control. (1981b). Kaposi's sarcoma and Pneumocystis pneumonia among homosexual men—New York City and California. *Morbidity and Mortality Weekly Report, 30*, 305–308.

Centers for Disease Control. (1986). *Reports on AIDS Published in the Morbidity and Mortality Weekly Report, June 1981 through February, 1986*. Springfield, VA: National Technical Information Service.

Centers for Disease Control. (1987). Revision of the CDC surveillance case definition of acquired immunodeficiency syndrome. *Morbidity and Mortality Weekly Report, 36*(Suppl. 1S), 1S–3S.

Centers for Disease Control. (1988). Transmission of HIV through bone transplantation: Case report and public health recommendations. *Morbidity and Mortality Weekly Report, 37*, 597–599.

Centers for Disease Control. (1990). AIDS and HIV infection in the United States: 1988 update. *Morbidity and Mortality Weekly Report, 38*, 1–38.

Centers for Disease Control. (1991). Mortality attributable to HIV infection/AIDS—United States, 1981–1990. *Morbidity and Mortality Weekly Report, 40*, 41–44.

Centers for Disease Control. (1992). 1993 revised classification system for HIV infection and expanded surveillance case definition for AIDS among adolescents and adults. *Morbidity and Mortality Weekly Report, 41*, No. RR-17.

Centers for Disease Control and Prevention. (1994). AIDS among racial/ethnic minorities—United States, 1993. *Morbidity and Mortality Weekly Report, 43*, 644–655.

Chiasson, M.A., Stoneburner, R.L., & Joseph, S.C. (1990). Human immunodeficiency virus transmission through artificial insemination. *Journal of Acquired Immune Deficiency Syndromes, 3*, 69–72.

Choi, K.H., Coates, T.A., Catania, J.A., Lew, S., & Chow, P. (1995). High HIV risk among gay Asian and Pacific Islander men in San Francisco. *AIDS, 9*, 306–307.

Chu, S.Y., Peterman, T.A., Doll, L.S., Buehler, J.W., & Curran, J.W. (1992). AIDS in bisexual men in the United States: Epidemiology and transmission to women. *American Journal of Public Health, 82*, 220–224.

Cochran, S.D., Mays, V.M., & Leung, L. (1991). Sexual practices of heterosexual Asian-American young adults: Implications for risk of HIV infection. *Archives of Sexual Behavior, 20*, 381–391.

Colebunders, R., Kapita, B., Nekwei, W., Bahwe, Y., Lebughe, I., Oxtoby, M., & Ryder, R. (1988). Breastfeeding and transmission of HIV. *Lancet, 2*, 1487.

Darrow, W.W., Echenberg, D.F., Jaffe, H.W., O'Malley, P.M., Byers, R.H., Getchell, J.P., & Curran, J.W. (1987). Risk factors for human immunodeficiency virus (HIV) infections in homosexual men. *American Journal of Public Health, 77*, 479–483.

Davey, R.T., Jr., Vasudevachari, M.B., & Lane, H.C. (1992). Serologic tests for human immunodeficiency virus infection. In V.T. DeVita, Jr., S. Hellman, & S.A. Rosenberg (Eds.), *AIDS: Etiology, Diagnosis, Treatment, and Prevention* (3rd ed., pp. 141–155). Philadelphia, PA: J.B. Lippincott.

Detels, R., English, P., Visscher, B.R., Jacobson, L., Kingsley, L.A., Chmiel, J.S., Dudley, J.P., Eldred, L.J., & Ginzburg, H.M. (1989). Seroconversion, sexual activity and condom use among 2915 HIV seronegative men followed up to 2 years. *Journal of Acquired Immune Deficiency Syndromes, 2*, 77–83.

Diaz, T., Buehler, J.W., Castro, K.G., & Ward, J.W. (1993). AIDS trends among Hispanics in the United States. *American Journal of Public Health, 83*, 504–509.

Diaz, T., & Klevens, M. (1997). Differences by ancestry in sociodemographics and risk behaviors among Latinos with AIDS. The supplement to HIV and AIDS Surveillance Project Group. *Ethnicity and Disease, 7*, 200–206.

Donegan, E., Stuart, M., Niland, J.C., Sacks, H.S., Azen, S.P., Dietrich, S.L., Faucett, C., Fletcher, M.A., Kleinman, S.H., Operskalski, E.A., Perkins, H.A., Pindyck, J., Schiff, E.R., Stiles, D.P., Tomasulo, P.A., Mosley, J.W., & the Transfusion Safety Group. (1990). Infection with human immunodeficiency virus type I (HIV) among recipients of antibody-positive blood donations. *Annals of Internal Medicine, 113*, 733–739.

Feinberg, M., & Greene, W. (1992). Molecular insights into human immunodeficiency virus type 1 pathogenesis. *Current Opinions in Immunology, 4*, 466–474.

Flaskerud, J. & Nyamathi, A. (1988). An AIDS education program for Vietnamese women. *New York State Journal of Medicine, 88*, 632–637.

Ford, W., Stoyanoff, S.R., Weber, M.D., & Kerndt, P.R. (1993). Differences in HIV risk behaviors and seroprevalence by country of birth among Hispanic men in Los Angeles County. *Abstracts of the Ninth International Conference on AIDS*, June 6–11, 2, 728 [abstract no. PO-C20-3067].

Friedland, G., Kahl, P., Saltzman, B., Rogers, M., Feiner, C., Mayers, M., Schable, C., & Klein, R.S. (1990). Additional evidence for lack of transmission of HIV infection by close interpersonal (casual) contact. *AIDS, 4*, 639–644.

Fujikawa, L.S., Salahuddin, S.Z., Palestine, A.G., Nussenblatt, R.B, Salahuddin, S.Z., Masur, H., & Gallo, R.C. (1985). Isolation of human T-lymphotropic virus type III from the tears of a patient with the acquired immunodeficiency syndrome. *Lancet, 2*, 529–530.

Gellert, G.A., Moore, D.F., Maxwell, R.M., Mai, K.K., & Higgins, K. V. (1994). Targeted HIV seroprevalence among Vietnamese in southern California. *Genitourinary Medicine, 70*, 265–267.

Goodman, E. (1986, August 1). It's no longer "us" and "them." *Los Angeles Times,* Pt. II, p. 3.

Gottlieb, M.S., Schroff, R., Fligiel, S., Fahey, J.L., & Saxon, A. (1982). Gay-related immunodeficiency (GRID) syndrome: Clinical and autopsy observations. *Clinical Research, 30*, 349A.

Gottlieb, M.S., Schroff, R., Schanker, H.M., Weisman, J.D., Peng T.F., Wolf, R.A., & Saxon, A. (1981). *Pneumocystis carinii* pneumonia and mucosal candidiasis in previously healthy homosexual men: Evidence of a newly acquired immunodeficiency. *New England Journal of Medicine, 305*, 1425–1431.

Groves, J.E. (1978). Taking care of the hateful patient. *New England Journal of Medicine, 298*, 883–887.

Hardy, A., Thornberry, O.T., & Dawson, D. (1990). AIDS knowledge among Hispanic American subgroups. *Abstracts of the Sixth International Conference on AIDS,* June 20–23, 3, 249 [abstract no. SC640].

Herek, G.M. (1990). Illness, stigma, and AIDS. In P.T. Costa, Jr. & G.R. VandenBos (Eds.), *Psychological Aspects of Serious Illness: Chronic Conditions, Fatal Diseases, and Clinical Care* (pp. 107–150). Washington, DC: American Psychological Association.

Hirayama, H., & Hirayama, K.K. (1986). The sexuality of Japanese Americans. *Journal of Social Work and Human Sexuality, 4*, 81–98.

Ho, D.D., Byington, R.E., Schooley, R.T., Flynn, T., Rota, T.R., & Hirsh, M.S. (1985). Infrequency of isolation of HTLV-III virus from saliva in AIDS. *New England Journal of Medicine, 313*, 1606.

Ho, D.D., Schooley, R.T., Rota, T.R., Kaplan, J.C., & Flynn, T. (1984). HTLV-III in the semen and blood of healthy homosexual men. *Science, 226*, 451–453.

Hoffman, P.N., Larkin, D.P., & Samuel, D. (1989). Needlestick and needleshare—The difference. *Journal of Infectious Diseases, 160*, 545–546.

Hollander, H. (1997). Initiating routine care for the HIV-infected adult. In M.A. Sande & P.A. Volberding (Eds.), *The Medical Management of AIDS* (5th ed., pp. 107–112). Philadelphia, PA: W.B. Saunders Company.

Hopewell, P.C. (1997). Tuberculosis in persons with human immunodeficiency virus infection. In M.A. Sande & P.A. Volberding (Eds.), *The Medical Management of AIDS* (5th ed., pp. 311–325). Philadelphia, PA: W.B. Saunders Company.

Horan, P.F., & DiClemente, R.J. (1993). HIV knowledge, communication, and risk behaviors among white, Chinese, and Filipino-American adolescents in a high-prevalence AIDS epicenter: A comparative analysis. *Ethnicity and Disease, 3*, 97–105.

Institute of Medicine. (1988). *Confronting AIDS: Update 1988.* Washington, DC: National Academy of Sciences.

Jacobson, M.A. (1997). Disseminated *Mycobacterium avium* complex and other bacterial infections. In M.A. Sande & P.A. Volberding (Eds.), *The Medical Management of AIDS* (5th ed., pp. 301–310). Philadelphia, PA: W.B. Saunders Company.

Jonsen, A.R., & Stryker, J. (Eds.). (1993). *The Social Impact of AIDS in the United States.* Washington, DC: National Academy Press.

Kelly, J.A., St. Lawrence, J.T., Smith, S., Hood, H.V., & Cook, D.J. (1987). Stigmatization of AIDS patients by physicians. *American Journal of Public Health, 77*, 789–791.

Kelly, J.J., Chu, S.Y., Diaz, T., Leary, L.S., & Buehler, J.W. (1996). Race/ethnicity misclassification of persons reported with AIDS. The AIDS Mortality Project group and the Supplement to the HIV/AIDS Surveillance Project Group. *Ethnicity and Health, 1*, 87–94.

Kitano, K.J. (1988). Correlates of AIDS-associated high-risk behavior among Chinese and Filipino gay men (thesis). University of California, Berkeley.

Kumar, P., Pearson, J.E., Martin, D.H., Leech, S.H., Buisseret, P.D., Bezbak, H.C., Gonzalez, F.M., Royer, J.R., Streicher, H.Z., & Saxinger, W.C. (1987). Transmission of human immunodeficiency virus by transplantation of renal allograft, with development of the acquired immunodeficiency syndrome. *Annals of Internal Medicine, 106*, 244–245.

Lafferty, J. (1991). Self-injection and needle sharing among migrant farmworkers (letter). *American Journal of Public Health, 81*, 221.

Laga, M., Taelman, H., Van der Stuyft, P., & Bonneux, L. (1989). Advanced immunodeficiency as a risk factor for heterosexual transmission of HIV. *AIDS, 3*, 361–366.

Levy, J. (1993). Pathogenesis of human immunodeficiency virus infection. *Microbiology Review, 57*, 183–189.

Levy, J.A. (1989). Human immunodeficiency viruses and the pathogenesis of AIDS. *JAMA, 261*, 2997–3006.

Lifson, A.R., O'Malley, P.M., Hessol, N.A., Buchbiner, S.P., Cannon, L., & Rutherford, G.W. (1990). HIV seroconversion in two homosexual men after receptive oral intercourse with ejaculation: Implications for counselling concerning safe sexual practices. *American Journal of Public Health, 80*, 1509–1511.

Loue, S., Lane, S., Lloyd, L.S., & Loh, L. (1999). Rephrasing the message: A new approach to HIV prevention in United States Southeast Asian communities. *Journal of Health Care for the Poor and Underserved, 10*, 100–121.

Loue, S., & Oppenheim, S. (1994). Immigration and HIV infection: A pilot study. *AIDS Education and Prevention*, 6, 74–80.

Magana, J.R. (1991). Sex, drugs, and HIV: An ethnographic approach. *Social Science and Medicine*, *33*, 5–9.

Maldonado, M. (1998). The HIV/AIDS epidemic among Latinos in the United States. *Update: National AIDS Minority Council, October*, 1–7.

Mandel, J.S., & Kitano, K.J. (1989). San Francisco looks at AIDS in Southeast Asia. *Multicultural Inquiry and Research on AIDS*, *3*, 1–2.

Marin, B.V., Tschann, J.M., Gomez, C.A., & Kegeles, S.M. (1993). Acculturation and gender differences in sexual attitudes and behaviors: Hispanic vs. non-Hispanic white unmarried adults. *American Journal of Public Health*, *83*, 1759–1761.

Martin, T. (1985, October). AIDS: Is it a major threat to blacks? *Ebony*, 9–96.

Masur, H., Michelis, M.A., Greene, J.B., Onorato, I., Vande Stouwe, R.A., Holzman, R.S., Wormser, G., Brettman, L., Lange, M., Murray, H.W., & Cunningham-Rundles, S. (1981). An outbreak of community-acquired *Pneumocystis carinii* pneumonia: Initial manifestation of cellular immune dysfunction. *New England Journal of Medicine*, *305*, 1431–1438.

Mays, V.M., & Cochran, S.D. (1987). Acquired immunodeficiency syndrome and black Americans: Special psychosocial issues. *Public Health Reports*, *102*, 224–231.

McMillan, S. (1996). Letter to the editor. *Science*, *271*, 1480.

Metler, R., Hu, D.J., Fleming, P.L., & Ward, J.W. (1994). AIDS among Asians and Pacific Islanders (A/PI) reported in the USA. In *Abstracts of the Xth International Conference AIDS/International Conference on STD*, Yokohama [abstract PCO325].

Moss, A.R., Osmond, D., Bacchetti, P., Chermann, J.C., Barre-Sinoussi, F., & Carlson, J. (1987). Risk factors for AIDS and HIV seropositivity in homosexual men. *American Journal of Epidemiology*, *125*, 1035–1047.

Murase, K., Sung, S., & Vuong, V. (1991). *AIDS Knowledge, Attitudes, Beliefs and Behaviors in Southeast Asian Communities in San Francisco*. The Center for Cross-Cultural Research and Social Work Practice, Department of Social Work Education, San Francisco State University.

Murphy, J., Muller, G., & Whitman, S. (1995). Epidemiology of AIDS among Hispanics in Chicago. *Journal of Acquired Immune Deficiency Syndromes and Human Retrovirology*, *11*, 83–87.

Najman, J.M., Klein, D., & Munro, C., (1982). Patient characteristics negatively stereotyped by doctors. *Social Science and Medicine*, *16*, 1781–1789.

New York City Commission on Human Rights. (1986, November). *AIDS and People of Color: The Discriminatory Impact*. New York: Author.

New York City Commission on Human Rights. (1987, August). *AIDS Discrimination and Its Implications for People of Color and Other Minorities*. New York: Author.

Oppenheimer, G.M. (1992). Causes, cases, and cohorts: The role of epidemiology in the historical construction of AIDS. In E. Fee & D.M. Fox (Eds.), *AIDS: The Making of a Chronic Disease* (pp. 49–83). Berkeley, CA: University of California Press.

Peterman, T.A., Stoneburner, R.L., Allen, J.R., Jaffe, H.W., & Curran, J.W. (1988). Risk of human immunodeficiency virus transmission from heterosexual adults with transfusion-associated infections. *JAMA*, *259*, 55–58.

Phillips, K.A. (1993). Factors associated with voluntary HIV testing for African-Americans and Hispanics. *AIDS Education and Prevention*, *5*, 95–103.

Popovic, M., Sarngadharan, M.G., Read, E., & Gallo, R.C. (1984). Detection, isolation, and continuous production of cytopathic retroviruses (HTLV-III) from patients with AIDS and pre-AIDS. *Science*, *224*, 497–500.

Porter, J., & Bonilla, L. (1991). The health belief model as a predictor of HIV-testing behavior among Latinos in the USA. *Abstracts of the Seventh International Conference on AIDS*, June 16–21, 1, 391 [abstract no. MD4006].

Price, R.W. (1997). Management of the neurologic complications of HIV-1 infection and AIDS. In M.A. Sande & P.A. Volberding (Eds.), *The Medical Management of AIDS* (5th ed., pp. 197–216). Philadelphia, PA: W.B. Saunders Company.

Rogers, M.F., White, C.R., Sanders, R., Schable, C., Ksell, T.E., Wasserman, R.L., Bellanti, J.A., Peters, S.M., & Wray, B.B. (1990). Lack of transmission of human immunodeficiency virus from infected children to their household contacts. *Pediatrics*, *85*, 210–214.

Roper, W., & Winkenwerder, W. (1988). Making fair decisions about financing care for persons with AIDS. *Public Health Reports*, *103*, 305–308.

Rosenberg, C.E. (1987). *The Cholera Years: The United States in 1832, 1849, and 1866* (2nd ed.). Chicago, IL: University of Chicago Press.

Rosenberg, P.S. (1996). Letter to the editor. *Science*, *271*, 1480–1481.

Saag, M.S. (1997a). Cryptococcosis and other fungal infections (histoplasmosis, coccidioidomycosis). In M.A. Sande & P.A. Volberding (Eds.), *The Medical Management of AIDS* (5th ed., pp. 327–342). Philadelphia, PA: W.B. Saunders Company.

Saag, M.S. (1997b). Quantitation of HIV viral load: A tool for clinical practice? In M.A. Sande & P.A. Volberding (Eds.), *The Medical Management of AIDS* (5th ed., pp. 57–74). Philadelphia, PA: W.B. Saunders Company.

Sabogal, F., Faigeles, B., & Catania, J.A. (1993). Data from the National AIDS Behavioral Surveys. II. Multiple sexual partners among Hispanics in high-risk cities. *Family Planning Perspectives, 25,* 257–262.

Sasse, H., Salmaso, S., Conti, S., & First Drug User Multicenter Study Group. (1989). Risk behaviors for HIV-1 infection in Italian drug users: Report from a multicenter study. *Journal of Acquired Immune Deficiency Syndrome, 2,* 486–496.

Schiller, N.G., Crystal, S., & Lewellen, D. (1994). Risky business: The cultural construction of AIDS risk groups. *Social Science and Medicine, 38,* 1337–1346.

Schoenbaum, E.E., Hartel, D., Selwyn, P.A., Klein, R.S., Darenny, K., Rogers, M., Feiner, C., & Friedland, G. (1989). Risk factors for human immunodeficiency virus infection in intravenous drug users. *New England Journal of Medicine, 321,* 874–879.

Shilts, R. (1987). *And the Band Played On: Politics, People, and the AIDS Epidemic.* New York: St. Martin's Press.

Singer, M., Flores, C., Davison, L., Burke, G., Castillo, Z., Scanlon, K., & Rivera, M. (1990). SIDA: The economic, social, and cultural context of AIDS among Latinos. *Medical Anthropology Quarterly, 4,* 72–114.

Singer, M., Jia, Z., Schensul, J.J., Weeks, M., & Page, J.B. (1992). AIDS and the IV drug user: The local context in prevention efforts. *Medical Anthropology, 14,* 285–306.

Stansell, J.D., & Huang, L. (1997). *Pneumocystis carinii* pneumonia. In M.A. Sande & P.A. Volberding (Eds.), *The Medical Management of AIDS* (5th ed., pp. 275–300). Philadelphia, PA: W.B. Saunders.

Stein, M.D., Piette, J., Mor, V., Wachtel, T.J., Fleishman, J., Mayer, K.H., & Carpenter, C.C.J. (1991). Differences in access to zidovudine (AT) among symptomatic HIV-infected persons. *Journal of General Internal Medicine, 6,* 35–40.

Subauste, C.S., Wong, S.Y., & Remington, J.S. (1997). AIDS-associated toxoplasmosis. In M.A. Sande & P.A. Volberding (Eds.), *The Medical Management of AIDS* (5th ed., pp. 343–362). Philadelphia, PA: W.B. Saunders.

Thiry, L., Sprecher-Goldberger, S., Jonckheer, T., Levy, J., Van de Perre, P., Henrivaux, P., Cogniaux-Lecler, J., & Clumeck, N. (1985). Isolation of AIDS virus from cell-free breast milk of three healthy virus carriers. *Lancet, 2,* 891–892.

Vanherns, P., Allard, R., Cooper, D.A., Perrin, L., Vizzard, J., Hirschel, B., Kinloch-de Loes, S., Carr, A., & Lambert, J. (1997). Acute human immunodeficiency virus type I disease as a mononucleosis-like illness: Is the diagnosis too restrictive? *Clinical Infectious Diseases, 24,* 965–970.

Vogt, M.W., Witt, D.J., Craven, D.E., Crawford, D.F., Witt, D.J., Byington, R., Schooley, R.T., & Hirsch, M.S. (1986). Isolation of HTLV III/LAV from cervical secretions of women at risk for AIDS. *Lancet, 1,* 525–527.

Ward, J.W., Petersen, L.R., & Jaffe, H.W. (1997). Current trends in the epidemiology of HIV/AIDS. In M.A. Sande & P.A. Volberding (Eds.), *The Medical Management of AIDS* (5th ed., pp. 3–16). Philadelphia, PA: W.B. Saunders.

Winkelstein, W., Lyman, D.M., Padian, N., Grant, R., Samuel, M., Wiley, J.A., Anderson, R.E., Lang, W., Riggs, J., & Levy, J.A. (1987). Sexual practices and risk of infection by the human immunodeficiency virus: The San Francisco Men's Health Study. *JAMA, 257,* 321–325.

Wofsy, C., Cohen, J., Hauer, L., Michaelis, B.A., Cohen, J.B., Padian, N.S., & Evans, L.A. (1986). Isolation of AIDS-associated retrovirus from genital secretions of women with antibodies to the virus. *Lancet, 1,* 527–529.

Wyatt, G.E. (1991). Examining ethnicity versus race in AIDS related sex research. *Social Science and Medicine, 33,* 37–45.

Ziegler, J.B., Cooper, D.A., Johnson, R.O., & Gold, J. (1985). Postnatal transmission of AIDS-associated retrovirus from mother to infant. *Lancet, 1,* 896–898.

13

Case Study Two
Diabetes Mellitus

Background

Diabetes is classified into five subtypes. Individuals with insulin-dependent diabetes mellitus, also known as IDDM or Type I diabetes, are dependent on exogenous insulin to prevent ketoacidosis and death (Berkow, 1987). This type of diabetes has been associated with histocompatibility antigens on chromosome 6. It is believed that environmental factors may induce the disease in susceptible individuals and that cell-mediated immune mechanisms are involved. Individuals with non-insulin-dependent diabetes mellitus, also referred to as NIDDM or Type II diabetes, may or may not use exogenous insulin but do not require it for their survival. Unlike IDDM, NIDDM often develops after the age of 30 and is associated with obesity. The third classification encompasses those persons who have diabetes that is associated with other conditions, such as pancreatic disease. Gestational diabetes occurs among women who develop glucose intolerance during pregnancy. In many instances, the glucose intolerance may cease with the end of the pregnancy. The final subclass consists of those individuals with impaired glucose tolerance (IGT) (Berkow, 1987). The discussion below focuses on NIDDM.

The Epidemiology of Diabetes

Incidence and Prevalence

The prevalence and incidence of diabetes varies across racial/ethnic classifications as they are currently constituted. For example, the prevalence of diabetes among blacks has been found to be 1.5 times that among whites (Harris, 1991; Roseman, 1985; Wetterhall et al., 1992). Brancati, Whelton, Kuller, and Klag (1996) found that the excess prevalence of diabetes among African-Americans appears to be greatest among those of lower socioeconomic status and concluded that African-American race is a strong independent risk factor for diabetes, especially among those of low socioeconomic status.

Hispanics have also been found to have a higher incidence of diabetes as compared to non-Hispanic whites (Gardner et al., 1984; Hamman et al., 1989; Hanis et al., 1983; Samet et al., 1988; Stern et al., 1981). A Colorado-based study, for instance, found an age-adjusted prevalence of NIDDM of 21 per 1,000 in white males, 44 per 1,000 in Hispanic males, 13 per 1,000 in white females, and 62 per 1,000 in Hispanic females (Hamman *et al.*, 1989). Across Hispanic groups, however, Cubans have been found to have a lower prevalence of diabetes than Puerto Ricans and Mexicans (Flegal *et al.*, 1991). The peak age-specific incidence among Hispanics occurs between the ages of 50 and 59, approximately one decade earlier than among non-Hispanic whites (Baxter *et al.*, 1993).

Despite the diversity across different Native American tribes, almost all tribes have been found to have a prevalence of diabetes substantially higher than that of the general U.S. population (Acton *et al.*, 1993; Carter *et al.*, 1989; Farrell *et al.*, 1993; Freeman, Hosey, Diehr, and Gohdes, 1989; Johnson and Strauss, 1993; Martinez and Strauss, 1993; Muneta, Newman, Wetterall, and Stevenson, 1993; Murphy *et al.*, 1992; Rith-Najarian, Valway, and Gohdes, 1993; Sugarman and Percy, 1989). The prevalence of diabetes has been found to be higher among various Asian and Pacific Islander groups as compared to whites (Fujimoto *et al.*, 1987; Sloan, 1963). The prevalence of NIDDM has been found to be higher among migrant Asians than among those in the country of origin. This has led to the hypothesis that Asians may constitute a vulnerable population and, when exposed to certain environmental factors associated with westernization, will be more likely to develop insulin resistance and glucose intolerance (Fujimoto, 1992). Various researchers have specifically found that higher levels of physical activity and an Asian diet relatively higher in carbohydrates and lower in fat and animal protein are associated with a reduced prevalence of diabetes (Fujimoto *et al.*, 1994; Huang *et al.*, 1996).

The incidence and prevalence of diabetes-related complications also varies across groups. For example, the incidence of end-stage renal disease is higher across all nonwhite groups than in whites. Although it was assumed that NIDDM was not an important factor in the development of end-stage renal disease, several studies have found that a higher proportion of individuals with end-stage renal disease are minorities with NIDDM, rather than IDDM (Cowie *et al.*, 1989; Pugh, Medina, Cornell, and Basu, 1995). A recent North Carolina-based study found that blacks had a 12-fold increase in the risk of renal disease due to NIDDM as compared to whites (Tell, Hylander, Craven, and Burkart, 1996). Various risk factors for end-stage renal disease have been implicated, including hypertension, glucose intolerance, insulin resistance, salt sensitivity, and hyperlipidemia (Powers and Wallen, 1998). Familial clustering of end-stage renal disease has been noted in African-Americans with NIDDM (Freedman, Tuttle, and Spray, 1995).

Higher rates of retinopathy have been reported among African-Americans, Hispanics, and several Native American tribes as compared to whites (Haffner *et al.*, 1988; Harris *et al.*, 1993; Lee, Lee, Lu, and Russell, 1992; Nelson *et al.*, 1989). Severe retinopathy is associated with duration of the diabetes, insulin therapy, and hyperglycemia (Haffner *et al.*, 1988, 1993).

Amputations are more frequent among blacks as compared with whites (9.0 per 1,000 compared to 6.3 per 1,000, respectively) (Carter, Pugh, and Monterrosa, 1996). Pima Indians have 3.7 times more amputations than whites (Carter, Pugh, and Monterrosa, 1996). The incidence of lower-extremity amputation has been found to be even higher among Oklahoma Indians (Lee *et al.*, 1993). Risk factors for amputation include presence of medial arterial calcification, retinopathy or nephropathy, the absence of patellar tendon reflexes, and impaired great toe vibration-perception threshold (Mayfield, Reiber, Nelson, and Greene, 1996; Nelson *et al.*, 1988).

Clinical gallbladder disease has been found to be associated with NIDDM in Mexican-American men and women and in non-Hispanic white women (Haffner *et al.*, 1990). Diabetic status has also been found to be associated with increased prevalence of and greater severity of destructive periodontal disease (Emrich, Schlossman, and Genco, 1991). A history of diabetes is associated with the development of hepatocellular carcinoma, although the relationship is stronger with respect to IDDM (Yu, Tong, Govindarajan, and Henderson, 1991).

Symptoms of sensory neuropathy affect between 30 and 40% of diabetic patients. Unlike many other complications and symptoms, it appears to be equally prevalent among men and women and among Hispanics and non-Hispanic whites (Harris, Eastman, and Cowie, 1993; Sands, Shetterly, Franklin, and Hamman, 1997). Neuropathy is more likely to occur with increased duration of diabetes, hypertension, and hyperglycemia (Harris, Eastman, and Cowie, 1993).

Diabetes-specific mortality has also been found to be higher among all nonwhite groups as compared to whites. A recent study of mortality in Wisconsin found that mortality due to diabetes was significantly higher for Native Americans of both genders who were less than 75 years of age (Tavris, Malek, and Dellinger, 1998). Increased mortality due to diabetes has been reported among other Native American tribes, including the Navaho (O'Connor, Crabtree, and Nakamura, 1997). Mexican-American elderly have also been found to be at higher risk of dying of NIDDM as compared to their non-Hispanic counterparts (Espino, Parra, and Kriehbiel, 1994). Diabetes has been linked to coronary heart disease (Haffner, Morales, Stern, and Gruber, 1992; Howard et al., 1995) and to early death from ischemic heart disease (Will and Casper, 1996).

Risk Factors

Higher incidence and prevalence of diabetes has been found to be associated with lower levels of exercise, higher percentage of fat calories in the diet, obesity, duration of obesity, and low birth weight (Cowie et al., 1993; Everhart, Pettitt, Bennett, and Knowler, 1992; Sugarman, Hickey, Hall, and Gohdes, 1990). Various environmental factors have been implicated in the development of NIDDM, including early exposure to cow's milk and low-level nitrate exposure through drinking water (Kostraba, Gay, Rewers, and Hamman, 1992).

An increased risk of NIDDM has been noted among those with family histories of NIDDM (Fujimoto et al., 1991), prompting significant investigation of genetic factors involved in the development of NIDDM (Elbein et al., 1996; Erlich et al., 1993; Stern, 1991; Taylor et al., 1996).

It has been hypothesized that the development of diabetes may be related to a thrifty genotype and/or increased acculturation, while reduced prevalence of diabetes may be associated with the "descending limb" of modernization. The "thrifty genotype" hypothesis posits that a highly efficient storage mechanism for calories developed so that calories could be stored in times of plenty and be available during periods of famine. However, when food supplies are constant, the thrifty genotype is believed to lead to obesity and NIDDM (Carter et al., 1996).

A relationship between the "ascending limb" of modernization and risk behaviors for diabetes has also been posited. These behaviors include the increased consumption of total calories, dietary fat, and refined sugars; the decreased consumption of fiber and complex carbohydrates; and a more sedentary lifestyle. Conversely, as individuals become more assimilated they may seek out a healthier lifestyle and thereby decrease their risk of developing diabetes (Stern et al., 1991).

Protective Factors

Exclusive breastfeeding for the first 2 months of life has been found to be associated with a significantly lower rate of NIDDM, providing some evidence to support the hypothesized association between early exposure to cow's milk and later development of NIDDM (Kostraba *et al.*, 1993; Pettitt *et al.*, 1997). Decreased risk of NIDDM has also been noted among those engaging in moderate or high-level physical activity (Adler, Boyko, Schraer, and Murphy, 1996) and, among Alaska Natives, those with daily diets high in omega-3 fatty acids, such as seal oil and salmon (Adler, Boyko, Schraer, and Murphy, 1994).

Cultural Factors in Diabetes Care

Relatively little research has been conducted with respect to cultural factors affecting the management of diabetes. Zaldovar and Smolowitz (1994) found in their study of non-Mexican-American Hispanic adults with diabetes that over three quarters of them believed that they had diabetes because it was the will of God. Almost one fifth believed that the use of specific herbs would cure their disease. Many expressed fatalis regarding the course of the disease. Taken together, these findings may indicate the role of fatalism and religious beliefs in the course of the disease.

Exercises

1. Early studies of HIV emphasized the increased risk of disease occurrence in specific ethnic communities, such as Haitians. Research has demonstrated an increased risk of NIDDM among numerous communities of color, including African-Americans, Native Americans, and Hispanics.
   a. Compare and contrast the public response to these two diseases and the response of these communities to the research.
   b. What factors explain any similarities or differences in response with respect to the two diseases?
2. Research has indicated that there may exist a gene or genes that are implicated in the development of NIDDM. Assume for the purpose of this question that there exists such a gene.
   a. What are the scientific, ethical, and political implications of such a finding? Consider in your discussion historical examples of our response to "genetic traits."
   b. Design a study to assess the relative contribution of the gene and environmental factors to the development of NIDDM. Consider the study design, the study population, inclusion and exclusion criteria, potential confounder and effect modifiers, and potential biases.

References

Acton, K., Rogers, B., Campbell, G., Johnson, C., & Gohdes, D. (1993). Prevalence of diagnosed diabetes and selected related conditions of six reservations in Montana and Wyoming. *Diabetes Care, 16,* 263–265.

Adler, A.I., Boyko, E.J., Schraer, C.D., & Murphy, N.J. (1994). Lower prevalence of impaired glucose tolerance and diabetes associated with daily seal oil or salmon consumption among Alaska Natives. *Diabetes Care, 17,* 1498–1501.

Adler, A.I., Boyko, E.J., Schraer, C.D., & Murphy, N.J. (1996). The negative association between traditional physical activities and the prevalence of glucose intolerance in Alaska Natives. *Diabetes Medicine, 13,* 555–560.

Baxter, J., Hamman, R.F., Lopez, T.K., Marshall, J.A., Hoag, S., & Swenson, C.J. (1993). Excess incidence of non-insulin-dependent diabetes mellitus (NIDDM) in Hispanics compared with non-Hispanic whites in the San Luis Valley, Colorado. *Ethnicity and Disease, 3,* 11–21.

Berkow, R. (Ed.), (1987). *The Merck Manual of Diagnosis and Therapy* (15th ed.). Rahway, NJ: Merck, Sharp & Dohme Research Laboratories.

Brancati, F.L., Whelton, P.K., Kuller, L.H., & Klag, M.J. (1996). Diabetes mellitus, race, and socioeconomic status. A population-based study. *Annals of Epidemiology, 6,* 67–73.

Carter, J., Horowitz, R., Wilson, R., Sava, S., Sinock, P., & Gohdes, D. (1989). Tribal differences in diabetes: Prevalence among American Indians in New Mexico. *Public Health Reports, 104,* 665–669.

Carter, J.S., Pugh, J.A., & Monterrosa, A. (1996). Non-insulin-dependent diabetes mellitus in minorities in the United States. *Annals of Internal Medicine, 125,* 221–232.

Cowie, C.C., Harris, M.I., Silverman, R.E., Johnson, E.W., & Rust, K.F. (1993). Effect of multiple risk factors on differences between blacks and whites in the prevalence of non-insulin-dependent diabetes mellitus in the United States. *American Journal of Epidemiology, 137,* 719–732.

Cowie, C.C., Port, P.K., Wolfe, R.A., Savage, P.J., Moll, P.P., & Hawthorne, V.M. (1989). Disparities in incidence of diabetic end-stage renal disease according to race and type of diabetes. *New England Journal of Medicine, 321,* 1074–1079.

Elbein, S.C., Bragg, K.L., Hoffman, M.D., Mayorga, R.A., & Leppert, M.F. (1996). Linkage studies of NIDDM with 23 chromosome 11 markers in a sample of whites of northern European descent. *Diabetes, 45,* 370–375.

Emrich, L.J., Schlossman, M., & Genco, R.J. (1991). Periodontal disease in non-insulin-dependent diabetes mellitus. *Journal of Periodontology, 62,* 123–131.

Erlich, H.A., Zeidler, A., Chang, J., Shaw, S., Raffel, L.J., Klitz, W., Beshkov, Y., Costin, G., Pressman, S., Bugawan, T., & Rotter J.I. (1993). HLA class II alleles and susceptibility and resistance to insulin dependent diabetes mellitus in Mexican-American families. *Nature Genetics, 3,* 358–364.

Espino, D.V., Parra, E.O., & Kriehbiel, R. (1994). Mortality differences between elderly Mexican Americans and non-Hispanic whites in San Antonio, Texas. *Journal of the American Geriatric Society, 42,* 604–608.

Everhart, J.E., Pettitt, D.J., Bennett, P.H., & Knowler, W.C. (1992). Duration of obesity increases the incidence of NIDDM. *Diabetes, 41,* 235–240.

Farrell, M.A., Quiggins, P.A., Eller, J.D., Owle, P.A., Miner, K.M., & Walkingstick, E.S. (1993). Prevalence of diabetes and its complications in the Eastern Band of Cherokee Indians. *Diabetes Care, 16,* 253–256.

Flegal, K.M., Ezzati, T.M., Harris, M.I., Haynes, S.G., Juarez, R.Z., Knowler, W.C., Perez-Stable, E.J., & Stern, M.P. (1991). Prevalence of diabetes in Mexican Americans, Cubans, and Puerto Ricans from the Hispanic Health and Nutrition Examination Survey, 1982–1984. *Diabetes Care, 14,* 628–638.

Freedman, B.I., Tuttle, A.B., & Spray, B.J. (1995). Familial predisposition to nephropathy in African-Americans with non-insulin dependent diabetes mellitus. *American Journal of Kidney Disease, 25,* 710–713.

Freeman, W.L., Hosey, G.M., Diehr, P., & Gohdes, D. (1989). Diabetes in American Indians of Washington, Oregon, and Idaho. *Diabetes Care, 12,* 282–288.

Fujimoto, W.Y. (1992). The growing prevalence of non-insulin dependent diabetes in migrant Asian populations and its implications for Asia. *Diabetes Research and Clinical Practice, 15,* 167–183.

Fujimoto, W.Y., Bergstrom, R.W., Boyko, E.J., Kinyoun, J.L., Newell-Morris, L.L. Robinson, L.R., Shuman, W.P., Stolov, W.C., & Tsunehara, C.H. (1994). Diabetes and diabetes risk factors in second- and third-generation Japanese Americans in Seattle, Washington. *Diabetes Research and Clinical Practice, 24*(Suppl.), S43–S52.

Fujimoto, W.Y., Leonetti, D.L., Kinyoun, J.L., Newell-Morris, L., Shuman, W.P., Stolov, W.C., & Wahl, P.W. (1987). Prevalence of diabetes mellitus and impaired glucose tolerance among second-generation Japanese-American men. *Diabetes, 36,* 721–729.

Fujimoto, W.Y., Leonetti, D.L., Newell-Morris, L., Shuman, W.P., & Wahl, P.W. (1991). Relationship of absence or presence of a family history of diabetes to body weight and body fat distribution in type 2 diabetes. *International Journal of Obesity, 15,* 111–120.

Gardner, L.I., Jr., Stern, M.P., Haffner, S.M., Gaskill, S.P., Hazuda, H.P., Relethford, J.H., & Eifler, C.W. (1984). Prevalence of diabetes in Mexican Americans. Relationship to percent of gene pool derived from Native American sources. *Diabetes, 33,* 86–92.

Haffner, S.M., Diehl, A.K., Mitchell, B.D., Stern, M.P., & Hazuda, H.P. (1990). Increased prevalence of gallbladder disease in subjects with non-insulin-dependent diabetes mellitus. *American Journal of Epidemiology, 132,* 327–335.

Haffner, S.M., Fong, D., Stern, M.P., Pugh, J.A., Hazuda, H.P., Patterson, J.K., van Heuven, W.A., & Klein, R. (1988). Diabetic retinopathy in Mexican Americans and non-Hispanic whites. *Diabetes, 37,* 874–884.

Haffner, S.M., Mitchell, B.D., Moss, S.E., Stern, M.P., Hazuda, H.P., Patterson, J., van Heuven, W.A., & Klein, R. (1993). Is there an ethnic difference in the effect of risk factors for diabetic retinopathy? *Annals of Epidemiology, 3,* 2–8.

Haffner, S.M., Morales, P.A., Stern, M.P., & Gruber, M.K. (1992). Lp(a) concentrations in NIDDM. *Diabetes, 41*, 1267–1272.

Hamman, R.F., Marshall, J.A., Baxter, J., Kahn, L.B., Mayer, E.J., Orleans, M., Murphy, J.R., & Lezotte, D.C. (1989). Methods and prevalence of non-insulin-dependent diabetes mellitus in a biethnic Colorado population. The San Luis Valley Diabetes Study. *American Journal of Epidemiology, 129*, 295–311.

Hanis, C.L., Ferrell, R.E., Barton, S.A., Aguilar, L., Garza-Ibarra, A., Tulloch, B.R., Garcia, C.A., & Schull, W.J. (1983). Diabetes among Mexican Americans in Starr County, Texas. *American Journal of Epidemiology, 118*, 659–672.

Harris, E.L., Feldman, S., Robinson, C.R., Sherman, S., & Georgopoulos, A. (1993). Racial differences in the relationship between blood pressure and risk of retinopathy among individuals with NIDDM. *Diabetes Care, 16*, 748–754.

Harris, M.I. (1991). Epidemiological correlates of NIDDM in Hispanics, whites, and blacks in the U.S. population. *Diabetes Care, 14*, 639–648.

Harris, M., Eastman, R., & Cowie, C. (1993). Symptoms of sensory neuropathy in adults with NIDDM in the U.S. population. *Diabetes Care, 16*, 1446–1452.

Howard, B.V., Lee, E.T., Cowan, L.D., Fabsitz, R.R., Howard, W.J., Oopik, A.J., Robbins, D.C., Savage, P.J., Yeh, J.L., & Welty, T.K. (1995). Coronary heart disease prevalence and its relation to risk factors in American Indians. The Strong Heart Study. *American Journal of Epidemiology, 142*, 254–268.

Huang, B., Rodriguez, B.L., Burchfiel, C.M., Chyou, P.H., Curb, J.D., & Yano, K. (1996). Japanese-American men in Hawaii. *American Journal of Epidemiology, 144*, 674–681.

Johnson, L.G., & Strauss, K. (1993). Diabetes in Mississippi Choctaw Indians. *Diabetes Care, 16*, 250–252.

Kostraba, J.N., Cruickshanks, K.J., Lawler-Heavner, J., Jobim, L.F., Rewers, M.J., Gay, E.C., Chase, H.P., Klingensmith, G., & Hamman, R.F. (1993). Early exposure to cow's milk and solid foods in infancy, genetic predisposition, and risk of IDDM. *Diabetes, 42*, 288–295.

Kostraba, J.N., Gay, E.C., Rewers, M., & Hamman, R.F. (1992). Nitrate levels in community drinking waters and risk of NIDDM. An ecological analysis. *Diabetes Care, 15*, 1505–1508.

Lee, E.T., Lee, V.S., Lu, M., & Russell, D. (1992). Development of proliferative retinopathy in NIDDM. A follow-up study of American Indians in Oklahoma. *Diabetes, 41*, 359–367.

Lee, E.T., Lee, V.S., Lu, M., Russell, D., Bahr, C., & Lee, E.T. (1993). Lower-extremity amputation. Incidence, risk factors, and mortality in the Oklahoma Indian diabetes study. *Diabetes, 42*, 876–882.

Martinez, C.B., & Strauss, K. (1993). Diabetes in St. Regis Mohawk Indians. *Diabetes Care, 16*, 260–262.

Mayfield, J.A., Reiber, G.E., Nelson, R.G., & Greene, T. (1996). A foot risk classification system to predict diabetic amputation in Pima Indians. *Diabetes Care, 19*, 704–709.

McCance, D.R., Hanson, R.L., Pettitt, D.J., Bennett, P.H., Bishop, D.T., & Knowler, W.C. (1995). Diabetic nephropathy: A risk factor for diabetes mellitus in offspring. *Diabetologia, 38*, 221–226.

Muneta, B., Newman, J., Wetterall, S., & Stevenson, J. (1993). Diabetes and associated risk factors among Native Americans. *Diabetes Care, 16*, 1619–1620.

Murphy, N.J., Schraer, C.D., Bulkow, L.R., Boyko, E.J., & Lanier, A.P. (1992). Diabetes mellitus in Alaskan Yup'ik Eskimos and Athabascan Indians after 25 years. *Diabetes Care, 15*, 1390–1392.

Nelson, R.G., Gohdes, D.M., Everhart, J.E., Hartner, J.A., Zwemer, F.L., Pettitt, D.J., & Knowler, W.C. (1988). Lower-extremity amputations in NIDDM 12-year follow-up study in Pima Indians. *Diabetes Care, 11*, 8–16.

Nelson, R.G., Wolfe, J.A., Horton, M.B., Pettitt, D.J., Bennett, P.H., & Knowler, W.C. (1989). Proliferative retinopathy in NIDDM. Incidence and risk factors in Pima Indians. *Diabetes, 37*, 878–884.

O'Connor, P.J., Crabtree, B.F., & Nakamura, R.M. (1997). Mortality experience of Navajos with type 2 diabetes mellitus. *Ethnicity and Health, 2*, 155–162.

Pettitt, D.J., Forman, M.R., Hanson, R.L., Knowler, W.C., & Bennett, P.H. (1997). Breastfeeding and incidence of non-insulin-dependent diabetes mellitus in Pima Indians. *Lancet, 350*, 166–168.

Powers, D.R., & Wallen, J.D. (1998). End-stage renal disease in specific ethnic and racial groups: risk factors and benefits of hypertensive therapy. *Archives of Internal Medicine, 158*, 793–800.

Pugh, J.A., Medina, R.A., Cornell, J.C., & Basu, S. (1995). NIDDM is the major cause of diabetic end-stage renal disease. More evidence from a tri-ethnic community. *Diabetes, 44*, 1375–1380.

Rith-Najarian, S.J., Valway, S.E., & Gohdes, D.M. (1993). Diabetes in a northern Minnesota Chippewa tribe. Prevalence and incidence of diabetes and incidence of major complications, 1986–1988. *Diabetes Care, 16*, 266–270.

Roseman, J.M. (1985). Diabetes in black Americans. In *Diabetes in America* (VIII1–VIII24). Washington, DC: United States Department of Health and Human Services [NIH Publ. No. 85-1468].

Samet, J.M., Coultas, D.B., Howard, C.A., Skipper, B.J., & Hanis, C.L. (1988). Diabetes, gallbladder disease, obesity, and hypertension among Hispanics in New Mexico. *American Journal of Epidemiology, 128*, 1302–1311.

Sands, M.L., Shetterly, S.M., Franklin, G.M., & Hamman, R.F. (1997). Incidence of distal symmetric (sensory) neuropathy in NIDDM. The San Luis Valley Diabetes study. *Diabetes Care, 20*, 322–329.

Sloan, N.R. (1963). Ethnic distribution of diabetes mellitus in Hawaii. *JAMA, 183*, 419–424.

Stern, M.P. (1991). Kelly West lecture. Primary prevention of type II diabetes mellitus. *Diabetes Care, 14*, 399–410.

Stern, M.P., Gaskill, S.P., Allen, C.R., Jr., Garza, V., Gonzalez, J.L., & Waldrop, R.H. (1981). Cardiovascular risk factors in Mexican Americans in Laredo, Texas. II. Prevalence and control of hypertension. *American Journal of Epidemiology, 113*, 556–562.

Stern, M.P., Knapp, J.A., Hazuda, H.P., Haffner, S.M., Patterson, J.K., & Mitchell, B.D. (1991). Genetic and environmental determinants of type II diabetes in Mexican Americans. Is there a descending limb to the modernization/diabetes relationship? *Diabetes Care, 14*, 649–654.

Sugarman, J., & Percy, C. (1989). Prevalence of diabetes in a Navajo Indian community. *American Journal of Public Health, 79*, 511–513.

Sugarman, J.R., Hickey, M., Hall, T., & Gohdes, D. (1990). The changing epidemiology of diabetes mellitus among Navajo Indians. *Western Journal of Medicine, 153*, 140–145.

Tavris, D.R., Malek, L.L., & Dellinger, J.A. (1998). Age- and gender-adjusted comparison of Wisconsin native mortality with general Wisconsin population, for diabetes and diabetes-related causes of death—1986–1995. *Wisconsin Medical Journal, 97*, 58–61.

Taylor, R.W., Printz, R.L., Armstrong, M., Granner, D.K., Alberti, K.G., Turnbull, D.M., & Walker, M. (1996). Variant sequences of the hexokinase II gene in familial NIDDM. *Diabetologia, 39*, 322–328.

Tell, G.S., Hylander, B., Craven, T.E., & Burkart, J. (1996). Racial differences in the incidence of end-stage renal disease. *Ethnicity and Health, 1*, 21–31.

Wetterhall, S.F., Olson, D.R., DeStefano, F., Stevenson, J.M., Ford, E.S., German, R.R., Will, J.C., Newman, J.M., Sepe, S.J., & Vinicor, F. (1992). Trends in diabetes and diabetic complications, 1980–1987. *Diabetes Care, 15*, 960–967.

Will, J.C. & Casper, M. (1996). The contribution of diabetes to early deaths from ischemic heart disease: U.S. gender and racial comparison. *American Journal of Public Health, 86*, 576–579.

Yu, M.C., Tong, M.J., Govindajaran, S., & Henderson, B.E. (1991). Nonviral risk factors for hepatocellular carcinoma in a low-risk population, the non-Asians of Los Angeles County, California. *Journal of the National Cancer Institute, 83*, 1820–1826.

Zaldovar, A., & Smolowitz, J. (1994). Perceptions of the importance placed on religion and folk medicine by non-Mexican-American Hispanic adults with diabetes. *Diabetes Education, 20*, 303–306.

Index